D1562610

Handbook of
Forensic Pathology

Handbook of
Forensic Pathology

Abdullah Fatteh

M.B., Ph.D., LL.B., D.M.J. (Clin.),
D.M.J. (Path.), M.R.C. Path., F.C.L.M.

Professor of Pathology, East Carolina University, Greenville, N.C.
Pathologist, Lenoir Memorial Hospital, Kinston, N.C.
Regional Forensic Pathologist, Office of Chief Medical Examiner
State of North Carolina
Former Associate Chief Medical Examiner, State of North Carolina, and
Associate Professor of Pathology, University of North Carolina, Chapel Hill, N.C.

J. B. LIPPINCOTT COMPANY
Philadelphia · Toronto

Copyright © 1973, by J. B. Lippincott Company

This book is fully protected by copyright and, with the exception of brief excerpts for review, no part of it may be reproduced in any form, by print, photoprint, microfilm, or by any other means, without the written permission of the publishers.

ISBN 0–397–50328–8

Library of Congress Catalog Card Number 73–14529

Printed in the United States of America

1   3   5   7   6   4   2

Library of Congress Cataloging in Publication Data

Fatteh, Abdullah.
  A handbook of forensic pathology.

  Includes bibliographies.
  1. Medical jurisprudence. 2. Violent deaths.
I. Title. [DNLM: 1. Forensic medicine.
2. Pathology. W700 F254h 1973]
RA1063.F27   614'.19   73–14529
ISBN 0–397–50328–8

Dedicated

to

Milton Helpern, M.D.
Geoffrey Mann, M.D.
Thomas Marshall, M.D.
Thomas Noguchi, M.D.

Foreword

Forensic pathology, the study and application of medical and pathology principles in determining the cause and manner of death in cases of violent, suspicious, unexplained, unexpected, sudden and medically unattended deaths, is a field of medical specialization that dates back to ancient civilizations. As long as there have been societies in which people could think and reason, there has been an awareness and understanding of the social necessity of determining how and why a particular individual died in those instances in which death was due to an obvious, suspicious or alleged act of foul play (homicide, accident, or suicide).

In past centuries, in the absence of sophisticated scientific equipment, advanced medical knowledge, and well developed technological skills, it was not possible for medical practitioners to determine all those things which are susceptible to objective evaluation and scientific validation today. Nonetheless, physicians and other scientists attempted to make these determinations to the best of their ability. These efforts ultimately gave rise in later years to organized teaching programs in forensic pathology at most university centers in Continental Europe.

Unfortunately, the development of forensic pathology in the United States has been comparatively slow, sporadic, and quite often superficial. This deficiency is being corrected in many jurisdictions at the present time, and hopefully, better medical-legal investigative facilities and technics will be uniformly adopted and utilized throughout the country before many more years pass.

Courses in forensic pathology at medical schools in the United States are relatively few in number, and most of these are quite inadequate and incomplete because of the limited time that is made available to the instructors. Outside of medical schools, there are only a few post-graduate seminars, lectures, and short courses sponsored from time to time by different professional organizations on various aspects of forensic pathology. However, for the most part, there simply has not been enough good authoritative material on the subject of forensic pathology made available to physicians, forensic scientists, attorneys, and law enforcement officials. There has been a definite need for an authoritative text which would readily present practical, timely, and concise information to individuals involved in official medical-legal investigation and other legal processes that require a knowledge and understanding of forensic pathology.

The Handbook of Forensic Pathology is indeed such a publication. The text is clear, articulate, and logically organized. The approximately 150 illustrations provide the reader with a unique opportunity to visualize many of the pathological entities which the author discusses in this book. Perhaps no other field of medical specialization requires the use of demonstrative evidence as much as forensic pathology, and the author, who is trained in law as well as in medicine and forensic pathology, was obviously well aware of this fact when he selected the excellent illustrations and other visual aids that are appropriately scattered throughout the 341 pages of this book.

The author has logically commenced this textbook with a chapter on scene investigation. The other 22 chapters cover basic, routine, uniform diseases, injuries, and other pathological entities encountered by medical examiners, forensic pathologists, coroners, clinical physicians, police officers, and other individuals involved in medical-legal investigation. In addition, infrequently seen, atypical, unique, and highly complex problems encountered in forensic pathology are also presented in a very lucid and effective manner by the author. Deaths from therapeutic mishaps, artefacts in forensic pathology and toxicology, and the "negative" autopsy are very valuable discussions which are not readily found, if at all, elsewhere in the scientific literature. The final chapter, in which the author deals with the pathologist as a witness should be of great practical interest and concern to attorneys and police officers, as well as forensic pathologists.

Abdullah Fatteh, the author of this handbook, is an outstanding, acknowledged expert in the field of forensic pathology. Dr. Fatteh is also an attorney and has had extensive educational background, training and practical experience in other related fields such as toxicology, medical jurisprudence, criminalistics, and firearms identification. Indeed, this very useful textbook is in great measure based upon actual medical-legal investigations and autopsies which Dr. Fatteh has been involved in throughout his professional career as an active, practicing forensic pathologist in Medical Examiner Offices.

Dr. Fatteh's contributions to the medical-legal literature are quite numerous, and his dedicated interest and involvement in various educational programs and other professional activities in the field of forensic pathology are well known among his colleagues and fellow practitioners of forensic sciences. He is indeed eminently qualified to have written this handbook of forensic pathology, which undoubtedly will become one of the most frequently used reference works in the libraries of Medical Examiner and Coroners' Offices, police departments, other governmental investigative agencies, and independent toxicology and crime laboratories. Attorneys in both the civil and criminal fields would do well to have this book available at all times, also, for it will prove to be a source of never ending scientific information to them in the evaluation, preparation and trial of personal injury cases such as medical malpractice and products liability, and the entire gamut of criminal cases, ranging from assault and battery to rape, vehicular fatalities, and homicide.

CYRIL H. WECHT, M.D.

Coroner, Allegheny County, Pennsylvania
Research Professor of Law and Director, Institute of
Forensic Sciences, Duquesne University
Clinical Assistant Professor of Pathology, University
of Pittsburgh School of Medicine
Director, Pittsburgh Institute of Legal Medicine
Past President, American Academy of Forensic Sciences
Past President, American College of Legal Medicine
Diplomate, American Board of Pathology (Anatomic, Clinical,
and Forensic Pathology)

Preface

The subject of Legal Medicine encompasses many specialties in the fields of Medicine and Law. Forensic Pathology is an important part of this wide field. In modern times, more and more attention is being paid to the role of the subspecialty of Forensic Pathology. The investigation of a crime resulting in death is incomplete without an adequate postmortem examination of the deceased. The number of insurance claims is increasing, and it is frequently of vital importance to determine the precise cause and manner of death. In the area of investigation of sudden, unexplained deaths, the contributions of forensic pathology are significant.

In every country of the world, there is some method of investigation of the deaths involving medicolegal considerations. The importance of autopsies is getting wider recognition and the incidence of investigations and autopsies is improving. There is, however, just a small number of full-time experienced Forensic Pathologists in each country and they do just a fraction of the total medico-legal work. Rather a bulk of the autopsy work is taken care of by hospital pathologists or general physicians whose principal interests are in laboratory pathology or in the field of their practice, and their involvement in Forensic Pathology is secondary and part-time. This book is primarily written for general pathologists and medical examiners.

With the discussion of every type of death, the findings at the scene of investigation and in the autopsy room are discussed. Therefore, not only the pathologists, but the law enforcement agency investigators would find helpful information pertaining to the scene investigation and gain insight into what Forensic Pathology can contribute. The medical students and residents would get appreciation of the problems surrounding the medicolegal investigations and autopsies, and discover clear guide on how to approach these cases. The members of the legal profession would derive a quick idea about what they could expect from the pathologist dealing with a forensic case.

The primary considerations in the book are observations and interpretations of the findings. Several illustrative cases are included to clarify certain situations. Procedures of investigations are discussed in detail and where appropriate check lists are included. Legal considerations are omitted since the laws vary from state to state and country to country. Therefore, anyone involved in the investigation of a death, be it a medical examiner, a pathologist, a coroner, a police surgeon or a law enforcement officer in any country of the world would easily be able to utilize the factual and basic information which is supplemented by lists of pertinent references.

No attempt is made to include the details of techniques for toxicological analyses of various poisons. Newer techniques are coming up and the old ones rapidly become outdated. However, great care is taken to apprise the investigator about the techniques of collecting samples for analyses and about the storage of these samples. Information about the type of samples and amounts required for certain poisons is included. The signs and symptoms of some of the poisons are briefly described so that the pathologist, if he has the clinical history, can evaluate the autopsy findings in proper light. The fatal doses and fatal concentrations of various poisons in different biological materials are presented so that the pathologist will have a ready guide to interpret the results he gets from the toxicologist.

It is the author's earnest hope that the students and practitioners of Pathology, Law and Law Enforcement sciences will find the information presented here of use.

ABDULLAH FATTEH, M.B., PH.D., LL.B.

Acknowledgements

Considerable help has been obtained directly or indirectly from many colleagues while I worked in the Department of Forensic Medicine of the Queen's University of Belfast, the Department of Legal Medicine of the Medical College of Virginia, the Office of the Chief Medical Examiner of Virginia, the Armed Forces Institute of Pathology in Washington, the Office of the Chief Medical Examiner of North Carolina and the Department of Pathology of the University of North Carolina in Chapel Hill. Without the encouragement and help of these colleagues this work would not have been possible. The author is specially indebted to Dr. Page Hudson and Dr. David Wiecking who spent considerable amount of their valuable time reviewing the manuscript critically. Their excellent suggestions are a part of the text. The author gratefully acknowledges his indebtedness to Dr. Arthur McBay who rendered valuable advice on the toxicology section. I am also grateful to many of my colleagues for their contributions of illustrative material.

For permission to use printed material and illustrations from my previously published works I wish to thank the following:

Appleton-Century-Crofts, Educational Division, Meredith
Corporation for text and photographs in Chapters 17 and 21
(From Fatteh. In Wecht, ed. Legal Medicine Annual 1972.)

Callaghan and Company for text in Chapter 21

Military Medicine for Figure 16-2

Medicine, Science and the Law for Figure 14-5

S. S. Kind, Editor: Journal of Forensic Science Society for Figure 8-18

H. A. Shapiro, Editor: Journal of Forensic Medicine for Figures 8-15 (*Bottom*) and Figures 8-22 (*Bottom*)

I am thankful to the British Medical Journal and Professors Moir and Fraenkel for their permission to reproduce Figure 11-8.

I wish to extend my deep appreciation to William Brinkhous who prepared majority of the illustrations in the book. Thanks are also due to Thomas Thuma for preparing illustrations in Chapter 3.

Collection and checking of references is always a difficult task. This work was made easy by Mrs. Jo Ann Bell who worked hard and provided quick service. I am grateful to her.

To Dr. Wallace R. Wooles, dean of the medical school at the East Carolina University and to my colleague Dr. S. W. Nye I am indebted for their cooperation in securing facilities.

For secretarial assistance I must commend Mrs. Jacqueline Brown. She was careful and patient under the most trying circumstances.

Every writer would know well that the contributions of the members of the family cannot be measured in words. My wife Mahlaqua and my children Sabiha, Faiz and Naaz provided with affection the one thing that a writer needs most—consideration.

Finally, it is with great pleasure that I extend my sincere thanks to the publishers, J. B. Lippincott Company. Their cooperation and generous courtesies at all times made the completion of this work a pleasant experience.

Contents

Color plates appear between pages 152–153

1. The Scene Investigation 1
  The Medical Investigator 1
  Documentation of the Facts 2
  Pronouncement of Death 3
  Record of Facts and Findings at the Scene of Death 4
  Identification of the Dead 5
  Cause of Death 5
  Manner of Death 5
  Time of Death 7
  Collection of Physical Evidence 7
  Statement at the Scene 10

2. The Medicolegal Autopsy: Special Procedures 11
  Preliminary Procedures 11
  Authorization for Autopsy 11
  History of the Circumstances of Death 11
  Initial Steps in the Autopsy Room 12
  External Examination 12
  Internal Examination 14
  Regional Examination 15
  The Head 15
  The Neck 15
  The Trunk 16
  Examination of the Exhumed Body 17
  Autopsy Protocol 18

3. Estimation of the Time of Death 20
  Cooling of the Body 20
  Livor Mortis (Lividity, Hypostasis) 22
  Rigor Mortis 23
  Decomposition 24

3. Estimation of the Time of Death—*(Continued)*
Other Physical Changes 25
Chemical Changes 27

4. Identification of the Dead 31
Clothes and Other Personal Effects 33
Fingerprints for Identification 33
External Markings and Stigmata 34
Hair and Identification 35
Dental Identification 40
Determination of Age 41
Case Studies 41
Identification of Bite Marks 43
X-rays and Identification 45
Identification by Internal Examination 45
Identification by Examination of the Blood 46

5. Examination of Skeletal Remains 48
Age 49
Sex 51
Race .... ̄.....60
Stature 63
Other Questions 63

6. Deaths from Blunt Force Injuries 66
Abrasions 66
Bruises 67
Lacerations 70
Regional Blunt Force Injuries 73
Head Injuries 73
Chest Injuries 76
Abdominal Injuries 77
Spinal Injuries 78
Injuries to the Extremities 80

7. Deaths from Cutting and Stabbing Wounds 82
Investigation of the Scene of Death 82

7. Deaths from Cutting and Stabbing Wounds—(*Continued*)
The Autopsy 84
Common Types of Cutting and Stabbing Wounds 86
        Suicidal Incised Wounds 86
        Homicidal Incised Wounds 89
        Accidental Incised Wounds 91
        Stab Wounds 93

8. Gunshot Wounds 97
Examination of the Scene 98
Anatomy of Guns 100
Examination of the Body 104
        Shotgun Wounds 107
        Rifled Gun Wounds 107
Suicidal Gunshot Wounds 113
Homicidal Gunshot Wounds 117
Accidental Gunshot Wounds 117
Concealed and Unusual Gunshot Wounds 117
Artefacts in Deaths from Gunshot Wounds 123

9. Asphyxial Deaths 131
Scene Investigation 131
        Cause of Death 131
        Manner of Death 132
        Time of Death 132
        Collection of Evidence 133
General Autopsy Findings 133
        Petechial Hemorrhages 134
        Congestion 137
        Pulmonary Edema 137
        Cyanosis 137
Strangulation 137
        Ligature Strangulation 138
        Manual Strangulation 140
        Accidental Strangulation 143
        Suicidal Strangulation 143
        Strangulation and Vagal Inhibition 144
Hanging 144
        Suicidal Hanging 144

 9. **Asphyxial Deaths**—*(Continued)*
       Accidental Hanging 146
       Homicidal Hanging 148
    Suffocation 149
       Smothering 149
       Choking 150
       Overlaying 150
       Traumatic Asphyxia 150

10. **The Diagnosis of Drowning** 154
    Investigation of Circumstances of Death and
       Examination of the Scene 154
    External Examination 156
    Internal Examination 158
    Obscure Cases 159
    Drowning in Skin and Scuba Diving 160
    Special Investigations in Drowning Cases 161
       Detection of Diatoms 161
       Chloride, Sodium, Potassium, Magnesium and
          Hemoglobin Studies 161
       Plasma Specific Gravity 163
       Electron Microscopic Studies 163
    Conclusion 164

11. **Deaths from Burns, Electrocution, Lightning** 166
    Burns 166
       Circumstances of Death 166
       Autopsy Findings 167
       How Does an Autopsy Help? 168
       Artefacts in Burned Bodies 175
    Electrocution 177
       Investigation of a Death 179
    Lightning 181

12. **Deaths from Heatstroke and Hypothermia** 184
    Heatstroke 184
    Hypothermia 186

13. **Sudden, Unexpected Natural Deaths** 189
    Causes of Sudden Death 190
    Trauma and Disease 193

14. **Stillbirths and Infant Deaths** 195
  Stillbirth 195
  Natural Deaths of Infants 196
      Crib Death Syndrome (Cot Death) 196
  Unnatural Deaths of Infants 199
      Battered Child Syndrome 199
      Suffocation, Strangulation, Drowning 205
      Cutting and Stabbing Wounds, Burns and Scalds,
          Poisoning 207

15. **Transportation Fatalities** 209
  Investigation of Automobile Accidents 209
      Examination of the Scene 209
      The Autopsy 210
      Reconstruction of the Crash 211
      Natural Death (at the Wheel) vs. Death from
      Injuries 211
      Homicide with the Automobile 214
      Suicide with the Automobile 216
      Driver Identification 217
      Alcohol and Drugs 218
      Conclusion 219
  Investigation of Aircraft Accidents 219

16. **Investigation of Deaths from Therapeutic Mishaps** 224
  Operative and Anesthetic Deaths 224
      Therapeutic Misadventure, Iatrogenic Disease 229
      Summary 233

17. **Artefacts in Forensic Pathology** 235
  Introduction 235
      Artefacts Introduced Between Death and Autopsy 235
      Artefacts Introduced During Autopsy 250
  Summary 252

18. **Negative Autopsy** 254
      Death from Fright or Shock 256

18. Negative Autopsy—*(Continued)*
Concealed or Apparently Insignificant Trauma 256
Lesions of the Nervous System 257
Lesions in the Neck 259
Lesions of Cardiovascular System 262
Lesions of the Adrenal Glands 267
Sickle Cell Disease 269
Decomposition 270
What to Do When the Autopsy Is Negative 271

19. Investigation of Poisoning Deaths 273
Examination of the Scene of Death 273
Autopsy on a Poisoning Death 275
Interpretation of Toxicological Results 278
Final Analysis of a Poisoning Case 279
Manner of Death 280

20. Consideration of Individual Poisons 283
Alcohols 283
Methyl Alcohol (Methanol, Wood Alcohol) 287
Ethylene Glycol 288
Isopropyl Alcohol 288
Amphetamines 289
Arsenic 290
Barbiturates 292
Cannabis (Marihuana) 295
Carbon Monoxide 296
Carbon Tetrachloride 299
Cyanides 302
Lead 304
LSD (D-Lycergic acid Diethylamide) 305
Morphine (Heroin) 307
Organophosphates (Parathion) 310
Propoxyphene Hydrochloride (Darvon) 312
Psychosedative Drugs 313
Phenothiazines 313
Meprobamate (Miltown, Equanil) 314
Imipramine (Trofranil), Amitriptyline (Elavil),
Desipramine (Pertofrane) 315
Salicylates 315

21. Artefacts in Forensic Toxicology 320
Introduction 320
Two Groups of Toxicological Artefacts 320
    Artefacts Introduced Between Death and the
      Postmortem Examination 320
    Artefacts Introduced During Autopsy 322
Discussion and Summary 323

22. Analytical Procedures: Simple Tests for Pathologists 325
    Alcohol 325
    Heavy Metals (Arsenic, Bismuth, Antimony,
      Mercury) 326
    Barbiturates 327
    Carbon Monoxide 327
    Cyanide 328
    Diatoms 329
    Ferrous Sulfate 330
    Isopropyl Alcohol 331
    Lead 331
    Methyl Alcohol 332
    Parathion 332
    Phenothiazines 332
    Salicylates 332
    Spermatozoa: Acid Phosphatase Test 333
    Strychnine 333

23. The Pathologist As a Witness 336
    Subpoena 336
    Preliminaries 337
    Court Attendance 338

Index 343

Handbook of
Forensic Pathology

1

The Scene Investigation

The scene investigation is of paramount importance in any medicolegal inquiry into a death. Indeed success or failure of the entire investigation may depend upon it. The visit to a scene of death crystalizes the circumstances surrounding it and adds substantially to the total knowledge of the case. Furthermore, an on-the-spot study of the circumstances of death prompts one to look for things that would not ordinarily come to mind if the scene were not visited.

Every natural death may not have to be investigated at the scene. However, it must be remembered that a death that may appear to be natural may, in fact, be the outcome of foul play. Therefore, if there is the slightest suspicion, one should examine the scene. A suspicious mind is a key to the detection of crime. Even with the most sophisticated methods and equipment for crime detection, many homicides go undetected because of the lack of suspicion and improper or inadequate investigation.[1] It is a good principle to treat a death as unnatural until convincing evidence proves it otherwise. In most jurisdictions throughout the world, about 20 percent of all persons die under circumstances that require an official medicolegal investigation to determine the cause and manner of death. About 10 percent of all deaths are caused by violence.[2] The types of death that usually require investigation by medical examiners, coroners or police surgeons in various jurisdictions of the world are:

1. Sudden in apparent good health.
2. Unattended by a physician.
3. Violent or unnatural.
4. Suspicious.
5. Unusual.
6. In prison or police custody.
7. In an operating room.

The Medical Investigator

In some countries, police officers investigate medicolegal cases. In England, for instance, a lay or medical coroner is in charge of such an investigation. In the United States, some states have adopted the modern

1

medical examiner system while other states still retain the coroner system. Whenever an autopsy is to be performed, the medical investigator, of course, steps in. The emphasis now leans justifiably, toward putting medical men in charge of all the investigations of deaths involving medicolegal questions, in cooperation with law enforcement officers.

When called upon to investigate a death, the role of a medical investigator is to:

1. Pronounce the person dead.
2. Help identify the decedent if his identity is not known.
3. Determine the cause of death.
4. Assist in determining the manner of death (i.e., whether it is natural, accidental, suicidal, or homicidal).
5. If unnatural, determine the means/agent causing death, such as knife, gun, poison.
6. Help establish approximate time of death.
7. If homicide, assist in identifying the person responsible for death.

When a death is reported by telephone, whether by a relative of the decedent, a funeral director, a police officer or just a passerby or witness to the death, it should first be determined whether the case is such that investigation at the scene is necessary. Every effort should be made to examine the body at the scene if the death appears suspicious.

Documentation of the Facts

In any medicolegal work, documentation of the facts is vitally important. Therefore, from the time the first call is received, records on the case should be maintained. First of all, the date and the time of the call and the name of the party calling should be noted. The name of the decedent, if known, and the address and telephone number of the place where the body is found should be asked for. After evaluating the initial information concerning the background and the circumstances of death, if it appears necessary the investigator should proceed immediately to the scene. In preparation for the investigation, it is advisable to carry a kit with the following articles:

1. Notebook and pen.
2. Camera with films and flashbulbs.
3. Syringe with 4-inch, size 15 needle and containers.
4. Thermometer with temperature range of $0°$ to $120°F$.
5. Measuring tape.
6. Pair of gloves.
7. Small plastic bags and labels.
8. Flashlight.
9. Stethoscope.

On arrival at the scene, the investigator must identify himself to the person present in charge of the remains. If there is suspicion of foul play he must call the police, if they are not already there, and work in cooperation with them. Then he can proceed with the investigation systematically along the following lines:

1. Obtain information about the circumstances of death and the background of the decedent.
2. Make observations about the overall scene (e.g., room, surroundings, clothes, etc.).
3. Photograph the scene and the body before anything is moved, and if indicated, after the body is moved.
4. Examine the body carefully.

The investigator should spend a few moments carefully observing the entire scene without unnecessarily disturbing it while the police work on other aspects of the case such as the search for fingerprints. He should not handle the weapon such as a gun or knife carelessly lest he erase the assailant's fingerprints and put his own on it. If the case is a homicide and the determination of time of death seems important, rectal temperature of the decedent should be obtained and observations made about weather conditions at the site the body was found. All the facts and findings at the scene should be recorded on a form such as that shown on page 4.

From the examination of the scene and of the body, the doctor may be able to draw several conclusions pertaining to the ultimate goals of the investigation which are described below.

Pronouncement of Death

At the scene of death, one of the first functions of a medical investigator or a coroner is to make sure that death has in fact, taken place. In most cases, the stiffening of the body and even the beginning of decomposition indicate death. In case of recent death, however, care should be exercised before the person is declared dead—absence of respiration and heartbeat; absence of reflexes, and changes in the eyes, such as clouding of the cornea and absence of corneal reflexes are some of the signs that should be checked before making the diagnosis of death. A mere check of the pulse may be misleading, for a person who is in a state of shock from any cause or one who is electrocuted or a victim of drowning may be alive with no pulse. In an elderly person the pulse may be feeble and imperceptible and a casual examination and pronouncement of death may result in an embarrassing situation, as illustrated in the following example:

In 1964, a physician was called to examine an elderly man at his home. The doctor saw the man lying in bed motionless, quickly checked the man's heart-

RECORD OF FACTS AND FINDINGS AT
THE SCENE OF DEATH

Date and Time of Call: Called by:

Name of Decedent: Age: Race: Sex:

Place of Death (Address):   Type of Premises:

Date and Time of Scene Investigation:

Type of Death (e.g., homicide, accident, etc.):

Body Identified by:

Circumstances of Death: 1. Past Medical History:
                         2. Events Leading to Death:
                         3. Time and Date Decedent
                            Last Seen Alive:
                         4. Time and Date Body Found:

Description of Body: 1. Approximate Height and Weight:
                      2. Clothing:
                      3. Injuries—Fatal and nonfatal:
                      4. Livor:
                      5. Rigor:
                      6. Body Temperature (Rectal
                         Temperature):

Probable Cause of Death:

Probable Manner of Death:

Rough Sketch of the Scene:

Name of Person Authorized to Move the Body:

beat by placing his hand on his chest and felt the radial artery. He declared the man dead and authorized the removal of the body to a morgue for autopsy. In the autopsy room, while the remains were being placed on the table, this author heard a gurgling sound and noticed a slight swallowing movement. The man was rushed to a hospital and lived for two more months.

Identification of the Dead

In most cases identification of the dead is not a problem. No one is expected to solve a difficult identification at the scene. However, a careful examination of the scene can reveal many clues. For instance, if the remains are skeletonized or the body is decomposed it is necessary to look for evidence such as personal effects. Frequently, one is able to pull out a wallet, papers or other identifying materials from the pockets of the decedent's clothes. If after the scene investigation, the identification of the dead person remains uncertain, further inquiries and a complete autopsy should be carried out. The details of such investigations are discussed more fully in Chapters 4 and 5.

Cause of Death

The medical history of the decedent (e.g., a history of heart attacks) and the absence of any injuries, or the possibility of poisoning, as deter-mined by the scene investigation, may indicate that the death is natural. Many jurisdictions in the United States and elsewhere do not call for autopsies on deaths that appear to be natural. In such instances, the death certificate may be issued at the scene and the body released. If, however, the cause of death is not obvious, an autopsy should be authorized and done. Many times, especially with violent deaths, the cause of death may be obvious (e.g., stab wound or gunshot wound). Such an injury at a concealed unexposed site may escape detection by a casual observer. Therefore, a thorough examination of the body, not forgetting the exami-nation of the back of the body, should be a routine practice at the scene of death. Toxicological analyses and histological studies may also be required.

Manner of Death

The examination of the scene can be of great assistance in determining the manner of death. While investigating a scene of death, it is always a good habit for the investigator to ask himself whether this death was the result of natural causes or whether it was an accident, a suicide or a homicide. The consideration of this question will go a long way in dealing with cases where the manner of death is not clear. Although a death may appear natural in every respect, other possibilities such as poisoning or concealed trauma should be kept in mind. The person who appears to have died from natural causes may have actually died accidentally from acute alcohol poisoning or from the combined effects of alcohol and drugs such as sleeping pills. Also, he may have committed suicide by using drugs, or in a rare circumstance there may have been criminal poisoning.

If the death is obviously the result of violent means, the scene observations should be carefully analyzed to determine the manner of death. If there is the slightest suspicion of foul play, the case should be treated as homicide until proved otherwise. There are often circumstances which can lead to false conclusions, as the following case history illustrates:

> A 23-year-old married man who had always enjoyed good health and lived a "normal sexual life" was found dead in a room locked on the inside hanging by a rope from a beam in the ceiling. His wife assumed he had committed suicide. However, at the scene, the lower half of the body was nude and the upper half partially covered with female clothes including a brassiere. Between the rope and the skin of the neck was a handkerchief. In the closets and cabinets in a room in which he had never permitted anyone to enter were female clothes and several photographs of nude women.

This, of course, was an *accidental* death from auto-erotic sexual activity. Figure 1-1 illustrates some of the features of such a death.

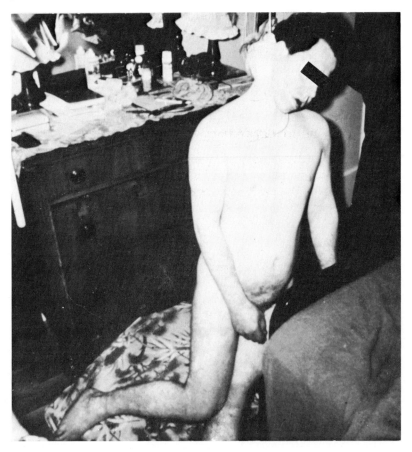

Fig. 1–1. Accidental death from autoerotic sexual activity.

In every part of the world, suicide bears a stigma. For this reason and for the reason of insurance claims, an attempt may be made by members of the family to conceal suicide and make it look as if death were accidental or natural. In such circumstances, the information given by the family members should be carefully evaluated and their reactions appropriately interpreted. There is also the possibility of alterations made at the scene prior to the arrival of the investigators. Similarly, in criminal cases, the criminal may alter the scene to conceal a homicide.

Time of Death

At the scene of death, a medical investigator is frequently asked at what time death occurred. The determination of the time of death of a homicide victim is often vital, since it may help exclude certain suspects and aid in limiting the investigation to a certain time period. Precise estimation of the time of death is extremely difficult to determine, television fiction presentations notwithstanding. Because of many variable factors, the estimation of time of death can be made only within broad limits. The best method of approach at the scene is a consideration of the combination of the circumstances of death, the history of the whereabouts of the decedent, the factors affecting the changes in the body after death, and the use of the available methods to determine the time of death. These methods are detailed in Chapter 3.

Collection of Physical Evidence

While the examination of the scene and the body is being made, attention should be paid to the collection of objects of evidential value. All evidence, even trace evidence, which is even remotely relevant to the investigation should be collected. The investigator should be particularly careful in collecting such evidence if the case is a homicide. After the measurements and the photographs are made and the fingerprints taken, the weapon, if found at the scene, should be taken into custody and placed carefully in a container. Other materials of evidential value such as hairs, fibers and objects or clothing on which there are stains should be collected in ample quantity and retained in transparent plastic bags. In a case of suspected poisoning, the bottles, boxes, vomit and even fecal matter at the scene should be collected. Every piece of physical evidence should be clearly labeled on the containers with the decedent's name, the description of the material, the name of the person collecting the evidence and the date it is collected. The chain of custody of all the materials collected can be a vital issue at a trial. Hence, every time the evidence is transmitted to another person, written receipt should be obtained. If the specimen or the sample is to be mailed to anyone, it should be sent by registered mail with return receipt requested. The following case illustrates the extent and the value of the collection of physical evidence:

One early morning, this author was summoned to a scene where a young male was found dead on an apartment floor with his face in a pool of blood-stained vomit. There was also evidence of diarrhea. On a nearby bed, a young woman was in a state of severe shock and was vomiting. She was immediately rushed to a hospital. In the room, there were numerous liquor bottles. These were collected. The autopsy on the man and the toxicologic analyses revealed that he had died from acute arsenic poisoning. The biological materials and the dozens of bottles collected from the scene showed the presence of arsenic. With the help of these observations, the woman was confirmed to be suffering from acute arsenic poisoning. The labels on the bottles helped find

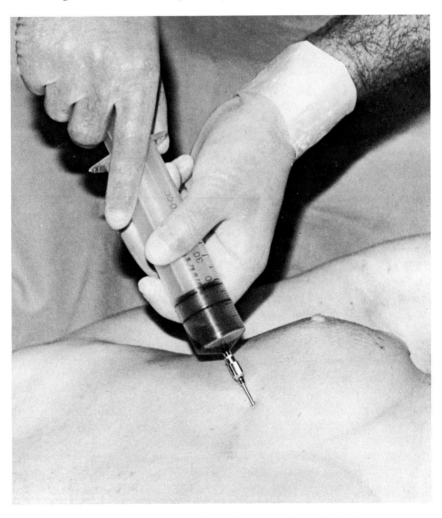

Fig. 1–2. The method of drawing blood from the body.

the source of the liquor and led to the arrest of an 80-year-old man who admitted to selling "moonshine" and to adding "white powder" to give "extra kick."

If the death appears natural and it is decided to conclude the investigation without an autopsy, it is advisable to retain samples of blood and/or urine from the body, lest a question of poisoning be raised at a later date. Blood can easily be withdrawn from the heart by inserting a 4-inch needle through the fourth or fifth left interspace and directing it backward, slightly to the right and slightly downward (Fig. 1-2). Similarly, a sample of urine can be obtained by introducing a needle into the bladder through the skin just above the pubic bone (Fig. 1-3). Such samples should always be drawn before the body is embalmed.

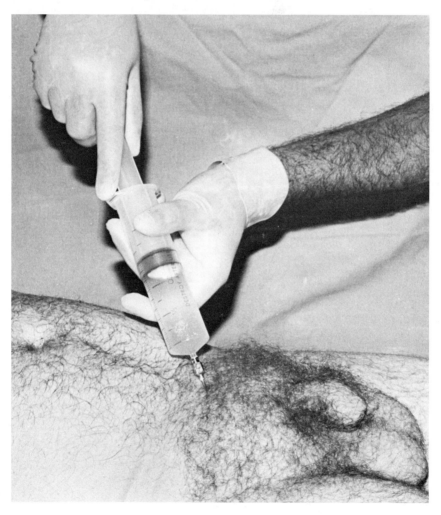

Fig. 1–3. The method of drawing urine from the body.

STATEMENTS AT THE SCENE

Occasionally, the scene of death is surrounded by curious observers and representatives from the news media. With the help of police, the area can be roped off so that unhindered investigation can be carried out. Always refrain from answering questions from the casual observer and great caution should be exercised in answering questions from the press. It is permissible to state the cause and manner of death if there is no doubt about them. However, if the circumstances are not clear, it is unwise to speculate publicly or to discuss theories about the motive of the criminal in a case of homicide. It is best to say that the investigation is not completed and that no conclusions have been reached. As far as the relationship with the law enforcement agents involved in the investigation is concerned, the medical investigator should cooperate fully, and freely exchange information.

One of the important by-products of a scene investigation is that the medical man is able to render pertinent advice to the police and other investigators regarding the earliest line of questioning and investigation to be followed after the body is found and before the postmortem examination is carried out.

REFERENCES

1. Havard, J.D.J.: Detection of Secret Homicide in Cambridge Studies in Criminology. vol. 11. MacMillan, London, 1960.
2. Snyder, L.: Homicide Investigation, ed. 2. Springfield (Ill.) Charles C Thomas, 1967.

2

The Medicolegal Autopsy: Special Procedures

PRELIMINARY PROCEDURES

The objectives of a medicolegal autopsy are different from those of a hospital autopsy. In an autopsy on a person dying under medical care the essential goals are to determine the cause of death and evaluate the treatment given during life. On the other hand, the main purposes of a medicolegal autopsy are to identify the body, to determine the cause and manner of death, to collect evidence in order to identify the object causing death and to identify the criminal. These differences in the ultimate aims of investigation account for the differences in the investigative procedures in the two types of cases. The procedures vitally important in the investigation of medicolegal cases are outlined in this chapter.

Authorization for Autopsy

The permit for performing an autopsy on a person dying under medical care is signed by the closest relative. The authorization for an autopsy on a medicolegal case depends on the local law. In jurisdictions with medical examiner systems, duly appointed medical examiners or the Chief Medical Examiner can legally authorize an autopsy; where the coroner system is retained the Coroner signs the permit. Before commencing the autopsy the pathologist must make sure that he has the authority to perform the autopsy. If the Coroner or the Medical Examiner has authorized an autopsy on a medicolegal case, objections from the members of the decedent's family should not be allowed to interfere with the pathologist's duties.

History of the Circumstances of Death

The pathologist must gather all the information about the circumstances of death prior to autopsy. Such information will guide him as to what

11

procedure to follow in performing the autopsy and what specimens to collect. Lack of such information may result in loss of vital evidence.

INITIAL STEPS IN THE AUTOPSY ROOM

The following procedures should form a part of the medicolegal autopsy, especially on a victim of homicide:

1. Photograph the remains in the condition received.
2. Collect trace evidence (hairs, fibers, glass, paint) and place in separate labeled containers.
3. Describe the clothing. Remove each article of clothing separately. (Do not cut the clothes.) Photograph the clothes to show defects caused by weapons such as bullets and knives.
4. Take x-rays of the body in the cases of firearm fatalities and in other cases when indicated.
5. Take a photograph of the face, after it is cleaned up, for identification purposes.
6. Record rectal temperature.
7. Obtain a sample of scalp hair by plucking tufts of hair with the hand or with forceps. (Do not cut the hair.)

EXTERNAL EXAMINATION

The external examination in a medicolegal case is far more important than in a hospital case. Of particular importance are the aspects of identification and injuries. External injuries not only reveal the nature of the object causing them but also indicate the severity of internal injuries. Other vital aspects related to external examination are the collection of specimens and the determination of the time of death. In view of the significance of the external examination it is imperative that nothing be left undone in any medicolegal case.

The general description of the body should include the age, sex, race, color of skin, height, weight, nutrition, muscle development, body build, bony frame, congenital and acquired deformities, scars, tattoos, moles, skin diseases and the distribution, nature and color of hair. A note should be made of the presence and distribution of lividity (hypostasis), rigor mortis and signs of decomposition. The eyes should be examined for color, size of pupils and the presence or absence of petechial hemorrhages. The mouth should be carefully examined for teeth and dentures, especially in cases in which the dental record is important. In males, a note should be made of whether or not the penis is circumcised.

The importance of the examination of external injuries in medicolegal cases cannot be overemphasized. Every effort should be made to record a verbal description, sketch the injuries on a body diagram and photograph them (Figs. 2-1 and 2-2). These records will serve a useful purpose later in court.

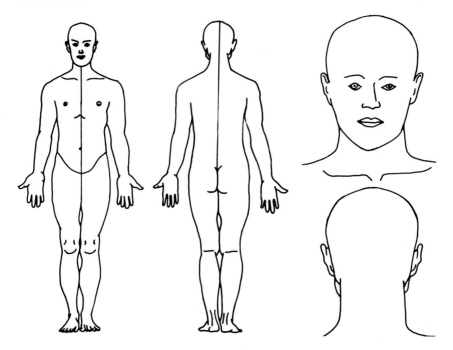

Fig. 2–1. (*Left*) A body diagram for recording findings of the external examination.

Fig. 2–2. (*Right*) A head diagram to record findings of the external examination.

The nature and the direction of abrasions, the color of bruises and the characteristics of lacerations and incised wounds should be noted with measurements. The position of injuries such as stab wounds and gunshot wounds should be related to distances from the top of the head, from the soles of the feet and from the midline. If the injuries are obscured by hair, as on the scalp, the area should be shaved. The inside of the lips may show bruising and lacerations caused by blows; the neck may reveal bruises and abrasions in the cases of hanging and strangulation; sexual assaults may be associated with injuries of the genitalia. The back should always be examined and the extremities should be searched for old or recent needle puncture marks. Injuries can escape detection unless care is exercised.

In homicides, after the wounds are documented by description, diagrams and photographs, they should be excised and retained.

In addition to collecting the trace evidence and the hair, swabs from the mouth, vagina and anus should be taken from the cases of suspected sexual assault before the internal examination is begun.

INTERNAL EXAMINATION

The incision shown in Figure 2-3 allows adequate exposure of neck organs when the skin is reflected, and yet the suture line is concealed when the corpse is dressed for viewing by relatives.

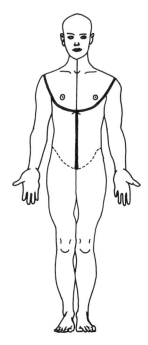

Fig. 2–3. A diagram of a primary autopsy incision.

Because the technique of internal examination of a medicolegal case also is essentially the same as that for a hospital case details about the removal and the examination of individual organs are not given in this book. It must be stressed, however, that *in a medicolegal case the autopsy must always be complete,* not omitting the examination of the brain, even though the cause of death is apparent elsewhere.

It is a good practice to obtain a blood sample from every medicolegal case. Blood can be easily drawn with a syringe from the right ventricle, pulmonary trunk or aorta. It is also advisable to determine the blood group of every homicide victim.

REGIONAL EXAMINATION

The Head

While the scalp is reflected its undersurface should be examined for bruises, because the evidence of blows on the head is most vividly evident on the undersurface of the scalp.

After the brain is removed in the usual way, the dura should be stripped from the skull to look for fractures. The best way to remove the dura is to hold a part of it with a wet towel and pull it away from the skull. Alternatively a clamp may be used.

In the cases of drowning, asphyxia and intracranial infections, the middle ears should be examined to check for hemorrhages and evidence of infection. For a quick gross examination of the middle ears the petrous bone forming the roof of the middle ears may be chiseled off. If histological examination is desired the bone should be sawed off around the middle ears.

The Neck

Medicolegally important conditions may be found in the neck. There may be significant injuries of the tissues and evidence of asphyxia due to strangulation or hanging. These findings and evidence of obstruction of the upper respiratory tract by choking on food or laryngeal edema are missed if the neck is not examined. Therefore, a complete medicolegal autopsy must include detailed examination of neck organs.

To remove the neck structures the skin is reflected up to a point a little above the hyoid bone. The structures are dissected away from the neighboring tissues on either side, the line of dissection being medial to the carotid vessels. If the tongue is to be removed with the neck organs, the knife is inserted under the lower jaw to sever the attachment of the tongue to the jaw. The tissues on either side under the arch of the jaw are cut to allow insertion of the fingers to hold the tongue and pull it down. After the tongue is pulled down, the tissues on either side of it are cut lateral to the tonsillar fossae, maintaining a downward pull on the tongue. Posteriorly the suprapharyngeal area should be cut transversely against the spine. The neck organs with the tongue, hyoid bone, soft palate, tonsils, pharynx, larynx, esophagus, trachea and the thyroid gland should be pulled downward, at the same time separating the structures from the spine. If the removal of the tongue is not necessary, an anteroposterior horizontal cut extending down to the spine may be made just above the hyoid bone and the neck structures removed to allow the examination of the pharynx, larynx, hyoid bone and the other structures below the level of hyoid bone.

The Trunk

Thorax and Abdomen. In all cases of suspected trauma to the chest (e.g., transportation fatalities, industrial accidents, traumatic asphyxia) and in persons with the history of asthma, the possibility of *pneumothorax* should be kept in mind. The presence of pneumothorax must be demonstrated before the chest wall is penetrated. To check for pneumothorax, a pocket is dissected between the chest wall and the skin and filled with water; the rib interspace is perforated with a knife or scissors under water. If under pressure air is present in the chest, it will bubble out of the perforation through the water.

If *air embolism* is suspected, the technique of opening the thorax and the abdomen should be modified so that the presence of air in the circulation can be demonstrated. Care should be taken not to cut any large vessels in the neck, chest and abdomen while opening the body cavities. After the abdomen is opened, the inferior vena cava, mesenteric and the adnexal vessels should be examined for the presence of air bubbles by puncturing the inferior vena cava under water. If air is present it will bubble out of water from the vessel. In the cases of air embolism the right ventricle of the heart invariably contains air. To demonstrate the presence of this air, the pericardium can be incised, the pericardial sac filled with water and the anterior wall of the right ventricle cut under water. Air bubbles will spurt out as soon as the ventricle is incised.

Abdominal Viscera. Because of its importance in medicolegal cases, a description of the nature and quantity of stomach contents should be recorded. If the abdominal viscera are to be removed separate from the thoracic organs, the esophagus should be ligated before it is cut to prevent loss of gastric contents. This procedure is particularly important in the cases of poisoning.

Genital Tract. Examination of the injuries of the female genital tract in the victims of sexual assault can be difficult. For proper evaluation of the injuries it may be necessary to remove the genital organs en masse.

To achieve satisfactory dissection the pubic symphysis is sawed and the pubic bones are separated. Dissection is made around the rectum, vagina and bladder and the tissues separated from the pelvic outlet. A circular cut is made around the vulval and anal orifices. The dissection is extended from around the pelvic outlet down to the circular cut around the external orifices. The uterus, cervix, vagina and vulva with bladder in front and rectum behind are removed in one block. After the bladder is dissected away the genital tract is laid open by making a single vertical cut through the anterior wall of the uterus and vagina.

EXAMINATION OF THE EXHUMED BODY

In criminal cases exhumation of the body for autopsy is usually carried out in order to gather additional information about the manner of death. In civil cases the purpose of exhumation is to aid in the settlement of dissected away the genital tract is laid open by making a single vertical compensation and liability for negligence.

Exhumation Authorization. Exhumation can be carried out only with proper authorization, and laws governing disinterment vary. In most places in the United States permits for exhumation in criminal cases are issued by a justice of a superior court. In a civil case in addition to the court order a written authorization must be obtained from the next of kin. In England the Home Secretary or the Coroner (only in his own jurisdiction) can authorize disinterment.

Autopsy Authorization. There must also be proper authorization for the pathologist to perform the autopsy. In civil cases the autopsy permit must be signed by the next of kin of the decedent; in criminal cases the authorization must come from the Medical Examiner or the Coroner who has jurisdiction over the case, or the pathologist should have a court order.

The Exhumation. The pathologist who is going to perform the postmortem examination should make every effort to attend the exhumation in order to satisfy himself as to the identity of the decedent. At the grave site he should note identifying features such as the headstone, nameplate on the casket, characteristics of the casket and the location of the grave. He should also make observations about the condition of the soil, water content, condition of the casket and of the body. If there is the remotest possibility of poisoning, the soil samples should be collected from the following positions at the site of disinterment: (a) The surface of ground above the coffin, (b) just above the coffin, (c) either side of the coffin, (d) under the coffin, (e) a remote area of the cemetery (control sample).

The Autopsy. In the autopsy room further efforts should be made to identify the remains. The funeral director or any person who knew the decedent during life can view the body to make identification. If the identity of the deceased remains in question, a complete investigation must be made along the lines discussed in Chapters 4 and 5.

External Examination. The description of the external examination should include a record of the identifying features, degree of decomposition, embalming incisions and trocar perforations. Photographs and, where indicated, x-rays of the body must be taken.

Internal Examination. The internal examination must be complete. Antemortem pathological changes may be affected by postmortem decomposition and embalming. It may be impossible to diagnose drowning, smothering, air embolism, pneumothorax and various other conditions. Although still identifiable, traumatic lesions, such as bullet and stab wounds may have altered in appearance. All important injuries should be excised at the autopsy and preserved. Care should be exercised in differentiating pathological lesions from postmortem artefacts (see Chap. 17).

Histological Examination. Tissues from various organs should be retained for histological examinations. The pathologist should bear in mind that histological details are well preserved in many embalmed bodies despite prolonged burial.

Toxicological Examination. For the toxicological examination, adequate material must be saved. In addition to portions of internal organs, samples of hair, skin, nails and bones should be kept. In spite of embalming, several of the poisons such as heavy metals, barbiturates and strychnine can be recovered from the biological materials.

AUTOPSY PROTOCOL

The findings of any medicolegal investigation and autopsy should be recorded at the time of examination of the body. The observations may be dictated or written down by the pathologist.

The autopsy report should include the details of identification of the body; date, time and place of examination; findings of external and internal examinations and the cause of death. A facsimile of the front page of the autopsy report used in the States of North Carolina and Virginia is shown in Figure 2-4. Such a format is recommended since it gives vital information at a glance. Details of the results of the external and internal examinations, x-rays, histological and toxicological studies, and opinions can be appended when a complete report is requested by any party.

The completed report should be sent to the person authorizing the autopsy.

REPORT OF AUTOPSY

DECEDENT _____Ringo_____R._____Rinker_____ Autopsy authorized by: Kenneth K. King, M.D., M.E.
                First name   Middle name   Last name   Name   Official Title

TYPE OF DEATH:		RIGOR	LIVOR	Body Identified by:
Violent or Unnatural ⊠	Unattended by a physician ☐	JAW ⊠ ARMS ☐	COLOR Purple	Body tag on left big toe
	Sudden in apparent health ☐	NECK ☐ CHEST ☐	ANTERIOR POSTERIOR ⊠	
Means: Gun	Unusual ☐ In prison ☐	BACK ☐ ABDOMEN ☐	LATERAL ☐	PERSONS PRESENT AT AUTOPSY
	Suspicious ☐	LEGS ☐	REGIONAL	Kenneth K. King, M.D.

AGE 25 RACE Negro SEX Male LENGTH 72" WEIGHT 170 lb EYES Brown PUPILS: R 6 mm. OPACITIES, ETC.
HAIR Black BEARD -- MUSTACHE Black CIRCUMCISED Yes BODY HEAT Cool L 6 mm.

NON FATAL WOUNDS, SCARS, TATTOOING, OTHER FEATURES: warm in flexures

An abrasion, 1 1/2 x 1", center of forehead.
See attached protocol, gunshot wound chart and x-rays.

PATHOLOGICAL DIAGNOSIS

---

1. Gunshot wound of chest:
   Perforation of fifth left rib anteriorly, perforation of anterior and posterior walls of left ventricle and pericardium 2" from apex.

2. Bilateral hemothorax: 1,000 c.c. blood left side, 200 c.c. right side.

3. Hemopericardium: 50 c.c.

4. Abrasion, forehead.

5. Adenoma, left adrenal.

Comment: A 0.22 calibre bullet lodged in subcutaneous tissues of back at the level of 9th interspace, 4" to the left of midline, was retrieved and retained.

Probable cause of death:
                    Gunshot wound of chest.

PROVISIONAL REPORT ☐
FINAL REPORT ⊠

A true copy:

_____ 1-1-73
   Chief Medical Examiner   Date

The facts stated herein are true and correct to the best of my knowledge and belief.
Jerry J. Joshua, M.D.
                                    Signature of Pathologist
10 a.m. to 1 p.m. 1/1/73   City Hospital
   Date and time of autopsy   Durham, N.C.
                                    Place of autopsy

Fig. 2–4. A facsimile of the front page of the autopsy report recommended for medicolegal cases; hypothetical data is filled in.

3

Estimation of the Time of Death

The pathologist involved in the investigation of medicolegal cases is frequently asked questions relating to the time of death. Accurate determination of the time of death is one of the most difficult problems to solve in forensic pathology. Literature on the various topics of medicolegal significance indicates that more efforts have been expended in the direction of solving this problem than on any other medicolegal problem. Despite extensive research no method is yet available which can accurately determine the time of death. The physical and chemical changes that occur in the body after death form the basis for the estimation of time of death. Therefore, in this chapter the discussion of such postmortem changes and their usefulness in estimating the time of death will go hand in hand.

COOLING OF THE BODY

Because the rate of cooling of the body after death is generally accepted as the most dependable criterion in estimating the lapse of time during the first 12 to 18 hours after death, much of the research has centered around the study of postmortem body temperature.

The most reliable temperature readings are obtained from the rectum without interfering with the body. Temperature readings from the liver after introducing a thermometer through an incision are also dependable. Axillary and oral temperatures are not recommended, however, because they are subject to wide fluctuations caused by environmental influences.

To obtain the rectal temperature a thermometer with a temperature range of 0 to 120°F, should be inserted 3 to 4 inches into the rectum and left there for 2 to 3 minutes. When the estimation of time of death is vital to a case, it is important to record the rectal temperature as soon as the body is found.

The average normal temperature at death is 99°F. It can vary, however, from person to person. Exercise or struggle prior to death may raise the rectal temperature up to 3 to 4 degrees. During sleep the rectal temperature is one or two degrees lower than it is during waking hours. With an infective process in the body, the rectal temperature at death may be markedly higher (e.g., a man who died from lobar pneumonia had the rectal temperature of 106°F. one half hour after death). On the other hand, in a victim of exposure the temperature may be in the low nineties. The rate of fall of rectal temperature from "normal" at the time of death also is affected by factors which slow the rate of cooling such as lack of ventilation, clothing and heavy bedclothes. Drop in rectal temperature is faster in the bodies of infants and elderly persons than in the bodies of young adults. The rate of cooling is twice as fast in water as in air.

There are several formulae which can be used in estimating the time of death with rectal temperatures.[2, 4, 15] No formula, unfortunately, gives consistently accurate results, partly because of various factors that modify the rate of cooling of a dead body. After a comprehensive research, Marshall and Hoare[14] evolved a formula which has been shown to be fairly accurate in determining the time of death during the first 18 hours after death. According to their formula, the unclothed body of an adult in an extended position, in an environmental temperature of 60°F. cools at the following rate:

> During first 3 hours after death—1°F. per hour
> During next 3 hours after death—2°F. per hour
> During next 3 hours after death—2°F. per hour
> During next 3 hours after death—1½°F. per hour
> Between 12 to 15 hours after death—1⅓°F. per hour

These authors indicate that the rate of cooling is 66 percent slower if the body is clothed.

Another formula that is simple and acceptable for making a *rough* estimate of the time of death is that proposed by Glaister and Rentoul[7] in which they assume that the body temperature at death is 98.4°F.

$$\frac{98.4° - \text{Rectal temperature}}{1.5} = \text{Number of hours since death}$$

In general, under normal circumstances, adults of average height and weight exposed to environmental temperatures of 60 to 70°F. the rate of cooling is approximately 2°F. per hour during the first 6 hours and approximately 1°F. per hour thereafter until the body temperature is the same as that of the environment. These deductions are applicable to death in a dry environment. However, the dead body in water cools twice as fast. No formulae based on experimental studies are available to determine the time of death of a person found in water. In general, a dead body in water cools at the rate of about 3 to 4°F. per hour in the first 12 hours and at the rate of 1½ to 2°F. per hour during the next 12 hours.

If thermometer readings are not available, a pathologist should remember that a body, warm at death, feels cool within 12 hours after death and is cold by 24 hours. A dead body in water will be cool in 3 to 6 hours and cold in 8 to 12 hours.

LIVOR MORTIS (LIVIDITY, HYPOSTASIS)

The apparent staining of skin in the dependent parts of the body is caused by the gravitational pooling of blood in the blood vessels. Body parts, such as the buttocks, which are in contact with the objects on which they are lying or areas pressed by clothing do not show livor mortis (Fig. 3-1). The settling of blood begins immediately after the cardio-vascular system fails and blood circulation stops. The staining of the skin of dependent parts, initially faint, becomes obvious within about a half hour after death and becomes marked in about 6 hours. This postmortem change has limited value in estimating the time of death.

A more important value of the observation of lividity is the determination of the position of the body after death. Obvious livor in the skin of the front of a body found lying on its back should indicate that the body was moved after death. Livor may disappear from the skin where it first appeared and reappear in dependent parts if the position of the

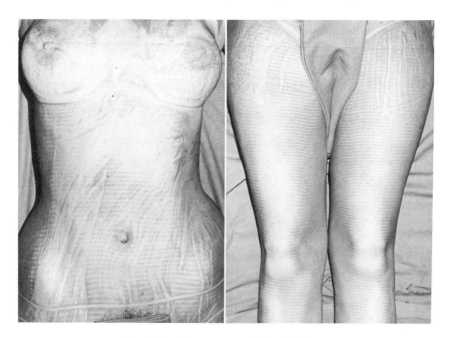

Fig. 3–1. Livor patterned by clothing.

body is changed, because blood is in a fluid state in the first 2 to 3 hours after death and again after about 12 hours postmortem. Sometimes the color of livor is also of significance; pink livor is seen in cases of carbon monoxide poisoning and brown in cases of poisoning with substances (nitrites, nitrates, aniline) causing methemoglobinemia. Refrigerated bodies or those found in cold places also show reddish-pink livor.

RIGOR MORTIS

After death adenosine triphosphatase breaks down, leading to increased accumulation of lactates and phosphates in the muscles. These salts cause stiffening and shortening of muscles, which is called rigor mortis.

Much reliance is placed by a practitioner at the scene of death and a pathologist in the autopsy room on the status of rigor to determine the time of death. It must, however, be stressed that postmortem stiffening of the body is not a reliable phenomenon in making an accurate estimate of the time of death. The times of appearance and disappearance of rigor are so uncertain, and it is so difficult to predict the degree of its development under a certain set of circumstances, that it cannot be relied upon to determine the time of death. At best, it can give but a rough estimate.

Rigor starts at the same time in all muscles of the body.[19] However, it becomes detectable earlier in some muscles than in others. Ordinarily the muscles of the face and the neck show rigor about 6 hours after death, in the muscles of the shoulders and upper extremities in the next few hours, in the trunk and then the muscles of the lower extremities in about 12 hours. If not broken, rigor persists for another 12 hours in the muscles of the whole body. After about 24 hours it begins to disappear, disappearing in about 12 hours in the same order as it appeared.

The reliability of rigor mortis as a criterion for timing of death is influenced by various factors such as metabolic processes of the body and environmental temperature. It develops faster and disappears more quickly when the metabolism is faster as a result of exercise or infections causing fever. The higher the environmental temperature, the quicker the rigor appears and the faster it disappears. In cold temperatures its appearance is delayed and it lasts much longer.

An investigator who relies on rigor mortis for the estimation of time of death should be aware of such conditions as cadaveric spasm (instant rigor) and freezing of the body, for these may mimic rigor mortis. Also, rigor may be obscured by heat stiffening of the body. Once rigor is broken, and this happens frequently from handling of the body after death, it leaves permanent laxity of the affected muscles. While evaluating

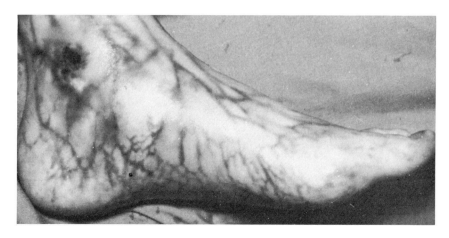

Fig. 3–2. Distended foot veins in a decomposing body. (See Color Plate.)

the status of rigor, the possibility of "broken" rigor should always be kept in mind.

DECOMPOSITION

Estimation of the time of death in a decomposed body is extremely difficult and the degree of decomposition can hardly be considered a reliable index. A body decomposes much faster in a warm atmosphere; whereas cold weather delays the process.

Estimation of the time of death in a body dead for several days can be as important as estimating the time of death in a recent death. The methods used for the period from 24 to 48 hours after death, although reliable for that period, give little help in dealing with bodies dead for longer periods. Therefore, late physical changes, such as decomposition, can sometimes be helpful in making a rough estimate of the time of death.

The abdominal viscera, especially the intestines, are usually the first to be affected by decomposition. This is reflected as a greenish staining of the skin in the flank regions of the abdomen in about 36 to 48 hours after death. Thereafter, decomposition becomes widespread as the anaerobic gas-forming organisms growing in the gastrointestinal tract lead to hemolysis of the blood. Purplish distended veins become obvious in shoulder areas, on the trunk and on the extremities (Fig. 3-2). Gas disrupts internal organs which show air sacs. The skin affected likewise begins to reveal blisters with or without slippage (Fig. 3-3 and 3-4). Such changes are ordinarily seen in bodies dead 3 to 5 days. In another day or two generalized swelling of the tissues begins and the face and the

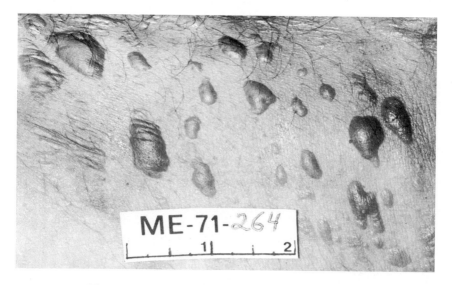

Fig. 3–3. Blister formation in a decomposing body.

abdomen become bloated and the eyeballs and tongue protrude. In a moist environment the tissues show, at this stage, disintegration and liquefaction. In a dead body, among the soft tissues the prostrate and uterus disintegrate last.

OTHER PHYSICAL CHANGES

In the absence of decomposition, drying of the tissues because of hot dry air can cause shriveling of the skin so that it becomes leathery and hard. This process is called *mummification*. With hot dry air it takes several weeks, sometimes months, for the body to mummify.

Another late change in a body is *adipocere formation* (saponification). Hydrolysis and hydrogenation of the subcutaneous fat causes adipocere which contains stearic and oleic acids with calcium soaps. Adipocere is a greasy, waxy, whitish, soft to firm material having a mouldy smell. Subcutaneous tissues in the face, female breasts and the buttocks most often show adipocere. The time of formation of adipocere is variable—a few weeks to several months—and it is greatly accelerated by moisture. In one body found in a damp place 6 weeks after death, almost all areas of the body showed adipocere; and in another, 4 weeks after death the breasts showed obvious adipocere. In dry exposed places or in dry graves, bodies do not show saponification of the tissues for several months. Embalming of the body delays saponification substantially.

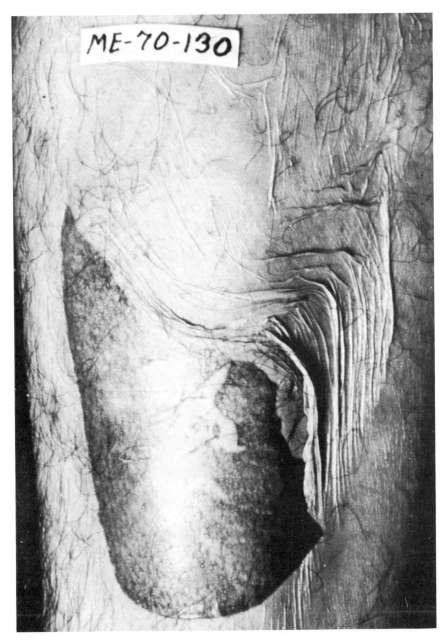

Fig. 3–4. Skin slippage in a decomposing body. (See Color Plate.)

Kevorkian[11] studied postmortem changes in the retina in 51 cases with the help of an ophthalmoscope. He claims that ophthalmoscopy is a "new and fairly accurate approach to the problem of estimation of time of death in unknown cadavers." He obtained perfect estimations (within 10 minutes) in 29 percent of the cases and the average error per case was only 1.2 hours.

It is important to note the quantity, state of digestion and character of the stomach contents at every autopsy for the findings may contribute to the determination of the time of the last meal and perhaps indirectly in the determination of the time of death. Fluids usually leave the stomach within 2 hours, semi-solids in 2 to 3 hours and solids in 4 hours.

Hair ceases to grow after death, whereas during life it grows at the rate of 0.4 mm. per day.[8] Note should be made of the length of the beard on a dead body so that an estimate of the time of the last shave can be made.

CHEMICAL CHANGES

In recent years attempts have been made to arrive at an accurate estimation of the time of death by investigating the biochemical changes occurring in body fluids after death. These have not, however, revealed an accurate and reliable method.[3]

Postmortem changes in the constituents of *blood* have been studied from time to time. The evaluation of the pH of blood, hematocrit studies and postmortem estimation of glucose levels have not brought rewarding results. No useful information has been obtained from the investigations of enzymes such as transaminase, lactic dehydrogenase, phosphatase and amylase.

Schleyer investigated other aspects of blood chemistry.[17] He suggests that serum concentrations not exceeding 14 mg. amino acid nitrogen per 100 ml. or 5 mg. creatine per 100 ml. point to death not more than 12 hours previously and that a serum creatine concentration not exceeding 11 mg. per 100 ml. shows that not more than 28 hours have elapsed since death. He also indicated that inorganic phosphorus in the serum in a concentration greater than 15 mg. per 100 ml. usually indicates a postmorten interval exceeding 10 hours.

The *cerebrospinal fluid* (CSF) has also been studied by several investigators. Some of the older studies have been reviewed by Mant.[13] Mason, Klyne and Lennox[16] studied potassium levels in postmortem samples of blood. Their results indicate that the time of death could be estimated only to within ± 8 hours of the actual time. Schourup's[18] investigations of CSF indicate that in the first 15 hours after death the lactic acid concentration rises from 15 mg. percent to over 200 mg. percent, the non-

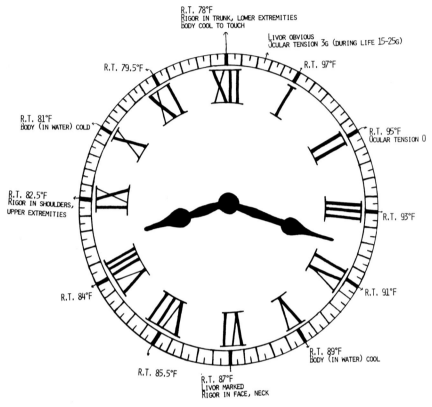

Fig. 3–5. Postmortem clock: Findings at 1 to 12 hours after death; R. T. =
rectal temperature.

protein nitrogen from 15 to 40 mg. percent and the amino acid from 1 to
12 mg. percent. Lundquist[12] did not find Schourup's method of any help.
Schleyer[17] made a study of amino acid nitrogen, creatine and nonprotein
nitrogen components of CSF and drew the following conclusions:

Amino acid nitrogen less than 14 mg.%: Death less than 10 hours
previously
Creatine less than 5 mg.%: Death less than 10 hours previously
Nonprotein nitrogen less than 80 mg.% : Death less than 24 hours
previously

A sample of CSF can be easily obtained from a corpse by tapping the
cisterna magna.

Vitreous and aqueous fluids in the eyeball in a dead body are usually
free from contamination and it is easy to withdraw up to 2 ml. of fluid
from each eyeball with a No. 20 needle and syringe. These facts have

led investigators to make chemical studies of these fluids. For instance, Jaffe[10] and Sturner[20] investigated potassium levels in the vitreous humor and Gantner[6] estimated the ascorbic acid levels. The results, however, have not proved to be an advance over other methods.[1] Similarly, the studies of enzyme changes in organs have been fruitless.[9]

From the above discussion is is clear that no method is yet known which can help determine the precise time of death. The estimate should be based on careful evaluation of all findings. In order that a pathologist may find all the useful information at a glance, a "postmortem clock" is constructed for the important period of the first 12 hours after death (Fig. 3-5). The findings indicated at various hours are, of course, subject to variations.

REFERENCES

1. Adelson, L., Sunshine, I., Rushford, N. B., and Mankoff, M.: Vitreous potassium concentration as an indicator of the postmortem interval. J. Forensic Sci., 8:503, 1963.
2. DeSaram, G. S. W., Webster, G., and Kathirgamatamby, N.: Postmortem temperature and the time of death. J. Crim. Law Criminol., 46:562, 1955–56.
3. Fatteh, A.: Estimation of time of death by chemical changes. Medico-legal Bulletin No. 163, Office of the Chief Medical Examiner, Richmond, 1966.
4. Fiddes, F., and Patten, T. D.: A percentage method for representing the fall in body temperature after death. J. Forensic Med., 5:2, 1958.
5. Gantner, G. E., Sturner, W. Q., Caffrey, P. R., and Brenneman, C.: Ascorbic acid levels in the post mortem vitreous humor: their use in the estimation of time of death. J. Forensic Med., 9:150, 1962a.
6. Gantner, G. E., Sturner, W. Q., Caffrey, P. R., and Brenneman, C.: Ascorbic acid levels in the post mortem vitreous humor: their use in the estimation of time of death. J. Forensic Med., 9:156, 1962b.
7. Glaister, J. and Rentoul, E.: Medical jurisprudence and toxicology. ed. 12, London, E. & S. Livingstone, 1966.
8. Gonzales, T. A., Vance, M., Helpern, M., and Umberger, C. J.: Legal Medicine, ed. 2. Appleton-Century-Crofts, New York, 1954.
9. Grech, J. L., and Parr, C. W.: The assessment of the time of death by enzyme assays. Proc. Third Internat. Meeting in Forensic Sciences. London, 1963.
10. Jaffe, F. A.: Chemical postmortem changes in the intra-ocular fluid. J. Forensic Sci., 7:231, 1962.
11. Kevorkian, J.: The fundus oculi as a "postmortem clock." J. Forensic Sci., 6:261, 1961.
12. Lundquist, F.: Physical and chemical methods for the estimation of the time of death. Acta. Med. Leg. Soc., 9:205, 1956.
13. Mant, A. K.: *In* Simpson, C. K.: Modern Trends in Forensic Medicine. London, Butterworth & Co., 1953.
14. Marshall, T. K., and Hoare, F. E.: The rectal cooling after death and its mathematical expression. J. Forensic Sci., 7:56, 1962.

15. Marshall, T. K.: The use of the cooling formula in the study of post-mortem body cooling. J. Forensic Sci., 7:189, 1962.
16. Mason, J. K., Klyne, W., and Lennox, B.: Potassium levels in the cerebro-spinal fluid after death. J. Clin. Pathol., 4:231, 1951.
17. Schleyer, F.: In Methods of Forensic Science. vol. 2 London, Interscience. 1963.
18. Schourup, K.: Dodstidsbestemmelse. Copenhagen, Dansk Videnskabs For-lag. 1950.
19. Shapiro, H. A.: Rigor mortis. Brit. Med. J., 2:304, 1950.
20. Sturner, W. Q., and Gantner, G. E.: The postmortem interval. A study of potassium in the vitreous humor. Am. J. Clin. Pathol., 42:137, 1964.

4

Identification of the Dead

Identification of a living person is rarely a problem. When the identity of a living criminal is in question, the medical man is seldom involved in the investigation. But in matters related to identification of the dead, the role of the pathologist is important.

It is necessary to identify a dead body not only for humanitarian reasons or to settle the questions of divorce, inheritance and insurance but also in cases of criminal death so that murder can be solved and the murderer apprehended.

The identity of the deceased is hindered if the body is in an advanced state of decomposition and skeletonized or if it is burned or mutilated. Occasionally severe injuries sustained in automobile and industrial accidents or plane crashes obscure identifying features. The loss of skin and body tissues after death caused by insects, animals and marine life also create identification problems for the pathologist.

Most dead bodies are easily identified, by someone who knew the decedent, from the facial appearance, the color of the hair and eyes, the general body build and the clothing. Identification of the deceased may be made by the next of kin from photographs of the body. If these means are of no avail, a systematic investigation is necessary.

In order to establish the identity of a dead person observations should include the consideration of the following features:

Clothes and personal effects, age, race, height, weight, color of eyes, fingerprints, deformities, scars, tattoos, hair, teeth, internal examination, and blood groups.

An external examination of the body permits only a rough estimate of age. The age of a fetus and of an infant can be estimated fairly accurately from the length of the body, eruption of teeth and from the study of ossification centers. Approximate lengths of the embryo and fetus at various periods of gestation are given in Table 4-1 and the periods of eruption of the deciduous teeth in Table 4-2. The appearance of the centers of ossification in various bones is also a useful criterion in determining the age of an infant (Table 4-3). The determination of age in an adolescent and adult is discussed in Chapter 5.

TABLE 4-1. Determination of the Intrauterine Age of the Embryo and Fetus from Its Length.

Month of Gestation	Crown-heel Length of Fetus in Inches
Embryo	
1	½
2	1
3	3½
4	6
Fetus	
5	10
6	12
7	14
8	16
9	18–20

TABLE 4-2. Periods of Eruption of the Deciduous Teeth.

	Periods of Eruption in Months	
Tooth	Upper Jaw	Lower Jaw
Central Incisor	7–8	6–8
Lateral Incisor	8–10	7–9
Canine	15–20	15–20
First Molar	12–15	12–15
Second Molar	20–30	20–30

TABLE 4-3. Appearance of Centers of Ossification of Bones in the Embryo and Fetus.

Bone	Month
Clavicle	1½
Shafts of Long Bones	2
Ischium	3
Pubis	4
Calcaneum	5
Sternal Manubrium	6
Talus	7
Lower End of Sternum	8
Cuboid	9

Questions concerning the sex and stature of the decedent usually arise when skeletonized remains are found. These aspects are presented in Chapter 5.

In the following paragraphs miscellaneous features helpful in the identification of a dead body are discussed. In practice, the release of information about the unidentified body to the news media sometimes serves a useful purpose, since it is one of the best ways to reach relatives of a missing person who can identify the body.

CLOTHES AND OTHER PERSONAL EFFECTS

The majority of the problems of identification are solved if there are clothes and personal effects found on the body. Because police investigators do not usually examine the remains if the body is in an advanced state of decomposition, the pathologist should very carefully examine the materials found. All the personal effects must be retained so that they can be shown to the relatives for positive identification.

If the clothes are in unsatisfactory condition, they may first be washed. The description of the clothes should contain notes on the type of garment, its color, its measurements (collar sizes, trouser lengths) and the nature of the fabric. Tears, cuts or holes should be noted as well as the number, color and position of buttons. Laundry marks and tailor's labels are also invaluable in establishing identity.

All the pockets in the clothing must be examined for identifying papers. A wallet or pocketbook with driver's license, social security card, credit cards and photographs can quickly clinch the identity of the person carrying them.

Rings, wristwatches, keys, necklaces, belts and footwear may also carry identifying marks. In one instance a bunch of keys was found with the body. One of the keys opened a door and another an old suitcase belonging to a missing person. This find, together with the identification of laundry marks on the clothes and other circumstantial details, led to the identification of the body as that of the missing person.

FINGERPRINTS FOR IDENTIFICATION

Fingerprints not only can lead to the identification of a murderer and the murder weapon but also can help in the identification of a dead body. Of all the means of identification fingerprints are the most reliable, because they remain unaltered throughout life. No two fingerprints are alike (no two identical fingerprints have been found in the world) and the chance of two fingerprints being identical is one in ten thousand million million.[6]

When fingerprinting is desired it is best to secure the services of the identification bureau of the local police department. They not only take fingerprints but also follow up on the search and consult the files of the FBI and other organizations that would have fingerprints.

If the gloves of epidermis have separated from the fingers they should be carefully retained, since satisfactory prints can easily be obtained from them. The pathologist at the scene of death should ensure that the detaching epidermis from the fingers is not lost during the transportation of the body. Even if the epidermis is shed and lost, the process of fingerprinting should not be omitted because the exposed dermis will give the same prints as the epidermis, albeit at times less clear. If the fingers to be printed are sodden, wrinkled or mummified, their contour can be made even by injecting liquid paraffin or even formalin or water within the tissues of the palmar aspect of the terminal phalanx of each finger. Richardson and Kade have described an innovation for softening and eliminating wrinkles and crevices of decayed and mummified fingers.[19]

In the case of an unidentified infant or child palm prints and footprints may also serve a useful purpose.

EXTERNAL MARKINGS AND STIGMATA

When faced with a problem of establishing the identity of a body, the external examination can reveal vital clues. Careful search for scars, tattoos, birthmarks, moles, skin diseases, skeletal deformities and calluses should be made. Even with advanced decomposition many of these features can still be detected.

Scars of different sizes and shapes may be located on various parts of the body. When scars are found their measurements, directions and positions on the body should be accurately recorded. Even an appendectomy scar, or midline scars on the abdomen and scars in the groin, often help settle the question of identity when considered in conjunction with other evidence. The finding of an unusual scar (Fig. 4-1) or a scar in an unusual location is also helpful in the investigation.

> The body of an elderly woman was found in a shallow grave at the border of a cemetery. The body was in an advanced state of decomposition and considerable adipocere had formed. External examination revealed three scars on the back between the shoulder blades. After reading the description of the body and the clothing in a newspaper, a young woman came to view the body. She was able to identify the body as her mother's from the scars on the body, despite the fact that she could not recognize the clothing. The scars were the result of an earlier stabbing by a man who was charged with her murder and admitted to shooting her.

Tattoos can be reliable means of identification. Tattoos showing initials and dates may provide ready basis for identification. Small tattoos in the form of dots, crosses and letters are as important as the large ones. The more unusual the location and the design of the tattoo, the greater is its value in identification (Fig. 4-2). The remarkable aspect of tattoos is that

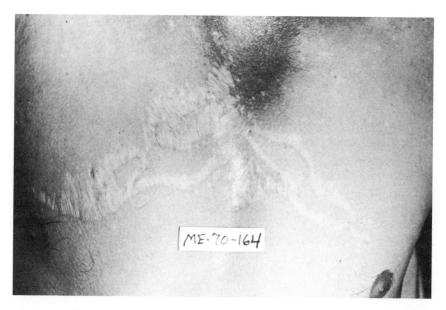

Fig. 4–1. An unusual scar caused by the removal of a tattoo.

they become more distinct and obvious when skin slippage occurs in decomposed bodies. Documentation of tattoos should include the description of the colors, size, shape and the location.

HAIR AND IDENTIFICATION

The examination of the hair not only helps in the identification of the dead body but also in the identification of the assailant, the weapon or the vehicle responsible for death. Therefore, a careful search should be made for hairs on the victim's hands and clothing, and on the weapon found at the scene of crime. The examination of the hair is essentially a task for the expert, but a few simple facts can assist the general pathologist in resolving some of the questions. From the examination of the hair one may be able to determine origin (i.e., human or animal), sex and age of the individual, area of the body from where the hair became detached, mode of separation of the hair, nature of the instrument cutting the hair, alterations caused by dyeing or bleaching, and trace elements.

Structural differences in human and animal hairs have been discussed by Niyogi.[16] Human hairs have narrow medulla, frequently interrupted with pigment which is concentrated in the outer cortex. Animal hairs have wider medulla with pigment concentration in the inner cortex. Cortical matter is more developed in human hairs than in animal hairs.

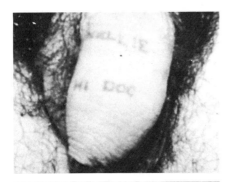

Fig. 4–2. Unusual tattoos. *Top,* An uncommon tattoo site. (Courtesy of David K. Wiecking, M.D.) *Center,* Skin slippage at the tattoo site on a decomposed body caused it to be more distinct. *Bottom,* Some of many unusual tattoos on a body.

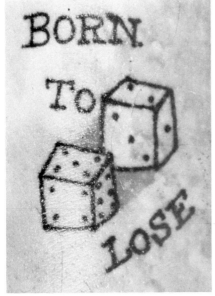

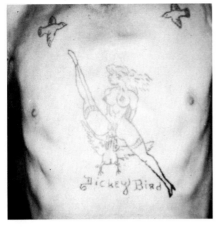

Fetuses have fine colorless hairs with no medulla. In infants and children the hairs are darker than in fetuses and a few hairs contain medulla. At puberty the hairs are longer and darker and many of them contain medulla. Adult hairs have maximum pigmentation and all of them have medulla. Aging causes graying of hair in some and loss of scalp hair begins in the second or third decade. Changes in the hairs due to age are most conspicuous in the scalp hairs.

In general, hairs of men are darker, thicker and more wiry than those of women. Montanari and his colleagues described a histological method by which Barr bodies in the epithelial cells of the hair follicles can be examined.[13] They found Barr bodies in the root bulbs in the proportion of 6 ± 2 percent in male hairs and in the proportion of 29 ± 5 percent in female hairs. Only rarely can positive determination of sex be made from hairs.

Body hairs show some regional features. Hairs of the head are soft, and round or oval on the transverse section; pubic hairs are curly and oval; eyebrow hairs are stiff, tapering and triangular or reniform; mustache hairs are usually triangular. A method of embedding hair for histologic sectioning has been described by Rosen and Kerley.[20]

Hairs which fall out naturally have normal root ends, while pulled hairs have distorted roots. Cut hairs show square ends, whereas burned hairs show shriveling and vacuolization. Dyed hairs show increased pigmentation but the pigmentation is decreased in bleached gray hairs.

The detection of trace elements in the hair by neutron activation analysis can help identify the source of the hair. Perkons and Jervis studied trace element concentration data for eighteen constituents in human hair.[17] From their work it becomes evident that comparison or differentiation between two or more otherwise similar hair samples can be made.

DENTAL IDENTIFICATION

Those aspects of dentistry which play a part in solving medicolegal problems, such as the establishment of the identity of a dead person or of the criminal, are included in the science called Forensic Dentistry or Forensic Odontology.

Teeth are by far the most durable of all human tissues and may be preserved even after the body is destroyed by decomposition, fire or chemicals. Therefore, the examination of the teeth, jaws and dentures is particularly helpful in identifying the victims of fire, airplane crashes and other mass disasters. Details of eruption, growth, disease and dental work can establish the identity of the deceased if dental charts made during life are available for comparison. Whenever the identity of the deceased or the assailant needs to be established, the examination of the teeth, dentures, jaws and bite marks must form an integral part of the autopsy. The autopsy surgeon may record the findings himself but it is always advisable to procure the services of a dentist. The examiner should pay particular attention to the following points:

1. The number, position and peculiarities of existing teeth and whether they are deciduous or permanent.
2. The number and situation of missing teeth and whether they were lost before or after death and whether the loss is recent or old.
3. The condition of teeth with reference to color, cleanliness, erosion, attrition, cavities, gum recession.
4. The details of dental work such as extractions, fillings, crowns, bridges and corrective appliances.
5. The details of dentures and jaws.

X-rays of the jaws may reveal additional information. If x-rays taken before death are available, comparison with x-rays made postmortem should be made. Observations made at the autopsy should be recorded on a dental chart such as the one in Figure 4-3. In burned remains the examination of the teeth may not be easy because of charring of the tissues. The pathologist should not hesitate to excise the tissues to expose the teeth. In serious criminal cases entire jaws may be excised and retained for further study and comparison tests.

Determination of Age

Age can be determined fairly accurately in children from the state of the dentition. The times of eruption of deciduous and permanent teeth provide a ready guide to age (Tables 4-2 and 4-4).

The determination of age from the examination of teeth is much more difficult after all permanent teeth have erupted. Miles has found the study

TABLE 4-4. Periods of Eruption of the Permanent Teeth.

Tooth	Period of Eruption in Years
Central Incisor	7
Lateral Incisor	8
Canine	11
First Premolar	9
Second Premolar	10
First Molar	6
Second Molar	12
Third Molar	17–25

RECORD OF DENTAL EXAMINATION

Name of Decedent:_____ Age:____ Race:____ Sex:_____

Autopsy Number:_____ Date of Autopsy: _____

Examination Requested by:_____ Examination Performed by:_____

Antemortem Dental Record Obtained from:_____ Date of Record:_____

Right   Left

Maxilla

Mandible

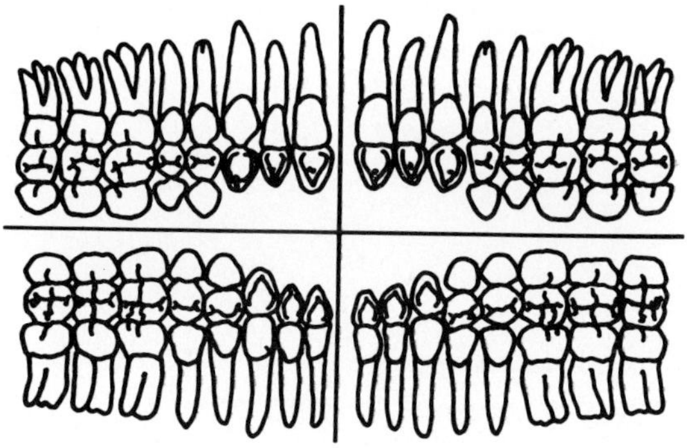

Right Maxilla: Left Maxilla:
1.   1.
2.   2.
3.   3.
4.   4.
5.   5.
6.   6.
7.   7.
8.   8.

Right Mandible: Left Mandible:
1.   1.
2.   2.
3.   3.
4.   4.
5.   5.
6.   6.
7.   7.
8.   8.

General Comments:

Signature of Examiner: Address of Examiner:

Fig. 4–3. A dental chart that can be used for recording findings in medicolegal cases.

of formation of third molars helpful in determining the age in adolescents and young adults.[12] Gustafson uses the following six criteria to help determine the age of an adult with an accuracy of ± 3 to 6 years—attrition, secondary dentine, changes in paradentium, cementum apposition, transparency and resorption.[8]

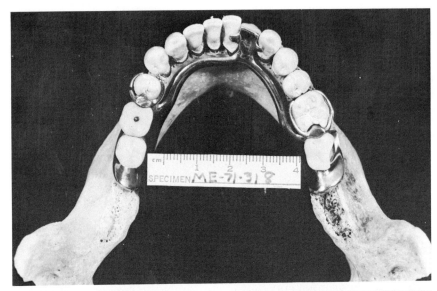

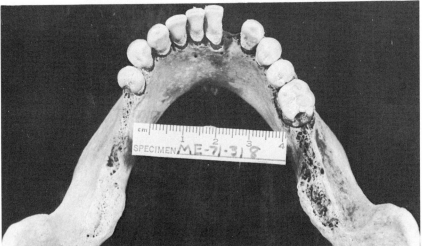

Fig. 4–4. *Top,* Identification of the dental plate by a relative of the decedent led to identification of the body. *Bottom,* Removal of the lower jaw and/or photographs of the jaw enable comparison with antemortem dental records.

Case Studies

In the past the *teeth* and the *dentures* have been some of the important means of identification as the following famous case illustrates.

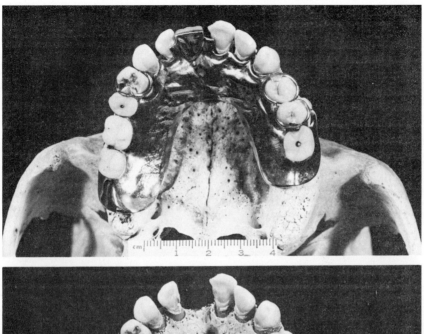

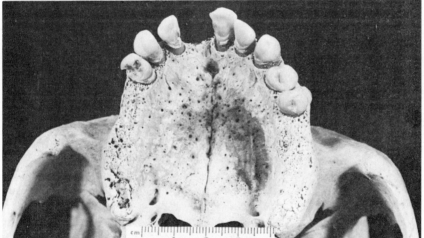

Fig. 4–4 (*Cont.*) *Top,* A dental plate in the upper jaw. *Bottom,* Upper jaw.

After Professor Webster murdered Dr. Parkman he attempted to destroy the victim's head in a furnace to erase all evidence that could lead to the identification of the deceased. However, the remains of a denture were found among the ashes and a dental surgeon was able to identify the dental material as belonging to Dr. Parkman.[1]

A second well-known case also was solved by the identification of dentures.

In the "Acid Bath" case the murderer, Haigh, shot a woman and immersed her body in commercial sulphuric acid for 2 to 3 days. When the sludge was sieved, a pair of acrylic-resin dentures were found. These were still fairly

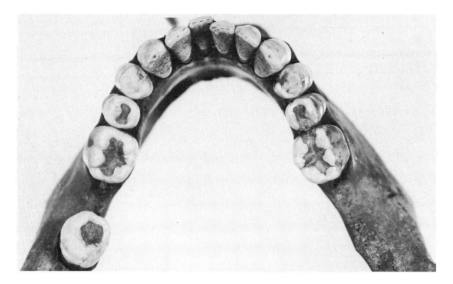

Fig. 4–5. Dental fillings in the lower jaw led to the identification of the deceased.

well preserved and a dental surgeon could recognize them as those that were made for the victim.[18]

In a recent case *dental plates* proved very informative.

A decomposed, partially skeletonized unidentified body was found in the woods. A supposed relative of the decedent was able to identify the dental plates found with the body (Fig. 4-4). This led to retrieval of dental charts on the deceased. The examination of the records and the decedent's teeth revealed twenty-three points of similarity.

In another instance dental *fillings* led to the identity of the deceased.

A skeletonized body was found in a shallow grave in the woods. Examination revealed extensive dental work and a healed fracture of the mandible. The findings corresponded to the data on a missing serviceman. The dental and medical records from an army hospital revealed details of cavity work identical to those found in the decedent's jaws (Fig. 4-5). The man had died from a gunshot wound of the head.

Residual roots can be of value also in identification as illustrated in the following case.

In the case of "Luton Sack Murder" the victim, a woman, was found strangled, trussed up naked in sacks in a river. One of the factors that helped confirm her identity was x-rays of her edentulous jaws which revealed residual roots. A local dentist had records identical with the victim's residual dentition and dental casts identical with those made from the body of the woman.

Identification of Bite Marks

The analysis of bite marks has become an important part of forensic odontology. In many instances the criminal has been identified from bite marks that he left on the body of the murdered victim or in the food materials at the scene of the burglary. Whenever bite marks are found on a body they should be described in detail and photographed (Fig. 4-6). Impressions of the bite marks made in plaster or silicon before shrinking of the tissues occurs can be extremely useful for comparison with the impressions made by the suspect's teeth.

In recent years interest in forensic odontology has grown sharply and numerous publications on the subject have appeared. The works of Luntz, Gustafson, and Furuhata and Yamamato are recommended for additional reading.[4, 8, 10]

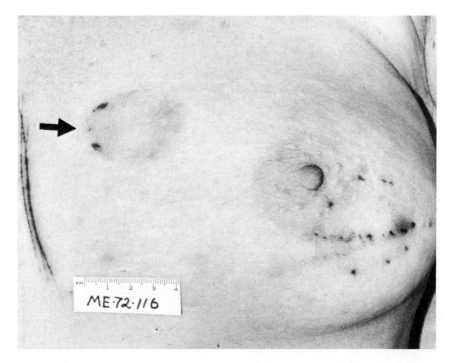

Fig. 4–6. Bite marks on the breast. Investigation of bite marks may lead to the identification of the assailant.

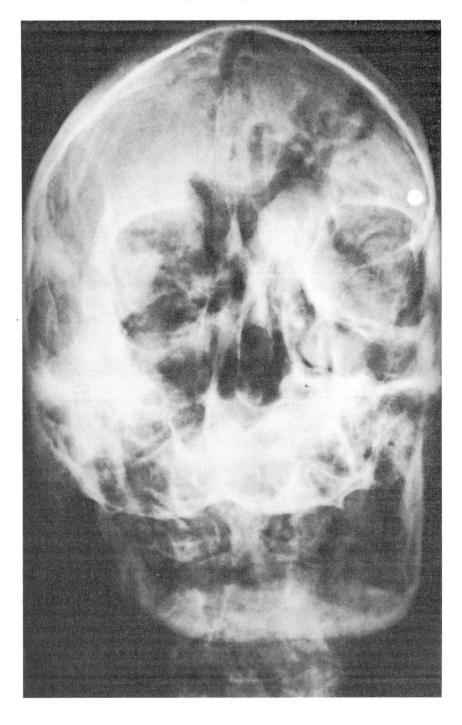

X-rays and Identification

X-rays can be of help in solving the problems of identification. They can give clues to the age, height and sex of a person. X-rays will also detect old fractures and abnormalities of the bones. The role of radiology in the identification of the victims of mass disaster is well illustrated by the investigation of the Noronic steamship tragedy.[22]

Mann and Fatteh described a case in which the identity of a murder victim was made for legal purposes by postmortem x-rays which showed a fracture of the zygomatic arch caused earlier by a bullet. The antemortem x-rays were available for comparison.[11]

In another case, x-rays of a markedly decomposed body of a man led to the detection of a BB shot in the orbital region (Fig. 4-7). The history of accidental shooting and lodgement of the shot in the eye, together with other clues, led to positive identification of the deceased. X-rays may help in differentiating human bones from animal bones. In one instance, an infant and some pigs, dogs and cats were burned in a wooden house. The bones of the infant were easily detected after all the bones were x-rayed.

Identification by Internal Examination

Internal examination of the body may reveal identifying features. For instance, identification of internal genitalia would establish the sex of the individual. Despite advanced decomposition, disease conditions such as gallstones, renal concretions and calcified leiomyomata will be identifiable. Chronic disease processes (e.g., silicosis, asbestosis) and congenital anomalies (e.g., horse-shoe kidney) diagnosed during life may be present. Surgical defects (e.g., burr holes) and surgical prostheses, such as plates in the skull and nails in the hip, would be significant. In a rare instance a pregnancy may help in identification. The value of an internal abnormality lies in being able to compare it to such an abnormality known to be present in a missing person.

In some cases, microscopic examination of the tissues may be required to identify the genital organs in order to determine the sex of the individual. Histological examination of even small specimens may help determine the human origin of the material, as well as the sex, race and age of the individual.[3] Microscopy may also enable identification of human material such as feces.[5]

Fig. 4–7. (*Opposite*) The finding of BB shot in the eye during a routine x-ray examination led to identification of the deceased.

IDENTIFICATION BY EXAMINATION OF THE BLOOD

The examination of blood may also help determine the identity of a person. This can be done by (a) determining the blood types and (b) sexing the blood cells.

Comparison of blood types of the dead body is possible, of course, only if the results of the blood grouping tests made during life are available. Even so the blood types, if matching, can give only supportive evidence, not conclusive. Matching of rare blood types may help establish the identity.[14] If only a part of the body is found, blood grouping may assist in the process of identification. If it is not apparent that the material is human, it is necessary first to make a positive identification. To do this the precipitin test should be performed.[23]

One may be able to determine the sex of the individual from the examination of the blood. The characteristic feature of female blood is a small drumstick-like projection from the nucleus in many of the neutrophils.

In medicolegal practice, the blood available for examination is not always in a fresh state. It is frequently in the form of dry spots, smears or pools and this makes blood typing difficult. In recent years several methods have been developed to group dried blood stains.[3, 9, 15]

REFERENCES

1. Dilnot, G.: The trial of Professor John White Webster. London, Bles, 1928.
2. Finck, P. A.: Histologic examination of trace evidence. J. Forensic Sci., *10*:253, 1965.
3. Funk, H. J., and Towstiak, W.: A practical method for detecting ABO agglutinins and agglutinogens in dried bloodstains. J. Forensic Sci., *10*:455, 1965.
4. Furuhata, T., and Yamamato, K: Forensic Odontology. Springfield, Ill., Charles C Thomas, 1967.
5. Giertsen, J. C.: Faecal matter in stains—their identification. J. Forensic Med., *8*:99, 1961.
6. Glaister, J., and Rentoul, E.: Medical Jurisprudence and Toxicology. Edinburgh, E & S Livingstone, 1966.
7. Gustafson, G: Microscopic examination of teeth as a means of identification in forensic medicine. J.A.D.A., *35*:720, 1947.
8. Gustafson, G.: Forensic Odontology. New York, American Elsevier Publishing Co., Inc., 1966.
9. Kirk, P.: Individuality of dry blood. J. Forensic Med., *8*:34, 1961.
10. Luntz, L., and Luntz, P.: Handbook of Dental Identification, Philadelphia, J. B. Lippincott, 1973.
11. Mann, G. T., and Fatteh, A. V.: The role of radiology in the identification of human remains. J. Forensic Sci. Soc. *8*:67, 1968.

12. Miles, A. E. W.: Dentition in the estimation of age. J. Dent. Res., *42*:255, 1963.
13. Montanari, G. D., Viterbo, B., and Montanari, G. R.: Sex determination of human hair. Med. Sci. Law, *7*:208, 1967.
14. Mourant, A. E.: The Distribution of the Human Blood Groups. ed. Oxford, Blackwell Scientific Publications, 1954.
15. Nicholls, L. C., and Pereira, M.: A study of modern methods of grouping dried blood stains. Med. Sci. Law, *2*:172, 1962.
16. Niyogi, S. K.: A study of human hairs in forensic work—a review. J. Forensic Med., *9*:27, 1962.
17. Perkons, A. K., and Jervis, R. E.: Trace elements in human head hair. J. Forensic Sci., *11*:50, 1966.
18. R. v. Haigh: Trial of J. G. Haigh, *In* Hodge, Lord DonBoyne (ed.): Notable British Trials. Edinburgh, 1949.
19. Richardson, L., and Kade, H.: Readable fingerprints from mummified or putrefied specimens. J. Forensic Sci., *17*:325, 1972.
20. Rosen, S. I., and Kerley, E. R.: An epoxy method of embedding hair for histologic sectioning. J. Forensic Sci., *16*:236, 1971.
21. Simpson, K.: The Luton sack murder. Police J., *18*:263, 1945.
22. Singleton, A. C.: The roentgenological identification of the victims of the "Noronic" disaster. Am. J. Roentgenol., *66*:375, 1951.
23. Wiener, A. S., and Gordon, E. B.: Examination of blood stains in forensic medicine. J. Forensic Sci., *1*:89, 1956.

5

Examination of Skeletal Remains

Identification of mutilated or skeletonized remains is a specialized field requiring the services of a number of investigators. The general pathologist would rarely be involved in the investigation of skeletal remains. Should the services of experts not be available in such cases, however, the pathologist can render substantial help with the broad knowledge of the principles of investigation and some general knowledge of the human skeleton.

When skeletal remains are found, the first important question to be answered is whether the remains are human or animal. If the remains are human the examination should be conducted to determine the answers to the following salient questions.

Do the remains represent one or more bodies?
What is the age, sex, race and the height of the individual?
Is there any evidence of violence?
What is the cause of death?
How long has the person been dead?
Are there any features which can identify the deceased?
Are there any personal effects that can facilitate identification?

If the pathologist is notified about the finding of skeletal remains, he should visit the scene to supervise the collection of the material. Every bone found at the scene should be retained for examination. Careful search for other human materials such as skin, tissue, hair and nails should be made. Portions of clothing and other personal effects can be invaluable in determining the identity of the individual. Photographs of the site where the remains are found should be taken before and after the remains are moved.

After the skeletal remains are brought into the autopsy room or laboratory, the bones should be laid out so that the body can be reconstructed for systematic examination. If soft tissue is attached to the bones it may be removed by leaving the material in diluted Clorox (one part of water with one part of Clorox). If only bleaching of the bones is desired, more dilute Clorox (nine parts of water with one part of Clorox) should be used. X-rays of the remains may help identify metallic objects mixed with the bones, and they may also be useful in studying the epiphyses and the ossification centers. The personal effects and the human material found with the bones should be closely examined and described. For the examination of the skeletal material the pathologist should not hesitate to procure assistance from an anatomist or an anthropologist and a dental surgeon.

From the examination of the bones one is able to determine easily whether they are human or animal, and whether the remains represent one or more bodies. Further, the examination helps determine the age, sex, race and the stature of the individual. Special procedures that a pathologist can follow to identify skeletal remains have been discussed by Kerley.[4] A summary of some of the important aspects is presented below.

Age

The age of a child may be assessed from the size of the bones, the appearance of the ossification centers and the fusion of the epiphyses. The sizes of the bones readily indicate the general age of the individual. Study of the ossification centers provides more accurate estimation of age.

All long bone shafts are ossified at birth. There are only six epiphyseal centers in a newborn which are listed in chronological order of appearance and fusion of epiphyses in Table 5-1. This information, based on the work of Flecker,[3] is helpful in determining the age of persons up to 22 years of age.

TABLE 5-1. Order of Appearance and Fusion of Epiphyses.
(Modified from Flecker)[3]

At birth	Head of humerus, distal femur, proximal tibia, calcaneum, talus.
During first year	Hamate, capitate, head of femur.
During second year	Proximal phalanges of inner four fingers.
At 2 years	Inner four metacarpals, first metatarsal, proximal phalanges of toes, distal phalanx of hallux.
At 3 years	In females, patella, proximal fibula, second metatarsal, third metatarsal, middle phalanges of second, third and fourth toes, distal phalanges of third and fourth toes. In males, triquetrum, proximal phalanx of thumb, middle phalanges of middle and ring fingers, tarsal navicular, second cuneiform.
At 4 years	Fourth metatarsal. In females, head of radius; fusion of greater tubercle to head of humerus. In males, lunate.
At 5 years	Navicular, greater trochanter. In females, distal ulna, lunate, triquetrum. In males, head of radius, proximal fibula; fusion of greater tubercle to head of humerus.

TABLE 5-1. (*Cont.*)

At 6 years	Medial epicondyle, distal ulna.
At 7 years	In females, distal phalanx of little finger; fusion of ischium and pubis.
At 8 years	Apophysis of calcaneus. In females, olecranon.
At 9 years	In females, trochlea, pisiform.
	In males, fusion of rami of ischium and pubis.
At 10 years	In males, trochlea, olecranon.
At 11 years	In females, lateral epicondyle. In males, pisiform.
At 12 years	In males, lateral epicondyle.
At 13 years	In females, fusion of ilium, ischium and pubis.
	In males, fusion of trochlea to lateral epicondyle.
At 14 years	In females, acromian, iliac crest, lesser trochanter; fusion of olecranon, upper radius, head of femur, distal tibia and fibula.
At 15 years	In females, fusion of medial epicondyle, proximal tibia. In males, acromian; fusion of ilium, ischium and pubis.
At 16 years	In males, fusion of lower conjoint epiphysis of humerus, medial epicondyle, olecranon, head of radius.
At 17 years	In both sexes, fusion of acromian. In females, fusion of upper conjoint epiphysis of humerus, distal ulna, distal femur, proximal fibula. In males, fusion of head of femur, greater trochanter, distal tibia and fibula.
At 18 years	In females, fusion of distal radius. In males, fusion of proximal tibia.
At 19 years	In males, fusion of upper conjoint epiphysis of humerus, distal radius and ulna, distal femur, proximal fibula.
At 20 years	In both sexes, fusion of iliac crest. In males, fusion of tuber ischii.
At 21 years	In both sexes, clavicle. In females, fusion of tuber ischii.
At 22 years	In both sexes, fusion of clavicle.

Determination of the age of an adult from the examination of skeletal remains is difficult. If the skull is available for examination, the study of cranial sutures may help in determining the age. The commencement and termination of the ectocranial and the endocranial sutures of the skull take place at specific times[7] (See Table 5-2). The suture closures, it must be stressed, at best help determine the age only in terms of decades.

If the pelvis is available for examination, the pubic symphysis should be carefully examined. According to Krogman the "pubic symphysis is probably the best single criterion of the registration of age in the skeleton."[7] The pubic symphysis is useful in determining age from the second to the fifth decade, and it can help determine age in five-year spans. The changes in the pubic bone, summarized in Table 5-3, are reliable indicators of age.[5, 14]

The degree of lipping of the margins of the vertebral bodies may give

TABLE 5-2. Estimation of Age From Suture Closures. Numbers Represent Years. C = Commencement of Suture Closure. CC = Completion of Suture Closure.

	Ectocranial				*Endocranial*			
	White Male		Negro Male		White Male		Negro Male	
Sutures	C	CC	C	CC	C	CC	C	CC
Sagittal	20	29	20	32	22	35	22	31
Coronal 1 and 2	26	29	23	32	24	38	24	38
Coronal 3	28	50	25	35	26	41	25	44
Lambdoid 1 and 2	26	30	23	31	26	42	23	46
Lambdoid 3	26	?31	?22	31	26	47	27	46
Spheno-frontal-orbital	28	46	21	35	22	64	20	44
Spheno-frontal-temporal	28	38	25	46	22	65	23	44
Spheno-temporal 1	37	?65	?50	—	31	64	40	41
Spheno-temporal 2	36	?65	?50	—	30	67	40	51
Spheno-parietal	28	38	28	46	29	65	23	49
Masto-occipital	28	32	27	31	30	81	25	46
Masto-occipital 3	26	33	26	31	26	72	17	30
Parieto-mastoid	39	?64	?50	—	37	81	33	51
Squamous	38	?65	?50	—	37	81	40	49

some indication of age.[13] In old age the changes in the mandible are of some significance. As old age advances the angle of mandible begins to open out and becomes more and more obtuse, while the alveolar ridges progressively subside.

Sex

With experience the chances of determining sex from the skeletal remains are 100 percent with the entire skeleton available, 95 percent with only the pelvis, 92 percent with the skull, 98 percent with the pelvis and skull, 98 percent with the pelvis and long bones and 80 percent with only long bones.[6] This indicates the relative importance of various bones in determining sex.

Sex differences in the male and the female *pelvis* are marked. Even in the fetus "significant sex differences" are present.[1] The sciatic notch index is probably the most useful criterion. The index is represented by

$$\frac{\text{Width of sciatic notch}}{\text{Depth of sciatic notch}} \times 100$$

In females the index is 5 to 6 and in males it is 4 to 5. Reynolds[11] has dis-

TABLE 5-3. Ten Phases in Age—Changes in the Pubic Symphysis. (Krogman)[5]

Phase	Symphyseal Surface	Ossific Nodules	Ventral Margin	Dorsal Margin	Extremities
First 18–19 years	Rugged horizontal grooves, furrows and ridges	None	None	None	No definition
Second 20–21 years	Grooves filling dorsally and behind	May appear on sym. surface	Ventral bevel begins	Begins	No definition
Third 22–24 years	Ridges and furrows progressively going	Present almost constantly	Beveling more pronounced	More definite dorsal plateau begins	No definition
Fourth 25–26 years	Rapidly going	Present	Beveling greatly increased	Complete dorsal plateau present	Lower commencing definition
Fifth 27–30 years	Little change	May be present	Sporadic attempt at ventral rampart	Completely defined	Lower clearer: upper extremity forming
Sixth 30–35 years	Granular appearance retained	May be present	Ventral rampart complete	Defined	Increasing definition upper and lower
Seventh 35–39 years	Texture finer; change due to diminishing activity	May be present	Complete	Defined	Carry on
Eighth 39–44 years	Smooth and inactive; no "rim"	May be present	No lipping	No lipping	Oval outline complete, extremities clearly outlined
Ninth 44–50 years	Rim present	May be present	Irregularly lipped	Uniformly lipped	Carry on
Tenth 50+ years	Erosion and erratic ossification		Broken Down		

cussed sex differences in the infantile pelvis. Sex differences in the adult male and female pelvis are summarized in Table 5-4. Figure 5-1 represents some of the salient differences.

The initial impression in sexing a *skull* is often the deciding factor.[7] General differences in the skulls of two sexes are included in Table 5-5. Particular attention should be paid to the forehead contour, orbits, supraorbital ridges, mastoids, glabella, and the mandible (Figs. 5-2 through 5-4). The foramen magnum is smaller in females than in males (Fig. 5-5). For vari-

TABLE 5-4. Sex Differences in the Adult Male and Female Pelvis. (Modified from Stewart)[12]

Trait	Male Pelvis	Female Pelvis
Pelvis As A Whole	Heavy, rugged, marked muscular markings	Less massive, smooth, muscular markings not prominent
Brim	Heart shaped	Circular, more spacious
True Pelvis	Relatively small	Spacious, shallow, oblique
Ilium	High, tends to be upright	Low, divergent laterally
Sacroiliac Articulation	Large	Small, more oblique
Pre-auricular Sulcus	Infrequent	Frequent, better developed
Greater Sciatic Notch	Small, close, deep	Large, wide, shallow
Acetabulum	Large, directed laterally	Small, directed anterolaterally
Ischiopubic Rami	Slightly everted, convex above	Markedly everted, concave above
Obturator Foramen	Large, oval	Small, triangular
Body of Pubis	Triangular	Quadrangular
Symphysis	High	Low
Subpubic Angle	V-shaped, narrow	U-shaped, wide
Sacrum	Long, narrow, evenly curved, may have more than 5 segments	Short, broad, markedly curved at S_{1-2} and S_{3-5}, as a rule has 5 segments

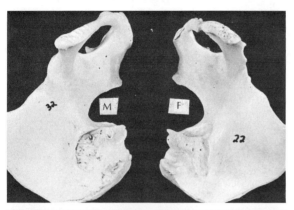

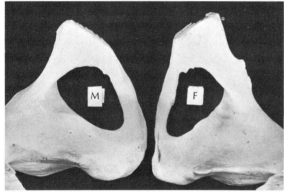

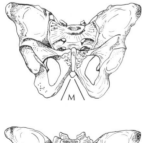

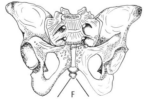

Fig. 5–1. Sex differences in the pelvis. *Top,* Small, close, deep sciatic notch in male (M); large, wide, shallow notch in female (F). *Center,* Large, oval obturator foramen in male (M); small, triangular foramen in female (F). *Bottom,* Narrow, V-shaped subpubic angle in male (M); wide, U-shaped angle in female (F).

ous measurements and other details the reader is referred to the *Human Skeleton in Forensic Medicine* by W. M. Krogman.[7]

The male *long bones* are longer and sturdier and with more prominent muscle markings than the female bones (Figs. 5-6 and 5-7). The measure-

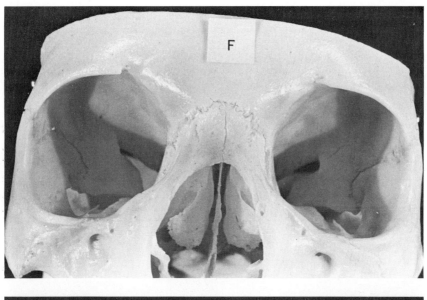

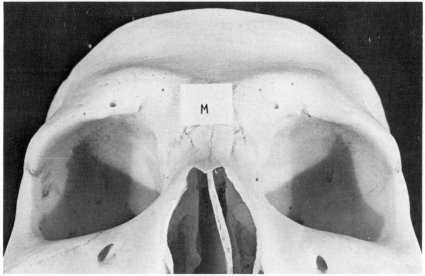

Fig. 5–2. *Top,* Male skull showing square orbits with large, thick, round supraorbital ridges. *Bottom,* Female skull showing round orbits with small, thin, sharp supraorbital ridges.

ments that are of great value in determining sex are the total length of the long bone, diameter of the head of the humerus, diameter of the femoral head and condylar breadth and width of the femur. Pertinent data are presented in Tables 5-6[6] and 5-7.[2] Parsons drew the following conclusions con-

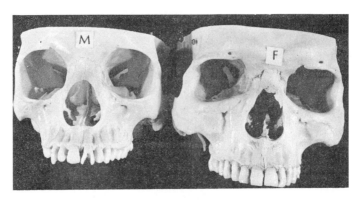

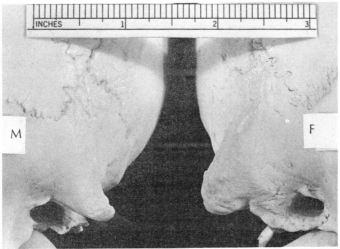

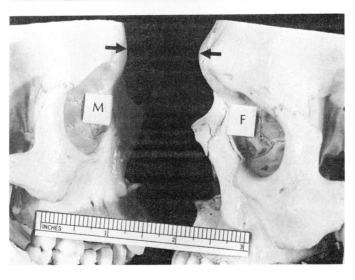

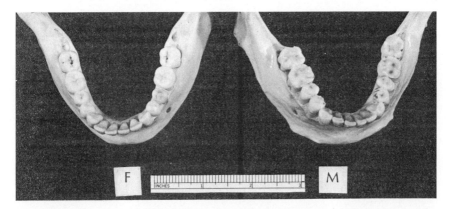

Fig. 5–4. Sex differences in the mandible. Smooth, pointed, v-shaped chin in female (F); rough, u-shaped chin in male (M).

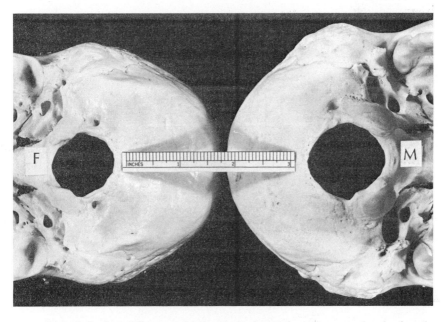

Fig. 5–5. Sex differences in the skull. Small foramen magnum in female (F); large in male (M).

Fig. 5–3. (*Opposite*) Sex differences in the skull. *Top,* Round orbits in female (F); square orbits in male (M). *Center,* Large, rough, blunt mastoid processes in Male (M); small, smoother, pointed processes in female (F). *Bottom,* Prominent, rough glabella in male (M); smooth, nonprotruding glabella in female (F).

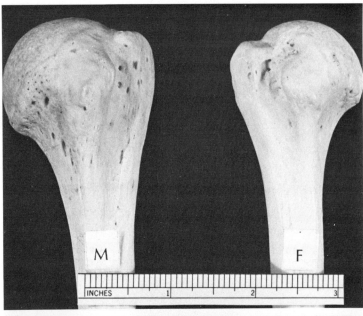

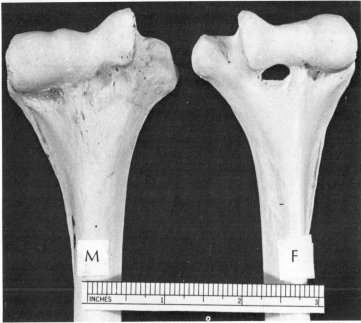

Fig. 5–6. *Top,* Sex differences in the humerus. Larger head and prominent muscle markings in the male (M); smaller, smoother head
in female (F). *Bottom,* Note the prominent muscle markings
in the male humerus (M).

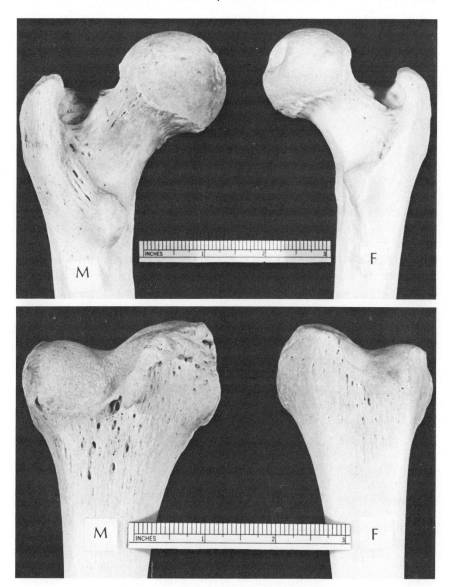

Fig. 5–7. *Top,* Sex differences in the femur. Note the smaller, smoother head in the female femur (F). Compare the muscular markings. *Bottom,* Note the differences between the muscular markings and the condylar widths in the male (M) and female (F) femurs.

cerning the femur from various measurements of 31 male and 16 female bones.[9, 10]

Maximum length: 450 mm. + = Male
                     400 mm. − = Female
Diameter of head: 48 mm. + = Male
                     44 mm. − = Female
Condylar breadth: 75 mm. + = Male
                     70 mm. − = Female

Race

The only two bones that can provide a reliable clue to race are the skull and the pelvis. Experts can determine the race of the skull in 85 to 90 percent of the cases and of the pelvis in 70 to 75 percent of the cases. In Table 5-8 salient differences in the Caucasoid and the Negroid skulls

TABLE 5-5. Sex Differences in the Skull. (Modified from Krogman)[6]

Trait	Male Skull	Female Skull
Size of Skull	Large	Small
Muscle Markings	Prominent	Not prominent
Supra-orbital Ridges	Medium to large, thick	Small, thin
Orbits	Square with thick, round margins	Round with thin, sharp margins
Forehead	Steep	Round, full
Frontal Eminence	Small	Large
Parietal Eminence	Small	Large
Occipital Area	Rough, markedly protruberant	Smooth, less protruberant
Mastoid Processes	Large, rough, blunt	Small, smooth, pointed
Occipital Condyles	Large	Small
Foramen Magnum	Large	Small
Palate	Large, broad, U-shaped	Small, parabola-shaped

TABLE 5-6. Relative Lengths of Long Bones in Males and Females. (Krogman)[6]

Bone	Length in mm. (Male)	Length in mm. (Female)	Male-Female Ratio
Femur	491	434	88.5
Tibia	409	359	88.0
Fibula	388	351	90.5
Humerus	336	317	94.5
Radius	255	220	86.4
Ulna	276	236	85.5

TABLE 5-7. Diameters of Heads of Humerus and Femur in Males and Females. Study of Two Hundred White Males and Two Hundred White Females. (Dwight)[2]

	Vertical Diameter of Humerus in mm.	Transverse Diameter of Humerus in mm.	Vertical Diameter of Femur in mm.
Male	48.76	44.66	49.68
Female	42.67	36.98	43.84
Difference	6.09	5.68	5.84

TABLE 5-8. Differences in the Caucasoid and the Negroid Craniofacial Traits. (Modified from Krogman)[6]

Trait	Caucasoid	Negroid
Skull Height	High	Low
Sagittal Contour	Rounded	Flat
Face Height	High	Low
Orbital Opening	Angular	Rectangular
Nasal Opening	Narrow	Wide
Lower Nasal Margin	Sharp	"Troughed" or "guttered"
Facial Profile	Straight	Downward slant
Palate Shape	Narrow	Wide

Examination of Skeletal Remains

TABLE 5-9. Formulae to Determine Stature from Measurements of Long Bones. (Trotter and Gleser)[16, 17]

Male Whites

Stature = 63.05 + 1.31 (femur + fibula) ± 3.63 cm.
Stature = 67.09 + 1.26 (femur + tibia) ± 3.74 cm.
Stature = 75.50 + 2.60 fibula ± 3.86 cm.
Stature = 65.53 + 2.32 femur ± 3.94 cm.
Stature = 81.93 + 2.42 tibia ± 4.00 cm.
Stature = 67.97 + 1.82 (humerus + radius) ± 4.31 cm.
Stature = 66.98 + 1.78 (humerus + ulna) ± 4.37 cm.
Stature = 78.10 + 2.89 humerus ± 4.57
Stature = 79.42 + 3.79 radius ± 4.66
Stature = 75.55 + 3.76 ulna ± 4.72

Female Whites

Stature = 50.12 + 0.68 humerus + 1.17 femur + 1.15 tibia ± 3.51 cm.
Stature = 53.20 + 1.39 (femur + tibia) ± 3.55 cm.
Stature = 53.07 + 1.48 femur + 1.28 tibia ± 3.55 cm.
Stature = 59.61 + 2.93 fibula ± 3.57 cm.
Stature = 61.53 + 2.90 tibia ± 3.66 cm.
Stature = 52.77 + 1.35 humerus + 1.95 tibia ± 3.67 cm.
Stature = 54.10 + 2.47 femur ± 3.72 cm.
Stature = 54.93 + 4.74 radius ± 4.24 cm.
Stature = 57.76 + 4.27 ulna ± 4.30 cm.
Stature = 57.97 + 3.36 humerus ±4.45 cm.

Male Negroes

Stature = 67.77 + 1.20 (femur + fibula) ± 3.63 cm.
Stature = 71.75 + 1.15 (femur + tibia) ± 3.68 cm.
Stature = 72.22 + 2.10 femur ± 3.91 cm.
Stature = 85.36 + 2.19 tibia ± 3.96 cm.
Stature = 80.07 + 2.34 fibula ± 4.02 cm.
Stature = 73.08 + 1.66 (humerus + radius) ± 4.18 cm.
Stature = 70.67 + 1.65 (humerus + ulna) ± 4.23 cm.
Stature = 75.48 + 2.88 humerus ± 4.23 cm.
Stature = 85.43 + 3.32 radius ± 4.57 cm.
Stature = 82.77 + 3.20 ulna ± 4.74 cm.

Female Negroes

Stature = 56.33 + 0.44 humerus − 0.20 radius + 1.46 femur + 0.86 tibia ± 3.22 cm.
Stature = 58.54 + 1.53 (femur + 0.96 tibia) ± 3.23 cm.
Stature = 59.72 + 1.26 (femur + tibia) ± 3.28 cm.
Stature = 59.76 + 2.28 femur ± 3.41 cm.
Stature = 62.80 + 1.08 humerus + 1.79 tibia ± 3.58 cm.
Stature = 72.65 + 2.45 tibia ± 3.70 cm.
Stature = 70.90 + 2.49 fibula ± 3.80 cm.
Stature = 64.67 + 3.08 humerus ± 4.25 cm.
Stature = 75.38 + 3.31 ulna ± 4.83 cm.
Stature = 94.51 + 2.75 radius ± 5.05 cm.

and facial features are presented. Todd has discussed racial differences apparent in the pelvis.[15]

Stature

Stature can be reconstructed from the length of bones. After the length of the long bones is obtained, one of the sets of published formulae should be used to calculate the height of the person. The formulae devised by Trotter and Gleser,[16] believed to be the best for general use in estimating stature, are reproduced in Table 5-9. For the reconstruction of stature it is best to measure the maximum length of all six long bones. The length of the femur and tibia should be measured in the oblique position, whereas the length of other bones should be obtained by taking a straight measurement of maximum vertical height.

Other Questions

The answer to the question as to how long the person has been dead depends to a large extent on the circumstances under which the remains were found. Weather conditions, status of the site of burial and the presence or absence of scavenging animals should be considered before hazard-

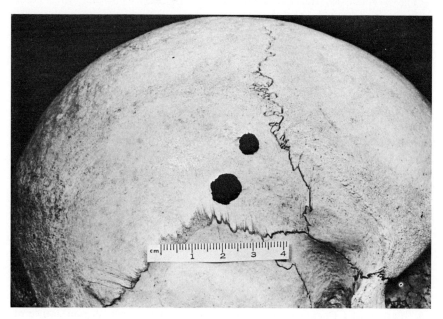

Fig. 5–8. Bullet holes in the skull. Discovery of antemortem trauma may indicate the cause and manner of death.

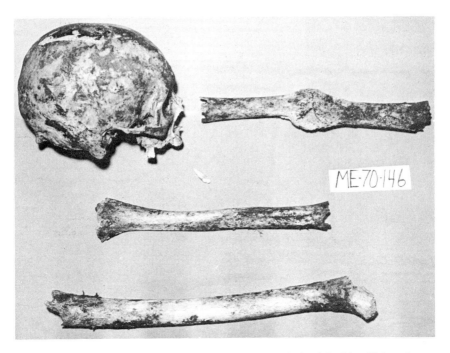

Fig. 5–9. Healed fracture of the humerus that helped in identifying the decedent.

ing a guess. In view of the many factors that can influence the degree of decomposition and the loss of body tissue, the doctor must guardedly offer a wide range of time of death.

In most instances, it is not possible to answer questions related to the possibility of violence or to the cause of death. Rarely does one detect the presence of missiles in the remains or discover evidence of trauma caused by bullets (Fig. 5-8). Fractures must be interpreted cautiously or else suspicion of foul play may be entertained. The finding of healed fractures may lead to the identification of the deceased (Fig. 5-9).

REFERENCES

1. Boucher, B. J.: Sex differences in the foetal sciatic notch. J. Forensic Med., 2:51, 1955.
2. Dwight, T.: The size of the articular surfaces of the long bones as characteristic of sex; an anthropological study. Am. J. Anat., 4:19, 1904–05.
3. Flecker, H.: Roentgenographic observations of the times of appearance of the epiphyses and their fusion with the diaphyses. J. Anat., 67:118, 1932–33.

4. Kerley, E. R.: Special observations in skeletal identification. J. Forensic Sci., *17:*349, 1972.
5. Krogman, W. M.: The human skeleton in legal medicine—medical aspects. *In* Levinson, S. A., (ed.): Symposium on Medicolegal Problems. Series 2. Philadelphia, J. B. Lippincott, 1949.
6. Krogman, W. M.: The Skeleton in forensic medicine. Grad. Med., *17:*(2 and 3), Feb.–March, 1955.
7. Krogman, W. M.: The Human Skeleton in Forensic Medicine. Springfield (Ill.), Charles C Thomas, 1962.
8. Maltby, J. F. D.: Some indices and measurements of the modern femur. J. Anat., *52:*363, 1917–18.
9. Parsons, F. G.: The characters of the English thigh-bone. Part I. J. Anat. Physiol., *48:*238, 1913–14.
10. Parsons, F. G.: The characters of the English thigh-bone. Part II. J. Anat. Physiol., *49:*335, 1914–15.
11. Reynolds, E. L.: The bony pelvic girdle in early infancy. Am. J. Phys. Anthropol., *3:*321, 1945.
12. Stewart, T. D. (ed.): Hrdlicka's Practical Anthropology. ed. 4. Philadelphia, Wistar Institute, 1952.
13. Stewart, T. D.: The rate of development of vertebral osteoarthritis in American whites and its significance in skeletal age identification. Leech, Johannesburg, *28:*114, 1958.
14. Todd, T. W.: Age changes in the pubic bone—1: the male white pubis. Am. J. Phys. Anthropol., *3:*285, 1920.
15. Todd, T. W.: Entrenched Negro physical features. Human Biol., *1:*57, 1929.
16. Trotter, M., and Gleser, G. C.: Estimation of stature from long bones of American whites and Negroes. Am. J. Phys. Anthropol., *10:*463, 1952.
17. Trotter, M., and Gleser, G. C.: A re-evaluation of estimation of stature based on measurements of stature taken during life and of long bones after death. Am. J. Phys. Anthropol., *16:*79, 1958.

6

Deaths from Blunt Force Injuries

Blunt force injury is the commonest type of injury seen in medicolegal cases. The variability in the appearances of the blunt force injuries and the diversity of objects causing them often compound the problems of interpretation of such injuries. A sharp cutting instrument causes an incised wound, but a single blunt object causes either an abrasion, a bruise or a laceration. Further, the laceration may resemble an incised wound. A far more significant fact is that the blunt force may not cause any external injury on the body and yet may be associated with fatal internal trauma. In many of the medicolegal cases a proper identification of each of these injuries is important, because the true significance of a particular injury and the nature of the object causing it cannot be assessed without recognizing the type of injury. For this reason the features of basic injuries—abrasions, bruises and lacerations—are described before the correlation of internal injuries and their significance is presented. The discussion of cutting and stabbing wounds is presented in Chapter 7.

While examining a body bearing evidence of blunt force trauma, every detail of the injuries must be noted. Sketches and photographs are invaluable. The following objectives of the investigation must be kept in mind:

1. Determination of the role of injury in causing death, whether the injury was a principal cause of death or a contributory factor.
2. Determination of the time of infliction of injury.
3. Determination of the manner of infliction of injury.
4. Identification of the object causing the injury.
5. Estimation of the degree of force involved.
6. Collection of trace evidence from the clothing and the body.

ABRASIONS

These are superficial injuries of the skin; the outer layers of skin are scratched or removed leaving a bare area with little or no hemorrhage. There is no splitting of the skin or bleeding under the exposed surface. If the area of abrasion is first rendered relatively ischemic by the pressure of the object causing it, the exposed surface is brownish and parchment-like. If any bleeding is present in an abrasion it is usually spotty because of the oozing of the capillaries.

Abrasions may be caused in various ways. Most commonly they are caused by friction between the body and a rough surface such as would happen in falls and in automobile accidents. Linear abrasions or scratches are caused by pointed objects such as thorns, wire-ends and pins. Elongated broad abrasions can be caused by friction of the skin with objects such as ropes and cords. A degree of pressure with friction against an object may result in abrasions depicting the pattern of the object.

Fatalities in which the examination of abrasions is important include cases of strangulation (abrasions caused by nails), hanging (rope marks), automobile accidents (imprints of tires and other objects), gunshot wounds (muzzle imprints), sexual assaults (abrasions of breasts and thighs) and those cases in which the recovery of trace evidence from the abrasions is vital.

Abrasions can easily be caused after death if the body is dragged. It is not always easy to differentiate antemortem from postmortem abrasions. If the abrasion is associated with bruising of the tissue it may be said that it was caused during life. Too much reliance should not be placed on whether the wound is wet (from blood and serum) or dry, for antemortem abrasions rapidly dry after death.

In any medicolegal investigation examination of the abrasions is important. Careful inspection of abrasions may reveal vital information. The following facts point up the significance of abrasions.

1. Abrasions initiate the suspicion of internal injuries and indicate the need for internal examination.
2. They may indicate the direction of force.
3. They may exhibit the pattern of the object causing the injuries.
4. They may contain trace evidence (hair, fibers, mud, sand, grass) helpful in identifying the object responsible for the injuries and from the nature of the trace evidence they may indicate the location (road, farm, beach) where the injuries were sustained.

Superficial decubitus ulcers and skin excoriations, such as diaper rash (Fig. 14-1), may resemble abrasions and must be carefully distinguished from injuries.

BRUISES

A bruise is a blunt-force injury consisting of escape of blood in a confined space following rupture of small blood vessels. The most frequently observed bruises are under the skin. Although bruises of the skin may appear spontaneously in persons with blood dyscrasias, a medicolegal investigator is primarily concerned with bruises caused by blunt force. Falls and automobile accidents are two common causes of bruises. A bruise will appear on any part of the body which is struck or compressed hard enough to rupture the subcutaneous vessels. The greater the degree of force the larger is the bruise likely to be. Bruises are more commonly seen on prominent parts of the body (e.g., around the eyes, on the knees, elbows and the wrists in the chronic alcoholic) and are usually round or oval but may be elongated or patterned on the structure of the objects causing them.

Some factors that influence the degree of bruising are:

1. Elderly persons and children who have loosely supported vasculature bruise more easily than do young adults.
2. Women, especially obese women, bruise easily because of the subcutaneous fat.
3. Persons in poor health and those with blood disorders are prone to easy bruising.
4. Loose tissue with poorly supported blood vessels (e.g., eyelids, external genitals) is predisposed to bruising with minor trauma (Fig. 6-1).

Soon after it is caused, a bruise is generally of reddish color, rapidly becoming purple. If the amount of bleeding under the skin is large, the bruise may appear blue. Within a few hours after infliction most of the bruises fall in the color shades of dark purple to dark blue. It takes usually 4 to 6 days for this color to change to greenish yellow. Bruises over a week old are usually yellowish. The discoloration of skin from bruising disappears within a month; smaller surface bruises may disappear in a week or two. In deeper tissue, bruising may persist for several weeks.

In general, a bruise can be considered a vital injury caused before death. It is possible, however, to rupture the subcutaneous tissues with blunt force after death. Although true infiltration of blood into the tissues does not occur in such circumstances, extrusion of blood from the ruptured blood vessels may cause discoloration of the overlying skin. Considerable force is required to produce "bruise" after death.[7] Postmortem pseudo-bruises rarely create problems of interpretation.[6] The significance of artefactual "bruises" is discussed in Chapter 17.

The areas of localized livor (hypostasis) should not be confused with bruises. If in doubt, incise the area. A bruise will show clotted blood infiltrating the tissue; the area of livor will show liquid blood flowing out freely from the cut blood vessels.

In the consideration of bruises the following facts should be remembered because of their medicolegal significance:

1. Bruises become more prominent as time elapses, especially after

death. They become even more prominent after autopsy. Drainage of blood from the vessels causes accentuation of the color in the bruised areas. Examination of the body several hours after the autopsy may reveal important previously invisible bruises.

2. A bruise is not necessarily produced at the point of impact of the object causing it. The seepage of blood from the torn vessels may cause skin discoloration next to or away from the point of impact.
3. A bruise may appear sometime after the infliction of injury.
4. Bruises may reveal the pattern of the objects causing them. Examples of patterned bruises are shown in Fig. 6-2 (tire marks) and Fig. 6-3 (necklace pattern).
5. Bruises in some areas, such as the scalp, may be missed if the area is not carefully examined. Bruises of deeper tissues may not be seen on external examination (e.g., blows or kicks on the abdomen or steering wheel impacts on the chest).
6. Bruises accompanying abrasions indicate the vital nature of abrasions.

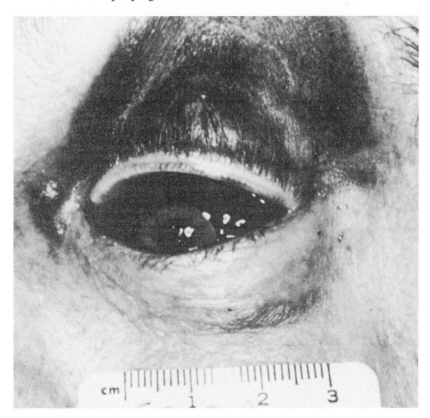

Fig. 6–1. Black eye. The looseness of the tissue predisposed to bruising.

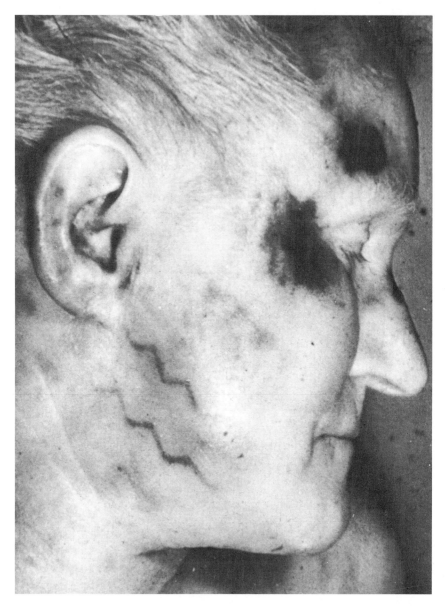

Fig. 6–2. A patterned bruise caused by a tire. (See Color Plate.)

LACERATIONS

A laceration is a tear of tissue. External lacerations involve tears of the skin and the subcutaneous tissues and may be caused on any part of the body, but they are more common in the skin covering the bones. They

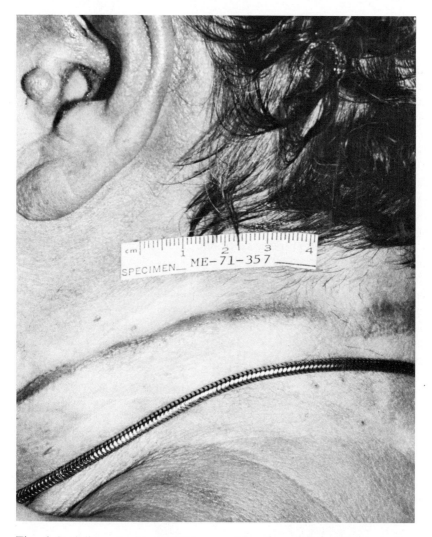

Fig. 6–3. A linear bruise caused by a necklace in a victim of strangulation.

may be caused by impact with a blunt force. Falls on such blunt objects as steps with edges, furniture, rough ground; automobile accidents; homicidal attacks with axes, hammers, iron bars, bottles; and kicking account for the majority of the lacerations seen in medicolegal practice. The mechanism of causation of lacerations is tearing of the skin or tissue due to a direct blow, or tearing of the tissue from stretching.

Most lacerations are easy to identify, for they have characteristic features. They have ragged margins and irregularly torn base. The structures in the base of a laceration, such as nerves and blood vessels (which can stretch to some extent), are frequently intact. Though the extremities of the laceration may be pointed or blunt, they too show minute tears in the margins. There is always a variable degree of bruising of the margins of the lacerations. Lacerations on some parts of the body, especially the scalp, may resemble incised wounds. The detection of bruising of the margins and the ragged nature of margins enable differentiation of such lacerations from true incised wounds which lack these features. Examination of the injury with a magnifying glass is invaluable in discerning these features.

It is important to remember that the shape of a laceration does not always correspond to the shape of the object causing it. For instance, injuries on the head caused by hammers with round or square striking face are usually crescent-shaped or triangular (Fig. 6-4). A laceration on the head caused by an iron bar is usually a linear tear with the width much smaller than the diameter of the bar.

External examination of the lacerations should be aimed at determining the nature of the object causing the injuries, the degree of force used and the likelihood of internal injuries. The shelving of the margins of the lacerations may indicate the direction of force. The injured area may contain foreign objects (glass, rust, soil, etc.) which can lead to the identification of the object responsible for the laceration. Likewise, if the weapon causing the injury is found, it may reveal the presence of a victim's hair, tissue and blood.

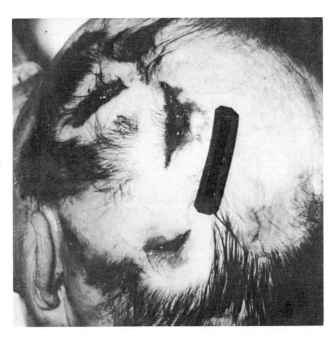

Fig. 6–4. Crescent-shaped lacerations of the scalp.

REGIONAL BLUNT FORCE INJURIES

External injuries such as abrasions, bruises and lacerations on a dead body frequently suggest the severity of internal injuries. It must, however, be emphasized that blunt force may not cause any external injury on the body and yet may be associated with fatal internal injuries. A complete external and internal examination of the body is important in the cases of blunt force injuries, for without it the true cause of death may not be established, the reconstruction of the events leading to death may not be possible, and miscarriage of justice may result. For proper understanding of the significance of these injuries a brief review of regional injuries from blunt force and their medicolegal aspects are included here.

Head Injuries

The medicolegal considerations of head injuries, as well as injuries to other parts of the body, include determination of the cause and manner of death, identification of the object causing the injuries, direction and degree of force, time of infliction of injury, the role of disease in the causation of injury, and the role of injury in the causation of disease. Because of their obvious significance these goals are repeated for emphasis.

Head injuries commonly result from automobile accidents, falls and fights.

External injuries often serve as indicators of the type of object used and of the direction of force. The severity of external injuries may be out of proportion to internal damage: a severely torn scalp may be accompanied by insignificant internal trauma; on the other hand, fatal cerebral injury may be present with little or no external injury. Because injuries in the scalp are not always obvious, the pathologist should not hesitate to shave the areas of suspected injuries (Fig. 6-5).

In the cases of head trauma, injuries of the undersurface of the scalp are the best indicators of blows on the head. Although the external examination of the scalp may not reveal any injuries, particularly in children (battered babies), when the scalp is reflected contusions from blunt force stand out and indicate the site of impact. The shape of the external injury of the scalp may point to the shape of the weapon.

The skull may or may not show any fractures. Even if the skull is not fractured there may be extensive brain damage. In children the skull is elastic and may not fracture even with severe trauma. The nature of the skull fracture can indicate the type of force; for instance, a localized depressed fracture may help gauge the shape and size of the object striking the head.

Fatal traumatic lesions that may be encountered in the practice of

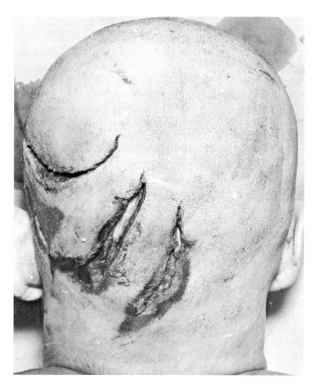

Fig. 6–5. Blunt force injuries (lacerations) of the scalp. Note the shaving of the head postmortem.

forensic pathology are cerebral concussion, cerebral contusions and lacerations and intracranial hemorrhages. Lindenberg has divided cerebral lesions in head trauma due to blunt force into two groups: primary lesions—caused by pressure and shearing and tearing forces, hemorrhages due to tearing of the vessels and necroses due to physical damage of the protoplasm; and secondary lesions—complications of "acute or subacute increased intracranial pressure due to hemorrhages, necroses and brain edema."[4] A short discussion of some of these lesions follows. For details the reader is referred to an excellent review of the subject by Courville.[2]

Cerebral concussion produced by severe shaking of the brain can cause death. At the autopsy no external injuries may be present and the examination of the brain will show little or no pathological change (see Chap. 18).

Cerebral contusion is the bruising of the cerebral cortex caused by sudden movements of the brain within the cranium as a result of blunt force. The bruises, usually wedge-shaped and located on the crests of the convolutions, are of two types: coup bruises—those found in the portion of the brain directly under the point of impact—and contrecoup bruises—those contusions found in the cerebral cortex in the region opposite the point of impact. Thus, a person struck on the right side of the head shows coup lesions in the cortex of the right temporal and parietal regions and contrecoup lesions in the cortex of the left parietal and temporal lobes. These contusions are frequently associated with severe cerebral edema which proves fatal. Grossly, the degree of flattening of the cerebral convolutions and the prominence and grooving of the unci with herniation indicate the degree of cerebral edema.

Lacerations. When the brain is lacerated the head trauma is usually severe and death rapid. Antemortem lacerations of the brain may not be easily recognized, since they are frequently not associated with hemorrhages. Artefactual tears caused during the removal of the brain may add to the difficulty of interpretation. Significant lacerations involve the base of the brain; lacerations of the midbrain, pons and medulla are serious. Cortical lacerations are always caused by a fractured skull and are easy to detect.

Extradural hemorrhage is the bleeding between the inner surface of the skull and the dura mater. Death from extradural hemorrhage is uncommon because the condition is amenable to treatment before serious pressure effects are caused. Most commonly such hemorrhages are a result of a rupture of the middle meningeal artery or one of its branches caused by a skull fracture across the course of the artery. If death results it is from pressure effects on the vital centers.

Subdural hemorrhage is bleeding between the dura mater and the pia-arachnoid. Whereas the extradural hemorrhage is arterial, the subdural hemorrhage is venous and is caused either by rupture of perforating veins, which cross the subdural space, or by rupture of one of the venous sinuses over the vertex. Cases of subdural hemorrhage are common in medicolegal practice. Questions that frequently arise are whether the hemorrhage was caused by a fall or was sustained in a fight; and if death is delayed after a fight or accident, whether the victim sustained additional head injury in the intervening time. The chronic alcoholic is prone to develop a subdural hematoma from a head injury. If an intoxicated individual sustains a head injury in a fall during a drunken state or while resisting arrest, signs of subdural hemorrhage may be masked by signs of acute alcohol intoxication. Under such circumstances imprisonment of the intoxicated person and his death in prison demand the most careful examination of the body. The findings must be interpreted in light of the circumstantial facts of the case.

Subarachnoid hemorrhage is bleeding in the space beneath the arachnoid membrane. The most common cause of subarachnoid hemorrhage is head trauma, but unlike other hemorrhages it is frequently due to natural causes.

Natural conditions frequently causing subarachnoid hemorrhages are rupture of congenital (berry) aneurysms and leaking of cerebral hemorrhages. In the investigation of a death from a subarachnoid hemorrhage, the examiner should strive to answer the following questions:

1. Was the hemorrhage caused by trauma?
2. Was the hemorrhage spontaneous from natural causes?
3. If a ruptured aneurysm is found, did the trauma precipitate the rupture?
4. If traumatic lesions are found, did the rupture of an aneurysm lead to these lesions from collapse?

While considering the possibility of injury as a cause of subarachnoid hemorrhage, it must be remembered that even minor trauma, sometimes without any evidence of external injury, can cause fatal subarachnoid hemorrhage.[8] Transmitted force from injuries to the neck can also cause subarachnoid hemorrhage. If an aneurysm is suspected to be the cause of subarachnoid hemorrhage, painstaking search for it must be conducted. The chances of success in finding the aneurysm are better if the brain is examined fresh. Failure to find an aneurysm does not necessarily mean that the cause of subarachnoid hemorrhage is trauma. In a series of 341 cases of spontaneous subarachnoid hemorrhage Simonsen was unable to demonstrate the origin of the hemorrhage in 93 of the (27%) cases.

Chest Injuries

Significant injuries to the chest involve the heart, aorta and the lungs.

Ribs are commonly fractured in automobile accidents and falls and often involve the lungs. Perforations of the lungs by broken rib ends frequently lead to fatalities from hemothorax, hemopneumothorax or pneumothorax. However, it is not necessary for the ribs to be fractured for hemothorax or pneumothorax to develop. With an elastic rib cage, as in children, compression of the chest can result in severe internal trauma without fractures of the ribs. To make the diagnosis of pneumothorax, the presence of air in the pleural cavities should be demonstrated by a procedure which is outlined in Chapter 2. Contusions of the lungs are commonly caused by blunt force injuries to the chest. Severance of the main bronchi caused by compression of the chest sometimes leads to mediastinal emphysema, a condition that can impede circulation and cause death. Similar embarrassment of circulation can occur from traumatic asphyxia (see Chap. 9). Thin-walled blebs on the surfaces of the lungs indicate rupture of alveolar sacs from pressure on the chest.

Fractured ribs also can cause perforations of the heart and rapid death from hemopericardium, or contusion of the myocardium resulting in delayed death (see Fig. 15-1). Even in the absence of rib fractures, serious injury to the heart may result from anteroposterior compression of the chest. With such compression, contusions and lacerations of the right artium are more common than those of the other chambers of the heart. If death results from a blow on the chest without causing any visible injuries, a meticulous autopsy is mandatory, since questions will be raised as to whether the injury could have caused coronary spasm, hemorrhage in the wall of the coronary artery or fatal arrhythmia of the heart.

One of the common causes of hemothorax is rupture of the thoracic aorta. Blunt force injury to the chest is invariably the cause of such a rupture. In the majority of the cases of a ruptured thoracic aorta, the point of rupture is about a centimeter distal to the origin of the left subclavian artery and the tear, as a rule, is circumferential in course. Occasionally, trauma may cause a partial tear of the aorta, resulting in a dissecting aneurysm.[5] Preexisting medial degeneration may also predispose the aorta to dissection of the coats, aneurysm formation and rupture with some degree of injury to the chest.

If there is an interval between injury and death, obvious questions will be asked as to whether death was caused by trauma or was accelerated by preexisting disease. For settling insurance claims and for determining the course of criminal proceedings arising from the death, correct answers to these questions are vital.

Abdominal Injuries

Injuries to the abdominal organs result either from localized blows or from crushing of the trunk such as occur with steering wheel impacts in automobile accidents or the falling of heavy objects on the body. Localized injuries result from kicks, fist blows and impacts with sharp and blunt objects. Internal injuries may or may not be accompanied by external evidence of violence.

The *liver* is injured by a crushing effect, direct blows or by broken ribs. Common liver injuries are surface contusions and lacerations. Surface lacerations are irregular, short and long, superficial tears which are not serious because bleeding from them is usually slow. If the liver is crushed, however, it has similar surface tears as well as much more extensive and serious lacerations within the depth of the liver tissue. These deep tears, which do not necessarily communicate with the lacerations in the surface, produce blood-filled cavitations within the liver that produce severe shock.

The *spleen* is injured easily with direct blows, or a crushing force or by broken ribs. Unlike the liver, the spleen bleeds rapidly if lacerated. In the absence of any marks of violence it is important to determine the precise cause of the rupture of the spleen. The facts that need to be established are whether the rupture was spontaneous due entirely to preexisting disease, whether trauma precipitated the rupture of a diseased spleen, or whether trauma was the sole factor in death.[9]

Injuries of the abdominal *aorta* deserve special attention. A difficult medicolegal problem of interpretation can arise when, for instance, an elderly person is found dead after a fall and the autopsy reveals a ruptured aortic aneurysm. The medical investigator should endeavor to provide an answer to the question of whether the fall caused the rupture or whether the rupture caused the collapse and fall.

When blunt force is applied to the abdomen, the *intestines* frequently escape injury because of their mobility. Displacement of the loops of intestines under pressure sometimes leads to tears in the mesentery with serious intra-abdominal hemorrhage. The surrounding structures are not injured unless there is severe generalized trauma. Rupture of the stomach or the urinary bladder is rare but is more likely if the stomach or the bladder is distended and direct localized force is applied.

To estimate the total blood loss, free blood in the abdomen should be measured. Also, the hemorrhage within the tissues should be taken into account since it can be substantial and can markedly accentuate the degree of shock.

Death from *delayed complications* of trauma (e.g., delayed hemorrhage from the spleen, peritonitis caused by injury of the viscus, renal failure, etc.) should be adequately investigated to establish or exclude the role of previous injury.

Finally, with a negative autopsy the possibility of reflex vagal inhibition from blows in the epigastric region should be considered.

Spinal Injuries

Injuries to the spine and the spinal cord can be caused in various ways. Flexion and extension (whiplash) injuries of the neck, with or without rotation, are common in automobile accidents. Direct blows on the neck or transmitted force from the mobility of the head or the body can cause serious spinal injuries. Injury of the cervical spine at the level of C2 to C4 and severance of the spinal cord occur in judicial hanging. Vertical compression of the spine may occur in falls on the feet from a height or from diving accidents. Falls from collapse as a result of disease may be associated with spinal trauma and should be properly identified.

Injuries of the spine consist essentially of fractures of the vertebrae and dislocations, the latter being more common.

The evaluation of spinal injuries can be difficult. In most instances there is no external evidence of trauma to the spine. Rarely would the position of the body clearly indicate the possibility of injury to the cervical spine

(Fig. 6-6). Pathologists should never fall into the trap of diagnosing the fracture of the cervical spine by simply twisting the neck. The neck of a dead body in which rigor has disappeared or has not set in may be markedly mobile even without a fracture of the spine; on the other hand, rigor of the muscles of the neck may restrict the mobility of a broken neck. The only right way of detecting the fracture of the cervical spine is by internal dissection.

Even internal dissection may occasionally result in negative findings (the difficulty in diagnosing the dislocation of the atlanto-occipital joint is discussed in Chapter 18). The fact that needs to be stressed concerns spontaneous reduction of a dislocation of the spine. A jerky motion of the head over the spine, for instance, may result in such an occurrence in the cervical region, leaving no trace of trauma to the bony structures.

Injuries of the spine may lead to laceration and contusion of the spinal cord which can cause rapid death. With a period of survival, hemorrhages in the spinal cord cause necrosis of the tissue. The important pathological change is edema of the spinal cord. If death results from spinal injury, it is usually from spinal shock, effect of trauma and edema of vital centers or delayed complications.

Concussion of the spinal cord can prove fatal. The changes in the spinal

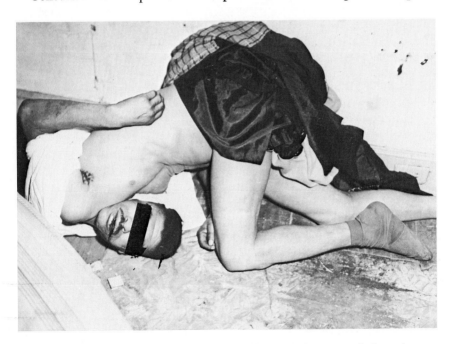

Fig. 6–6. The position of this body indicates a fracture of the spine. (Courtesy of John T. Daly, M.D.)

cord suggestive of concussion are softening of the spinal cord with foci of hemorrhages in its substance, focal areas of necroses and edema of the tissue. The axis cylinders of the nerve fibers and the myelin sheaths show histological alterations.[3] Whenever injury to the spinal cord is suspected, it should be removed for gross and microscopic examination.

Delayed complications. Injuries of the spinal cord may result in paraplegia and quadruplegia and death may not occur for days, months or years. Complications such as decubitus ulcers, respiratory tract infections, urinary tract infections with or without renal stones or septicemia may develop. Even if death is delayed by decades such cases should be investigated by medical examiners or coroners. A complete autopsy provides conclusive evidence concerning the role of the injury in causing death.

The importance of distinguishing antemortem fractures of the cervical spine from postmortem fractures is discussed in Chapter 17.

Injuries to the Extremities

Injuries to the extremities consist of fractures of the bones and bruising and laceration of the soft tissues, resulting either in immediate hemorrhage and shock or delayed complications. Such injuries are caused by direct or indirect blunt force or by crushing of the extremities such as occurs in industry, automobile accidents and falls.

For the evaluation of the injuries causing rapid death, the amount of blood loss and the progression of shock should be considered. If limbs are crushed while the person is alive, "crush syndrome" may develop in which the crushed extremities become swollen because of the extravasation of blood in muscle planes, the myoglobin is released and the blockage of renal tubules by myoglobin leads to renal shut down and death.

In the immediate postinjury period and during the first several days after the injury, fat or bone marrow can be released from the fractured bones and enter the blood circulation, resulting in fat or bone marrow embolism. Severe soft tissue trauma can also cause fat embolism. When fat embolization occurs, demonstration of fat in the blood vessels of the brain is necessary for death to be ascribed to fat embolism.

Immobilization of the patient induced by bone fracture is frequently associated with stasis of blood and phlebothrombosis in the immobilized extremity. Death from complicating pulmonary embolism is common. Sequelae of immobilization such as decubitus ulcers, hypostatic pneumonia and septicemia are also common. In elderly persons fractures of the femur sustained in falls lead to fatalities from such complications. Campbell[1] has presented a medicolegal evaluation of 582 cases of fractured hip and has rightly stressed the importance of differentiating those cases in which death is caused by injury from those in which the fracture plays no significant role or is only a contributory factor aggravating preexisting disease.

REFERENCES

1. Campbell, J. E.: The fractured hip in its relation to death. A medicolegal evaluation. J. Forensic Sci., *3:*401, 1958.
2. Courville, C. B.: Trauma to the central nervous system and its membranes. In Camps, F. E. (ed.) Gradwohl's Legal Medicine. Bristol, John Wright and Sons, 1968.
3. Davison, C.: General pathological considerations in injuries of the spinal cord. In Brock, S. (ed.): Injuries of the Skull, Brain and Spinal Cord, ed. 2, Baltimore, Williams & Wilkins, 1943.
4. Lindenberg, R.: General remarks on brain lesions in head trauma due to blunt force. Seminar in forensic pathology. J. Forensic Sci., *2:*213, 1957.
5. Marshall, T. K.: Traumatic dissecting aneurysms. J. Clin. Path., *11:*36, 1958.
6. Moritz, A. R.: Pathology of trauma. ed. 2, London, Henry Kimpton, 1954.
7. Polson, C. J.: The Essentials of Forensic Medicine. Springfield (Ill.), Charles C Thomas, 1965.
8. Simonsen, J.: Fatal subarachnoid hemorrhage in relation to minor head injuries. J. Forensic Med., *14:*146, 1967.
9. Stevens, T. J. T., and Hudson, R. P.: Spontaneous rupture of spleen in plasma cell leukemia. Can. Med. Assoc. J., *100:*31, 1969.

7

Deaths from Cutting and Stabbing Wounds

Medicolegally important incised wounds (cuts, slashes) are commonly homicidal and suicidal though they may occasionally be caused accidentally by falling on sharp objects. The majority of stab wounds (penetrating and perforating wounds) are homicidal; suicidal and accidental stab wounds are infrequent.

Incised wounds are made by cutting objects with sharp edges such as knives and razors. Stab wounds are caused by knives, daggers, scissors, bayonets, files, screwdrivers and even ice picks.

In most of the fatalities from accidentally sustained injuries, the circumstances of death are clear enough not to warrant undue concern. Essentially, therefore, the medical investigator is concerned with the problem of differentiating homicidal injuries from those self-inflicted.

Analysis of the findings at the scene of death, examination of the weapon, examination of the decedent's clothing and proper interpretation of the injuries on the body should form the basic components of the investigation of a death from cutting or stabbing wounds.

INVESTIGATION OF THE SCENE OF DEATH

At the scene of death the principal objective of the medicolegal investigation is the recognition of the manner in which the injuries were sustained. The examination of the scene and of the body disclose criteria which help differentiate a homicide from a suicide or an accident. In order to gather optimal information, the following procedure should be followed at the scene of death.

1. Obtain information about the circumstances of death from the police and witnesses at the scene (see Chap. 1).
2. If suicide is suspected, look for a suicide note and inquire about

the personal history of the decedent—social, financial, domestic and health problems, history of depression and suicide threats.

3. Make general observations about the scene. Note any evidence of struggle, such as overturned furniture or trampled ground.

4. Photograph the scene and make sketches before anything is moved.

5. Note whether the weapon is present or absent. If present, note the position of the weapon in relation to the body. If the weapon is in the decedent's hand, describe whether it is loosely held or tightly grasped. If the weapon is not near the body, search the general area for it. (If the weapon is grasped tightly in the hand which is in a state of instantaneous rigor, suicide is a certainty. The presence of the weapon held loosely in the hand does not rule out homicide, since the assailant may place the weapon in the decedent's hand to simulate suicide. If the weapon is absent or thrown away from the body, crime should be suspected.)

6. If the injuries are suspected to be accidental, identify the object causing them.

7. Describe the position of the body and the hands.

8. Describe the clothing and note any tears, missing buttons and so on. Ascertain whether the weapon penetrated the clothing or whether the clothing was displaced from the area of injury. (This may help differentiate a homicide from a suicide, since suicides usually inflict injuries on bare areas.)

9. Note the amount of bleeding at the scene. (A record of the extent of bleeding makes the evaluation of the injuries more accurate and also may give some indication as to the length of survival after the injury.)

10. Examine the body, including the back. Examine the hands and fore-arms for defense wounds (vide infra). Make note of injuries and record them on body diagrams.

11. Look for evidence of sexual assault. Tears of clothing and injuries of the genital organs should be noted.

12. If a weapon is found at the scene of death, handle it with extreme care with a view to preserving fingerprints, bloodstains, hair and fibers on it. Do not pick up the weapon carelessly with bare hands. Detach from the weapon and retain in appropriate containers any materials that are likely to be lost. Fingerprints on the weapon may lead to identification of an assailant in the case of homicide. If the weapon is soiled by the assailant's blood, blood grouping may help identify him. If the weapon causing the death is found away from the body, matching of the blood groups of the decedent with those of blood on the weapon help associate the weapon with the

death. Similarly, the study of hair, fibers and other trace evidence on the weapon may render help in the investigation.

13. Let the police handle the weapon. Request them to make the weapon available for the evaluation of injuries after it has been examined for fingerprints and trace evidence.

14. If the weapon is not found at the scene of death, advise the police about the type of weapon that is likely to have been used. (The dimensions of the external wounds indicate the approximate width of the blade of the weapon. The extremities of the wounds indicate whether the weapon has one or two cutting edges.)

THE AUTOPSY

In any medicolegal autopsy the establishment of the cause and the manner of death are principal issues. Depending on the mode of death, the autopsy can serve a number of important purposes. In the case of a death from cutting or stabbing wounds, the autopsy can help answer unanswered questions. With a view to answering various questions the pathologist would do well to proceed along the lines indicated below. The steps are listed not only to define the procedures to be followed in the autopsy room but also to indicate the purpose of each procedure.

1. Photograph the clothing and injuries on the body. Photographs are useful for testimony in court at a later date.

2. Record injuries by words and sketches. The descriptions should include the position, shape, length and the width of each wound, as well as the margins, base, extremities and direction of each injury. The injuries should be documented diagrammatically as described in Chapter 2. Such records can make the task of the pathologist in court more simple and lessen the chance for misinterpretation by other persons reading the reports.

3. Examine the injuries to determine whether they were caused before or after death. (This is not a simple problem. It might not be possible to say that the wound was caused before death unless obvious bruising is present in the margins of the wound. Reliable histological changes are not seen in wounds caused less than eight hours before death. It has been shown that the histochemical methods are better tools in differentiating antemortem wounds from those caused after death).[2]

4. Determine whether the injuries are, in fact, cuts and stabs or lacerations, and, if possible, the time of infliction of the injuries. (Incised

wounds have sharp margins and tapering extremities and do not show any obvious contusion of the margins. Lacerations, on the other hand, have ragged margins, which may show contusion, and their extremities are usually not tapering. A rough determination of the time of infliction of wounds is possible only if the wound has been inflicted several hours prior to death.[1, 5]

5. From the nature of external wounds, determine the kind of weapon that is likely to have been used.[4] Estimate the width of the blade and determine whether the weapon is likely to have one or two cutting edges, and whether it was sharp or blunt.

6. Collect foreign materials such as hair, grass, fibers and so on that may be in the wounds.

7. From the depth of the wounds estimate the minimal length of the blade of the weapon. (The best way to estimate the depth of the wound is by careful exploration of the track of the wound. Do not, however, insert the suspected weapon in the wound to gauge the depth. When estimating the minimal length of the blade of the weapon, the elasticity of the skin and the mobility of the underlying tissues must be taken into consideration.)

8. Determine the direction of the weapon within the body, since this may indicate whether the injury was self-inflicted, homicidal or accidental. Also, find out whether there was any rocking movement of the weapon.

9. If the injuries are homicidal, evaluate the position of the assailant in relation to the victim. The position of wounds and the direction in which they taper help assess this aspect. Look for defense wounds, since their presence indicates homicide.

10. Assess the findings to determine the rapidity of death or collapse and to estimate the ability of the victim to walk or to perform certain acts after being wounded.

11. If there are several wounds decide which one was fatal.

12. Record the findings suggesting sexual assault. Examine the external and internal genitalia in female victims and take swabs for examination for sperms and for acid phosphatase test.

13. Evaluate the role of contributing factors, such as preexisting disease or intoxication, in causing death.

14. If the suspected weapon is presented, determine whether the wounds found on the body are consistent with those caused by such a weapon.

15. If necessary, perform experiments with the weapon alleged to have been used to determine whether in fact it could produce injuries of the type found on the body and to estimate the force required to inflict such injuries.

COMMON TYPES OF CUTTING AND STABBING WOUNDS

A brief description of some of the more common types of cutting and stabbing wounds is included here to assist the pathologist in recognizing and interpreting "run-of-the-mill" cases.

Suicidal Incised Wounds

These wounds are usually found at classical sites—the neck, front of the wrist, front of the elbow and occasionally the groin (Fig. 7-1). Would-be suicides select one or more of these sites to sever the blood vessels (radial artery, carotid artery, femoral vessels) in order to bleed to death. A wound thus inflicted almost always presents a typical pattern.

Suicidal wounds on the wrists, elbows or groin are usually multiple, frequently superimposed and lie parallel to each other. They are superficial, in a majority of the cases being only skin deep, and expose the tendons and the blood vessels. The arteries are not often cut. Because multiplicity of the wounds and their superficial nature distinctly reveal the element of hesitation on the part of the victim, they are appropriately called "hesitation" or "tentative" wounds (Fig. 7-2). A single deep cut on the wrist is not consistent with suicide and hence should arouse suspicions of foul play.

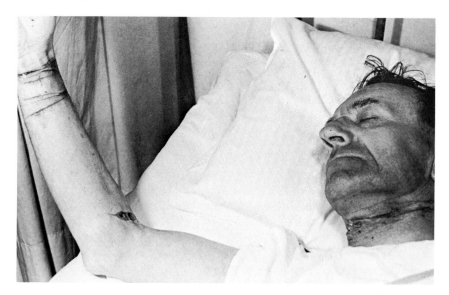

Fig. 7–1. Suicidal incised wounds at classical sites—wrist, elbow and neck.

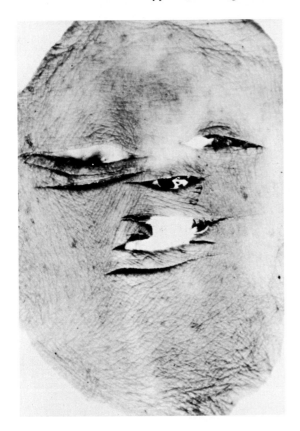

Fig. 7–2. Eight parallel "hesitation" or "tentative" wounds on the front of the wrist.

A young woman suffering from acute postpartum psychosis inflicted blows on the head of her 15-day-old newborn, cut the infant's wrists (Fig. 7-3) and strangled it to death.

Old scars of healed incised wounds indicating a previous suicidal attempt may be found at the site of recent cuts on the wrists.

Suicidal cutthroats also reveal characteristic multiple, parallel, superficial "hesitation" marks, but in addition to the fatal wound. The pattern of the wounds depends on whether the person used the right hand or the left. If the right hand was used, the wounds begin high on the left side of the neck, usually at the angle of the mandible, and pass downward across the front of the neck immediately above the thyroid cartilage, tapering off on the right side of the neck but at a lower level than on the left side. If the left hand was used the pattern is reversed (Fig. 7-4). The wounds are shallow on the sides of the neck and deep in the midline. Superficial linear cuts may be above or below the deep cut. Fatal wounds vary in depth. Incisions extending right up to the spine and laying the larynx open are not uncommon. Since the neck is stretched back at the time of the inflic-

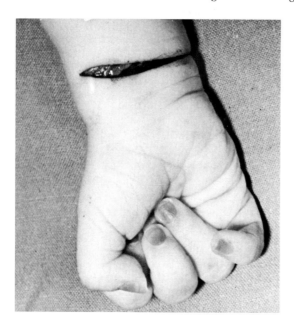

Fig. 7–3. A homicidal in-
cised wound of the wrist.

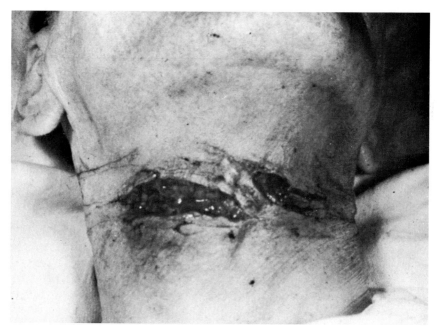

Fig. 7–4. A suicidal cutthroat. Note that the incisions are higher on the
right side. The decedent was left-handed.

tion of the wounds, the neck structures in the midline are easily cut. The suicide aims to cut the carotid arteries, but these frequently escape injury. Death results from venous hemorrhage, aspiration of blood and occasionally from air embolism.

In a victim of suicidal cutthroat, hesitation marks on other parts of the body are frequently seen. There may also be evidence indicating the use of drugs in an attempt to commit suicide.

> An elderly man was found dead with his head in a gas oven. He had died from carbon-monoxide poisoning. Examination of the body revealed several "hesitant" incised wounds on the front of the left wrist, front of the left elbow and on the neck. The stomach contained a mass of recently ingested white tablets. On toxicological analysis these were found to be aspirin and phenobarbital tablets.

Homicidal Incised Wounds

These wounds may be found on any part of the body as the result of active slashing by an assailant or the victim's trying to defend himself. These wounds always lack the planning of suicidal wounds and vary considerably in direction, depth and location. The two most common forms of homicidal incised wounds are cutthroat and defense wounds. A brief note on each of these follows.

Homicidal cutthroat is common. It is important to differentiate suicidal cutthroats from those homicidally inflicted. Each type presents characteristic features that allow proper identification of the manner of infliction. The homicidal wound on the neck is usually horizontal with both extremities of the wound in the same line as the middle section of the wound. The wound is usually a single deep cut and, since the neck is not stretched, the large blood vessels (carotid arteries and jugular veins) are frequently severed. Whereas the suicidal wound is invariably high in the neck, the homicidal wound may be anywhere on the neck. The cutthroat can be identified with certainty as homicidal if defense wounds are present and "hesitation" wounds are absent.

Defense wounds are slashes on the fingers, hands or forearm resulting from an instinctive reaction in self-defense. Wounds are seen commonly on the palms or palmar aspects of the fingers (Fig. 7-5). Wounds on the palmar aspects of the hands are usually caused by the grasping of the attacker's weapon; those on the back of the hand (Fig. 7-6) or on the forearm are caused by attempts to ward off the attack. With sharp weapons the wounds are clean-cut; with blunt weapons one may see bruises, abrasions and lacerations. If the weapon grasped by the victim has two sharp edges, wounds are present on the palm as well as on the palmar aspects of the fingers. A weapon with one cutting edge obviously causes wounds on

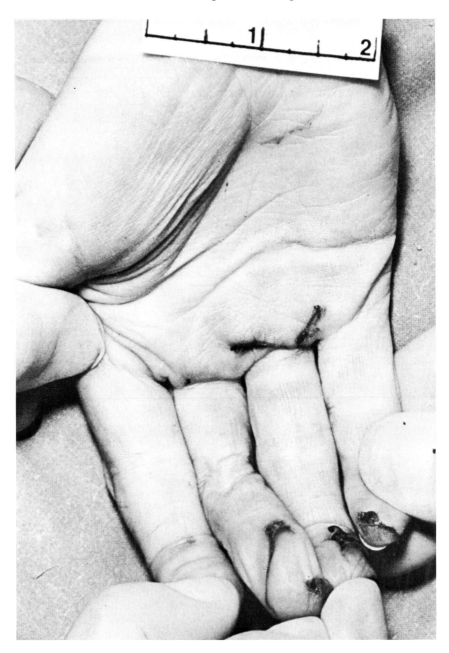

Fig. 7–5. Defense wounds.

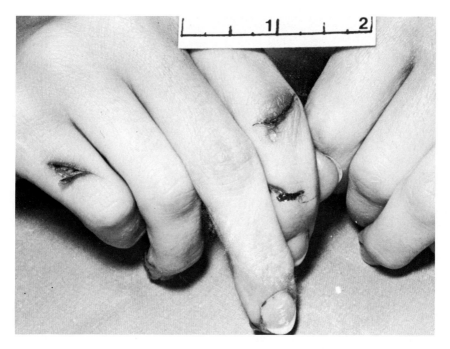

Fig. 7–6. Defense wounds on the back of the hand.

the side of the cutting edge. Multiple wounds are present if the victim loses the grasp of the weapon and makes repeated attempts to hold it or ward it off. Although the presence of defense wounds constitutes strong evidence in favor of homicide, the absence of such wounds does not rule out a homicidal attack. With a surprise attack the first serious wound may render the victim defenseless. Attacks from the back do not give the victim a chance to defend himself, nor will a person under the influence of alcohol or drugs or one rendered unconscious be able to defend himself. Under such circumstances defense wounds are lacking.

Accidental Incised Wounds

These wounds can be caused by falling on sharp objects such as broken glass when persons are involved in automobile accidents. Rarely do they present a problem in interpretation. If an accidental cutthroat (Fig. 7-7) arouses suspicions of foul play, the history of the circumstances of death will readily assist is determining the mode of infliction of such an injury. Gonzales *et al.* (1954),[3] and Smith and Fiddes (1955),[6] have described accidental neck injuries simulating homicidal cutthroat.

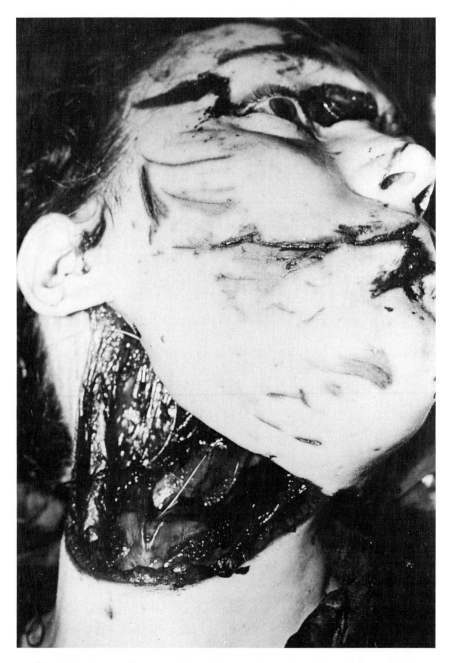

Fig. 7–7. An accidental cutthroat in a victim of an automobile accident.

Stab Wounds

Stab wounds are penetrating wounds with the depth of penetration greater than the surface width or breadth. The external appearance of the wound depends on the instrument causing it. If the weapon is sharp and pointed the wound is an elliptical slit with clean-cut margins. Relatively blunt weapons, such as pokers or screwdrivers, however, produce a slit with ragged margins. Both extremities of the wound are pointed if the weapon causing it has two sharp edges. An object such as a scissors blade causes a wound with one extremity pointed and the other blunt or square.

Deaths from homicidal stabbing are more common than those from suicidal stabs, and death from stab wounds must be considered a result of homicide until proved otherwise. The sites of the wounds and the multiplicity of the injuries easily distinguish a murder from a suicide. The investigator will have to rely on the facts of the circumstances of death to identify stab wounds caused accidentally.

Suicidal stab wounds are usually found in the heart area. Some individuals stab themselves in the epigastric area under the assumption that the heart is situated in that area. The suicide usually stabs once (rarely more than once), but unlike the suicidal cutthroat the wound is not associated with "hesitation" wounds in the area of stabbing or elsewhere. The suicide deliberately lifts the clothes to stab in a bare area and the weapon will be found still in the wound, in the decedent's hand or near the body unless the scene has been altered. It must be stressed that the finding of a single stab wound in the heart area does not prove suicide or exclude murder.

Homicidal stab wounds can be found anywhere on the body. A multiplicity of wounds suggests murder, and if they are in areas inaccessible to the decedent, they are certain to be homicidal. If multiple stab wounds are present, it is possible that some of them were inflicted after death. Such postmortem stabbing is more likely if the assailant is in an erotic sex frenzy.

> A prisoner in the tailoring shop of a prison suddenly attacked another prisoner with a pair of scissors. He stabbed his victim several times in the chest. Even after the victim was motionless the attacker continued to stab him in sheer frenzy despite efforts to control him. Only one of 46 wounds inflicted was fatal.

> In another case, a young married woman who was alone at home was stabbed by an unknown assailant. She was found dead with multiple stab wounds on the neck, chest, abdomen, arms, hands and the back (Fig. 7-8). The heart, lungs, spleen, intestines and the mesentery were penetrated by the weapon. There was no evidence of "sexual" assault.

Although homicidal stab wounds are more commonly multiple (Fig. 7-9), murder may be accomplished with a single wound. Death from a

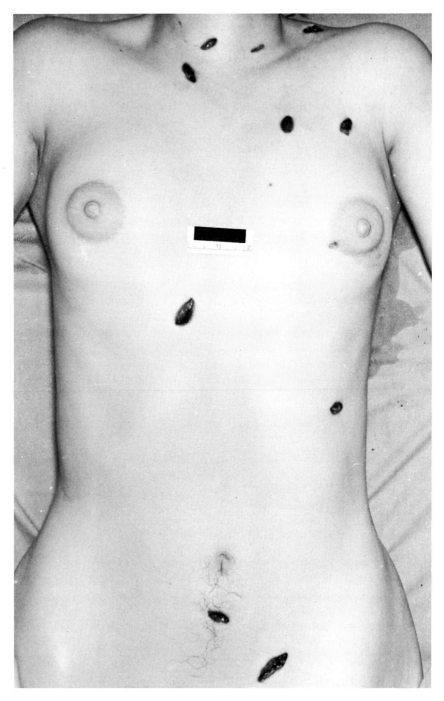

Fig. 7–8. Multiple homicidal stab wounds.

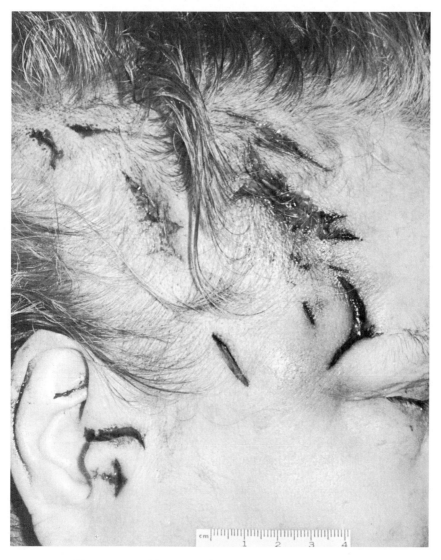

Fig. 7–9. Multiple homicidal stab wounds on the head.

single wound anywhere on the body must be carefully investigated to exclude homicide. If the stab wound is at a site away from the heart area ("elective" position chosen by suicides), it must arouse suspicions of homicide, especially if the weapon enters the body through the victim's clothing.

If a wound is caused by a thin-pointed object, such as a needle or ice pick, it may be so small that its true significance may not be appreciated without a careful autopsy.

A 69-year-old man was involved in a argument with his 49-year-old son. In a burst of anger the older man stabbed his son with an ice pick in the temple area. The younger man became unconscious and died on the way to the hospital. At the autopsy the only external injury on the body was a 4 × 2 mm. wound in the left temple region. Examination of the brain revealed massive subarachnoid hemorrhage at the base of the brain. Dissection of the arteries at the base showed a nick in the left middle cerebral artery. The ice pick had perforated the cranium and penetrated the brain. The tract of the wound was in a straight line extending from the external injury in the temple area to a point a little beyond the nick in the middle cerebral artery.

REFERENCES

1. Fatteh, A.: Vital Reaction—An Investigation of Skin Wounds. A Thesis Approved for the Degree of Ph.D. by the Queen's University of Belfast, Belfast, 1965.
2. Fatteh, A.: Histochemical distinction between antemortem and postmortem skin wounds. J. Forensic Sci., *11:*17, 1966.
3. Gonzales, T. A., Vance, M., Helpern, M., and Umberger, C. J.: Legal Medicine Pathology and Toxicology. ed. 2. New York, Appleton-Century-Crofts, 1954.
4. Rabinowitsch, A.: Medicolegal conclusions on the form of the knife used based on the shape of stab wounds produced. J. Forensic Med., *6:*160, 1959.
5. Raekallio, J.: Histochemical studies on vital and postmortem skin wounds. Ann. Med. Exp. Biol. Fenn., *39*(Supp. 6): 1, 1961.
6. Smith, Sir S., and Fiddes, F. S.: Forensic Medicine. ed. 10. London, J. & A. Churchill, 1955.

8

Gunshot Wounds

Gun related deaths are common throughout the world. In the United States, gunshot wounds rank among the leading causes of death. Approximately 25,000 persons die every year in the United States from injuries caused by firearms. In the state of North Carolina, with a population of 5 million, gunshot wounds accounted for 1001 fatalities in 1969 and 1025 in 1970 (2.5% of total deaths). Gunshot wounds were the seventh leading cause of death.[6]

With such a high incidence of firearm fatalities, the general pathologist is bound to be involved in the investigation of gunshot wounds. Many cases cannot be satisfactorily investigated without the help of the pathologist or medical investigator. The doctor, therefore, should be prepared with the knowledge of the procedures of investigation in such cases. In order to evaluate the wounds better he should also possess a working knowledge of the common types of firearm and ammunition.

As in any other medicolegal investigation of death, the study of a case of gunshot wound should aim at answering the principal questions concerning the cause and the manner of death, the time of death and the identification of the deceased. However, there are other questions involved in the case of gunshot wounds, many of which the medical man is expected to answer.[13] In answering such questions a systematic evaluation of a case of gunshot wound is suggested with the following points in mind:

1. Preservation and collection of evidence at the scene of death
2. Identification of the weapon
3. Discovery of the wounds and identification of gunshot wounds
4. Number and location of wounds in the clothing and on the body
5. Features of gunshot wounds and adjacent areas
6. Range of fire (contact, close, distant)
7. Angle of fire
8. Number of shots fired
9. Course of the projectile in the body
10. Retrieval of the bullet or pellets and determination of the type of gun

11. Retrieval of foreign materials (fabric, wadding, and so on) from the wound tract in the body
12. Period of survival
13. Identification of lethal injury
14. Recording of injuries for presentation in courts (reports, diagrams, photographs, x-rays)
15. Special investigations (fingerprints, blood type, toxicologic studies, histologic examinations, test firing, localization of gunpowder, and so on.)

The facets of investigation that can help the investigator accumulate all pertinent information are the examination of the scene of death, of the weapon and of the body and the ancillary investigations.

EXAMINATION OF THE SCENE

In a case in which death has resulted from gunshot wounds, examination of the scene helps determine whether the death was accidental, suicidal or homicidal.

In addition to the general aims of the scene investigation described in Chapter 1, specific aims of the examination of the scene in the cases of death from gunshot wounds are:

1. Study of the circumstances of shooting
2. Preservation of evidence (fingerprints on the weapon, gunpowder on hands)
3. Examination of the gun and the body, and recording of findings
4. Collection of evidence (gun, empty cartridges, shells, clothing, bloodstains, hair)
5. Preliminary advice on the line of further investigation

Circumstances of the Shooting. In a majority of the cases the circumstances of death become obvious at the beginning of the *conversation with the witnesses.* The *location of the shooting* (hunting area, locked room, entertainment spot) may give a ready clue to the manner of death. The *presence or absence of the gun* at the scene of death is an important factor. If the gun is present, suicide or accident are more likely; its absence should arouse suspicion of foul play. The possibility of alteration of the scene should always be kept in mind. The *type of the gun* that caused death and its condition may sometimes help draw conclusions about the manner of death. If suicide is thought to be a possibility, the *personal history of the decedent* can clinch the issue.

Preservation of Evidence. Before the examination of any scene of death is commenced, due consideration should be given to the aspect of preservation of evidence, particularly in the investigation of a gunshot wound fatality. If a crime is committed, the detection of fingerprints on the weapon (if present at the scene), on doorknobs and so on may solve the murder. Therefore, every care should be taken to preserve such evidence.

First of all, photographs of the scene, the body and the gun should be taken before anything is touched. Then the gun may be picked up for examination by holding it near the muzzle with gloved hands. The medical investigator should leave this part of the investigation to the detectives at the scene.

Another important precaution to be taken at the scene concerns the handling of the clothes and the body. If there is gunpower residue on the victim's hands it should be preserved by wrapping the hands in dry, clean plastic bags. For detailed examination in the autopsy room, the clothes should preferably be left on the body undisturbed. Specific instructions should be given to the funeral director who is going to move the body to the necropsy room not to unclothe it and especially not to embalm it (see Chap. 17).

Recording of Findings. Careful notes should be made of the details of the circumstances of death and of the observations made at the scene. These should be supplemented with appropriate photographs of the scene. The general appearance of the location of death should be described. If the gun is present at the scene, its position in relation to the body should be noted as well as its serial number, make, model, caliber, type of action and a description of the ammunition. Observations on the number of gunshot wounds, their positions in the clothing and on the body are important. Equally important are notes about the presence or absence of a burning effect, tattooing and powder residues on the clothing and around the wounds of the body.

Collection of Evidence. A preliminary examination of the gun may indicate how many shots were fired. This information together with the number of entrance wounds on the body may reveal the need for a search of spent bullets, including the ones that pass through the body. If any loose bullets are found they should be collected. If they are embedded in the walls, ceiling or furniture they should be extracted and retained. At the scene or in the autopsy room bullets should not be held with forceps. Bullets should be put in cardboard boxes, not in metal containers.

The type of bullets and their markings may help identify the gun. From some weapons spent cartridges are automatically ejected. These as well as shotgun shells should be carefully searched for at the scene. In the absence of a gun at the scene these cartridges and shells with their identifying information indicate the type of gun used and may lead to the identification of the particular gun that inflicted the wounds.

Preliminary Advice on the Line of Further Investigation. The presence of a medical investigator at the scene of a firearm death can contribute substantially to the overall investigation, since he is in the best position to interpret the wounds on the body. From examination of the body he can render advice on the time of death, time of infliction of wounds, range and angle of fire, and the type of gun used. If crime is suspected such advice helps police investigators plan and pursue a certain line of investigation and avert any lapse in the investigation that is likely to occur due to delay in the autopsy.

ANATOMY OF GUNS

Firearms are of two principal types: smoothbore and rifle.

Shotguns. Shotguns are smoothbore weapons; that is, the inside wall of the barrel is smooth. Shotguns are usually double-barreled, with the right barrel being a straight cylinder and the left "choked" or narrowed near the muzzle. Some shotguns have over-and-under double barrel. The choke is designed to keep the shot together over a longer distance. Examples of shotguns are the Browning autoloader, Mossberg Model 183K and Winchester Model 12, guns ordinarily used by sportsmen for hunting and designed to fire cartridges containing lead pellets. The shotgun can be "broken" open at a hinge near the breech for the removal of empty cartridge cases.

Shotguns are usually designated by the diameter of the barrel (bore); the unit of measure is the gauge and is determined by the number of solid balls of pure lead, each with the diameter of the barrel, that can be prepared from one pound of lead. If twelve balls can be made from one pound of lead, each ball exactly fitting the inside of the barrel of a shotgun, the gun is called a 12-gauge or 12-bore shotgun. This system of nomenclature does not apply to 0.410 gauge shotguns. The common bore gauges and their equivalents in inches are listed in Table 8-1.

Shotgun ammunition consists of *shells or cartridges* with variable characteristics. Shell cases may be made of brass, cardboard or plastic. The base of the shell is rimmed; the cap at the base contains a small quantity of powder charge which fires when the trigger strikes it. Inside the shell are powder charge, wads and pellets (Fig. 8-1). The powder commonly used today is smokeless powder. When the powder in the cap is ignited, the main bulk of the powder charge is also ignited and the wads and pellets are propelled out of the barrel. The force of ignition of the powder charge within a compressed space drives the shot, and with it are carried to variable distances flame, smoke and unburned powder.

Shotgun pellets have specific sizes and weights as shown in Table 8-2.

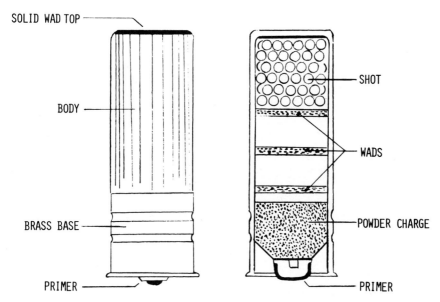

SOLID WAD TOP

BODY

BRASS BASE

PRIMER

SHOT

WADS

POWDER CHARGE

PRIMER

Fig. 8–1. The structure of a shotgun shell.

Data on buckshot is given in Table 8-3. The size of a pellet is difficult to measure after the shot is fired because most of the pellets become deformed. However, the pathologist can easily determine the type of shotgun used by weighing the pellets after they are cleaned and dried (see Table 8-2).

TABLE 8-1. Shotgun Gauges with Decimal Equivalents.

Shotgun (gauge)	*Decimal Equivalent* (in inches)
10	0.775
12	0.730
16	0.670
20	0.615
28	0.550
410	0.410

Rifled Guns. Rifled weapons are of two types: low velocity, short-barreled *pistols* and high velocity, long-barreled *rifles*. These guns bear a number of parallel but spiral lands (projecting ridges) and grooves (depressed spirals between the lands), on the interior of the barrel from breech to muzzle, referred to as rifling. The diameter of the gun bore is the distance between the two opposite lands. This distance, expressed in hundredths of an inch, is called the *caliber* (Fig. 8-2). The commonly used

TABLE 8-2. Size and Weight of Pellets Used in Shotguns.

Shot Number	Diameter of Pellet (in inches)	Number of Pellets Per Ounce	Weight of Each Pellet (in grams)
12	0.05	2385	0.0118
10	0.07	870	0.0325
9	0.08	585	0.0471
8	0.09	410	0.0691
7½	0.095	350	0.0810
6	0.11	225	0.1260
5	0.12	170	0.1667
4	0.13	135	0.2100
2	0.15	90	0.3150
BB	0.18	50	

TABLE 8-3. Size, Number and Weight of Pellets Used In Various Buckshots.

Buckshot Number	Diameter of Pellet (in inches)	Number of Pellets Per Shell	Number of Pellets Per Pound
4	0.24	27	340
3	0.25	20	300
1	0.30	16	175
0	0.32	12	145
00	0.33	9	130

rifled weapons have calibers of 0.22, 0.25, 0.32, 0.38 and 0.45 inch. Rifled weapons fire a single bullet. The rifling causes a spiraling motion of the bullet and imparts gyroscopic steadiness to it during its flight.

Of the short-barreled rifled weapons, the *revolver* is recognized by the way the ammunition is carried to the breech. A metal drum, usually having

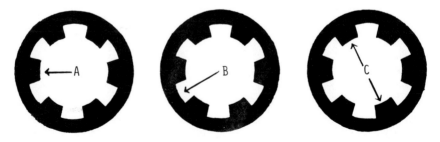

Fig. 8–2. The interior of a rifled gun. A—land, B—groove, C—caliber (distance between two opposite lands).

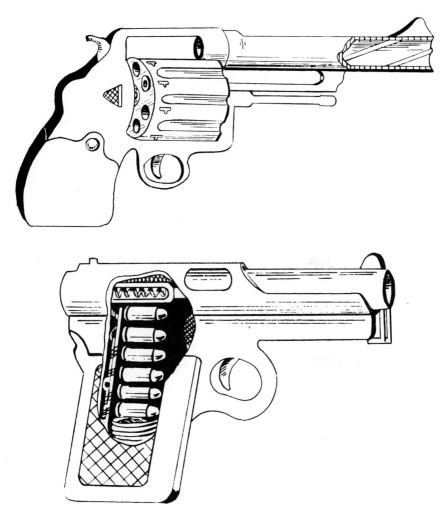

Fig. 8–3. *Top,* A revolver with a metal drum. *Bottom,* An automatic pistol with a magazine under the breech.

spaces for six cartridges, revolves each time the trigger is released, bringing into position the next live cartridge for firing. In the automatic *pistol* the cartridges are placed in a metal box (magazine) under the breech (Fig. 8-3). Each time the trigger is pulled the bullet in the breech is fired and the spent cartridge is automatically ejected. At the same time a spring mechanism pushes the next live cartridge into the breech ready to be fired. Examples of revolvers are 0.22 caliber Iver Johnson, 0.38 caliber S & W (used by police) and 0.45 caliber Webley-Fosberry; commonly used pistols are 0.22 caliber Webley and Scott, 0.25 caliber Colt and 0.45 caliber

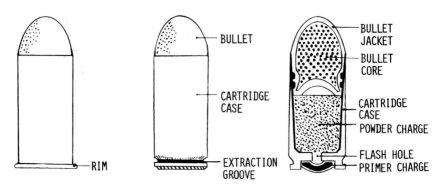

Fig. 8–4. The components of a pistol cartridge.

Colt. Other guns such as the so-called Saturday Night Special are commonly used in the United States.

Long-barreled *rifles* have a high velocity performance with a range of fire of up to 6000 to 7000 feet. Examples of rifles are 0.32 caliber Remington, Rifle U.S. and Winchester Models 70, 760 and M1898.

Ammunition for pistols consists of cartridges having either a rimmed base, used in the automatic pistol, or a base with a groove. The components of a typical pistol cartridge are the case, bullet, powder charge and primer charge (Fig. 8-4).

EXAMINATION OF THE BODY

Examination of the body helps identify wounds caused by firearms, differentiates entrance from exit wounds and determines the angle and range of fire. It also helps detect the features of suicidal, accidental and homicidal wounds. In the following paragraphs various features of wounds caused by shotguns and rifled weapons are discussed.

Shotgun Wounds

The nature of the entrance wound caused by a shotgun depends to a great extent on the range of fire.

Contact Wounds caused by shotguns with the muzzle pressed against the body of the decedent are usually round or oval. The margins of the wounds in the skin are usually clean cut, rarely ragged, and show contusion of the tissue which is blackened by gunpowder. There may be singeing of the margins by flame associated with the shot. Because shot and gases are blasted within the wound, the subcutaneous and deeper tissues show severe disruption. Contact wounds on the head are associated with greater disruption of the margins, and these wounds often show subsidiary linear tears in the skin extending from the margins of the principal wound. If a double-barreled weapon is used and it is held against the skin, the firing muzzle causes contusion and blackening. The imprint of the nonfiring muzzle may be left next to the gunshot wound in the form of circular abrasion (Fig. 8-5). With the gases entering the body, the blood and tissue along the tract of the shot show the presence of carbon monoxide.

Close-range Wounds caused when the muzzle is up to 24 inches from the body, but not pressed against the skin, depict certain identifiable characteristics. With a loose contact or with the muzzle up to 6 inches from the body, the wound is usually round or oval. The margins of the skin wound may be clean-cut or slightly ragged. There is some burning effect from the flame and blackening of the skin from smoke and unburned powder. The width of the zone of blackening increases with the increase in the distance of fire. The blackening due to smoke may be seen with ranges up to 15 inches. Tattooing by unburned powder may be seen in wounds caused by shotguns with the muzzle distance of up to 24 inches. The deeper tissues show marked disruptions and may show the presence of carbon monoxide.

Long-range Wounds are defined for the purpose of present discussion as wounds caused by shotguns from a distance of over 24 inches. Although a wound caused from a distance of 2 to 3 feet may be a single round hole, with increasing range of fire the pellets start to scatter and cause subsidiary

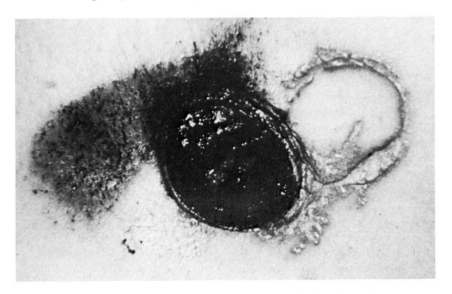

Fig. 8–5. A contact shotgun wound. Note the blackening from the escape of gases, and the imprint of the nonfiring muzzle.

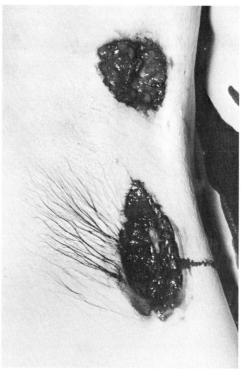

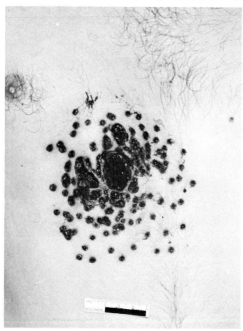

Fig. 8–6. Shotgun wounds in the axilla show crenations in the margins caused by scattering pellets. *Bottom,* This shotgun wound shows the scatter of pellets.

pellet holes. From a distance of 3 to 9 feet (1 to 3 yards) the shotgun produces a single large wound with crenations of the margins caused by the scattering pellets. Longer distances reveal a greater scatter of pellets which cause small wounds around the main wound. From the degree of the scatter of pellets a rough estimate of the range of fire can be made (Fig. 8-6). To make such an estimate, measure the distance between the two farthest pellets in inches minus one. The number thus obtained gives the range of fire in yards. This formula is applicable only if the barrel of the gun is unchoked. With a choke the spread of the pellets is over a smaller area.

Not all shotgun wounds have a similar appearance (Fig. 8-7). A shotgun wound may resemble a large stab wound. If the shotgun is held against the body, gases are blasted into the body with the shot. The rapid entry of the shot and the gases causes a momentary vacuum immediately below the skin that may result in the extrusion of soft tissues, such as fat, through the wound. In addition to the wound caused by the shot, other injuries caused by wadding may be present.[11] The interposition of heavy clothing may alter the appearance of skin wounds. If the shot passes through clothing, the defects in the clothes and the presence or absence of blackening and pellet holes should be described.

Exit Wounds are infrequently seen in deaths from shotgun wounds. If the exit wound is present it usually shows eversion of skin margins with disruption of the tissue and subsidiary tears in the skin. Features that are associated with entrance wounds (burning, tattooing, blackening) are, of course, absent.

In a case of shotgun injury the internal examination gives the precise cause of death. While carrying out this examination, every effort should be made to retrieve about a dozen pellets. The examiner must also look for wads and pieces of fabric from the clothing of the decedent in the cases of contact or close-range shotgun wounds (Fig. 8-8). The pellets and wadding may help identify the gun.

Rifled Gun Wounds

The characteristics of the wounds of entry caused by pistols, revolvers and rifles are for the most part alike. Specific features of wounds inflicted from various distances are described below.

Contact Wounds caused when the muzzle is pressed against the skin are circular, unless the shot is fired with the gun at an angle. There is usually a thin band of contusion in the margins of the wound. In the contused area the hair is singed in some cases and there is blackening of the subcutaneous tissue which is hemorrhagic and disrupted. Tattooing is minimal or absent. Contact wounds in areas where there is bone immediately under the skin show slightly different features. For instance, head wounds, more often

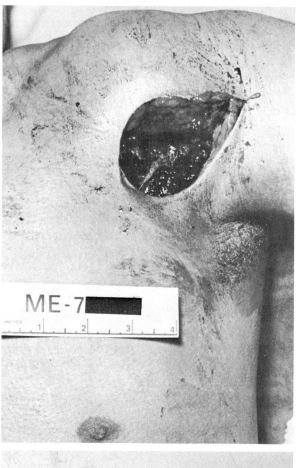

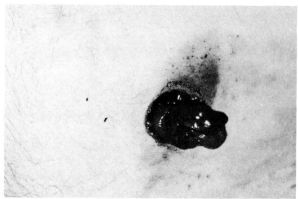

Fig. 8–7. *Top,* This shotgun wound resembles a stab wound. *Bottom,* Protrusion of fat from a gunshot wound.

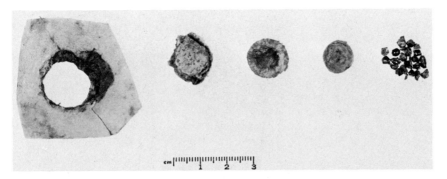

Fig. 8–8. Pellets, wads and fabric were removed from a gunshot wound.

than not, show subsidiary tears in the margins of the principal wound if the underlying bone is thick. If the bone is thin, as in the temple area, the wound of entry is usually round. In most cases, there is contusion of the wound margins and burning and blackening of the subcutaneous tissues. With a tight contact, the imprint of the muzzle may be present (Fig. 8-9). The attachment to the muzzle may leave an imprint, giving the appearance of an abrasion, caused by the nonfiring muzzle of a twin-barrel gun.

Close-range Wounds inflicted when the muzzle is in loose contact with the skin or from a distance of less than 2 feet, have fairly typical characteristics. With a perpendicular strike the wound is invariably round, unless there is bone immediately under the skin. Head wounds may show subsidiary tears. The flame effect, with singeing of the hair and scorching of the tissues, occurs if the distance of fire is no more than 6 inches. With a pistol or revolver the flame effect is observed if the range of fire is less than 3 inches. Smoke fouling is seen frequently with distances of up to 12 inches. Tattooing by unburned gunpowder particles is seen around the entrance wound if the gun is fired from a distance less than 24 inches (Fig. 8-10).

Long-range Wounds of entry caused by rifled weapons are round or oval holes with no flame effect, blackening or powder tattooing.

Entrance gunshot wounds in the skull are easy to differentiate from exit wounds. The skull is formed of an outer and inner table. When the bullet enters the outer table it causes a round entrance wound. When the same bullet exits from the inner table to enter the cranial cavity there is beveling, and the exit hole in the inner table is much larger than the hole in the outer table. If the bullet exits from the cranium it causes a smaller hole in the inner table and a larger one in the outer table (Fig. 8-11).

Frequently, entrance gunshot wounds reveal grayish staining of the margins of the wound by grease. This grease staining should not be interpreted as blackening of the skin from flame, smoke or gunpowder. Such staining is commonly seen in wounds inflicted from long ranges.

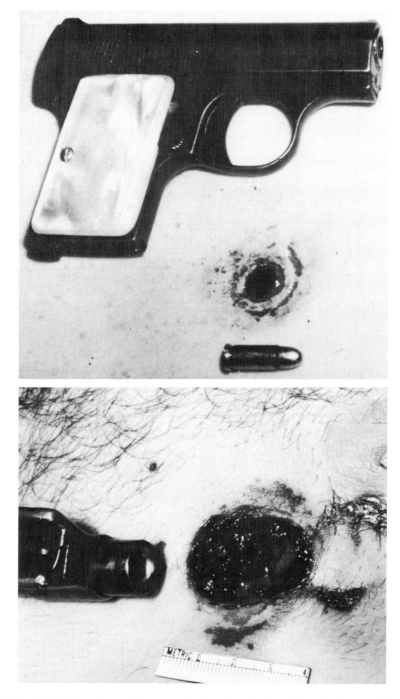

Fig. 8–9. *Top,* A gunshot wound showing the imprint of the muzzle. *Bottom,* A gunshot wound associated with an abrasion caused by the attachment on the muzzle.

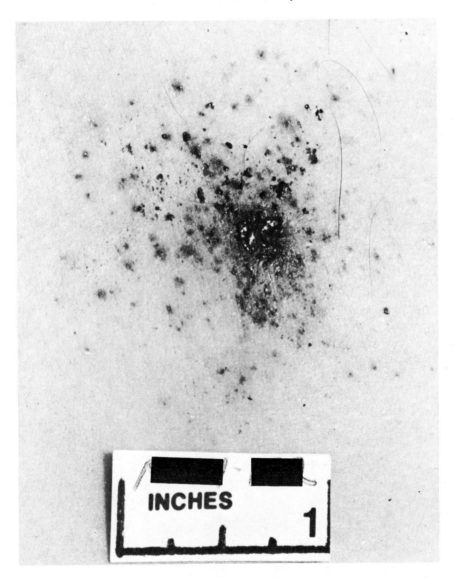

Fig. 8–10. Tattooing by gunpowder particles indicates that the range of fire was less than two feet.

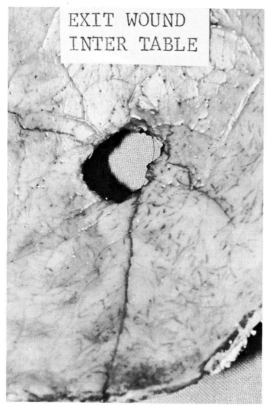

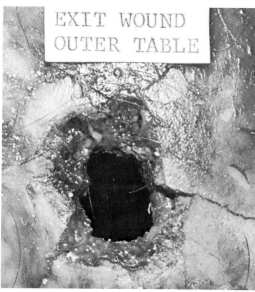

Fig. 8–11. *Top,* A bullet hole in the skull. *Bottom,* A bullet hole in the skull.

Examination of the entrance wounds can help in the determination of the angle of fire. If the gun is held obliquely against the skin, gases may escape from between the muzzle and the skin at a point where the muzzle is not in tight contact with the skin, causing a localized smoke effect (see Fig. 8-5). If the missile or shot strikes the body at an angle, the entrance wound shows abrading of the skin on the side where the missile first came in contact with the skin. For instance, if the right margin of the wound shows skin abrasion, the gun is most likely to have been fired from the right side.

Exit Wounds caused by rifled weapons are round or irregular with none of the features seen in entrance wounds. With small caliber weapons, exit wounds are slightly larger than entrance wounds. High velocity weapons may produce entrance wounds larger than exit wounds.

SUICIDAL GUNSHOT WOUNDS

Two facts should be kept in mind: Suicides elect classical sites and self-inflicted wounds are ordinarily contact or close-range wounds. Based on the results of our study of 844 suicides, the sites chosen to inflict suicidal wounds, in order of frequency, are the temple area (right temple by right-handed persons and left temple by left-handed persons), heart area, mouth and the center of the forehead.[10] The epigastrium and the area under the chin are also sometimes chosen by suicides.[2]

A contact wound in the temple area or in the dead center of the forehead with blackening of the skin margins poses no difficulty in interpretation, especially if supporting evidence in favor of suicide is available (Fig. 8-12). One must, however, be cautious in drawing conclusions about wounds which are not in the classical locations (Fig. 8-13). An entrance wound on the face must arouse suspicion of foul play, and in the case of a wound around the eye the possibility of crime should be ruled out before a verdict of suicide or accident is rendered. In rare instances suicidal gunshot wounds are found behind the ear but in such cases every care should be taken to rule out homicide.

In the following instance a suicidal gunshot wound was found at a site most presumptive of homicide—the vertex of the head.

A young man who was known to dislike guns bought a 0.22 caliber rifle to shoot himself. He found privacy in an unused cottage garage. Suspending a rope from a beam, he attached the gun pointing downward. By placing the muzzle at the back of his head, he pulled the trigger by means of a curtain rod curved at one end, shooting himself. This man had marital and financial problems, he had been depressed and he did leave a suicide note.

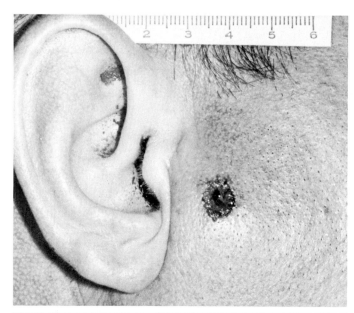

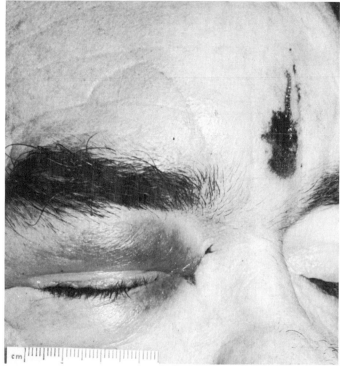

If a person shoots himself through the mouth, the entrance gunshot wound is in the posterior third of the palate and bears the classical features of a contact wound. The top of the head is frequently blown up but the tongue is never injured. Unless the entrance wound is searched and identified, a single exit wound in the head may be misinterpreted as an entrance wound.

The upper half of the neck, the area under the chin or jaw, is sometimes selected by suicides, particularly if they use long-barreled guns, because it is easier to stabilize the muzzle under the jaw or the chin. If a long-barreled gun is used, the trigger may be pulled either by a toe or by a mechanism, such as a string, tied to the trigger. Some are able to stretch the arm and pull the trigger with a finger. Such a gunshot wound is, as a rule, a contact one. Some suicides prefer to hold the muzzle under the rib cage; shooting themselves by placing the muzzle in the egigastrium or under the rib margins. An arrangement set up to pull the trigger is often found at the scene in such cases. If the victim holds the barrel near the muzzle to stabilize it against the skin, some of the smoke and gunpowder may soil the hand. However, similar powder and smoke soiling also may be seen in homicidal shootings if the victim attempts to hold the gun to push it away in self-defense (Fig. 8-14).

Suicidal gunshot wounds of the extremities are extremely rare. One young man bled to death after he blasted the femoral vessels by placing the gun against the front of the right thigh. He pulled the trigger with the left great toe.

Multiple suicidal gunshot wounds, though uncommon, do occur. In our series of 844 suicides, there were thirteen cases of multiple gunshot wounds. Eight of these showed two gunshot wounds in the chest in each case, two had both gunshot wounds in the head (temple area) and three had gunshot wounds in the head and chest. The autopsy in each case showed that one of the two bullets had caused nonfatal injuries. In some cases the circumstances of death are clear. This author has reported a case with two suicidal gunshot wounds in the temple area (Fig. 8-15) in which only a complete investigation provided conclusive answers.[8] Wood[16] investigated an unusual case with four suicidal gunshot wounds in the head.

> When an elderly recluse was not seen up and about in his apartment for a few days, his neighbors summoned police to investigate. On breaking open his apartment door, he was found dead lying on the bed. An old 0.32 caliber revolver was found on his body with very old ammunition. There were four

Fig. 8–12. (*Opposite*) *Top,* A suicidal gunshot wound at a classical site. *Bottom,* A suicidal gunshot wound in the center of the forehead. A black eye is commonly associated with gunshot wounds of the front part of the head.

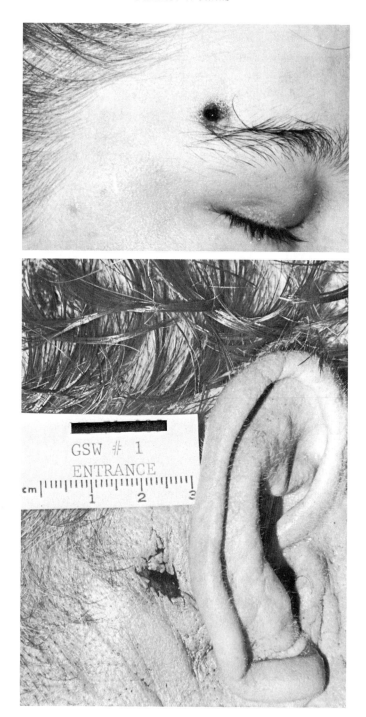

gunshot wounds on the head (Fig. 8-16). Two penetrated the scalp, one penetrated the skull and one entered the cranium. He had suffered from severe arthritis and in a suicide note that he had left he cited poor health as the reason for taking his own life.

Mason and his associates have reported a case in which a 74-year-old man shot himself in the head four times to commit suicide.[14]

HOMICIDAL GUNSHOT WOUNDS

These wounds could be seen on any part of the body and be inflicted from a variety of ranges. Wounds on the face, on the back and on any inaccessible part of the body should be presumed to be homicidal until accidental infliction can be ruled out. Although a majority of the homicidal wounds are inflicted from a range of more than an arm's reach, close-range wounds and even contact wounds may be homicidal. A homicidal contact gunshot wound at a site commonly elected by suicides can create considerable difficulty in interpretation. In cases with contact wounds at sites not used by suicides, the possibility of homicide must be kept in mind.

ACCIDENTAL GUNSHOT WOUNDS

Accidental shootings usually occur from careless handling of guns. Children, hunters and intoxicated individuals are common victims. The sites of the wounds and the ranges vary a great deal. In a majority of the cases the circumstances of death clarify the manner of death. However, when the circumstances are not clear, every detail of the case should be considered to rule out the possibility of suicide or homicide.

CONCEALED AND UNUSUAL GUNSHOT WOUNDS

Gunshot wounds may not always be obvious and they may not have distinctive characteristics.

If the body is covered with blood, the blood clots may obscure the firearm injury. In a case with multiple gunshot wounds the entrance wound in the chest was missed on a preliminary external examination. X-rays and

Fig. 8–13. (*Opposite*) *Top,* A gunshot wound immediately above the eye. Such a wound should arouse suspicion of foul play. *Bottom,* A homicidal gunshot wound behind the ear.

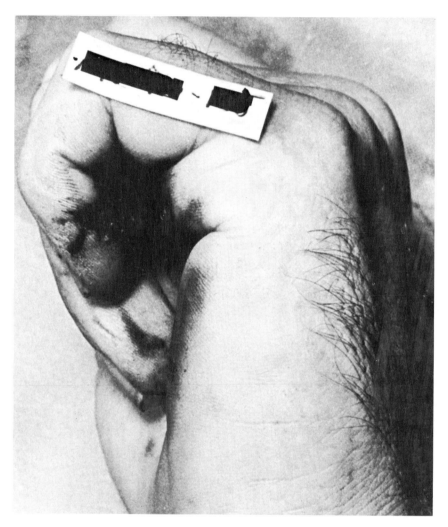

Fig. 8–14. A gunshot wound and gunpowder soiling of the hand.

the finding of one too many bullets led to further search and the discovery of the wound. In another case in which the body bore multiple gunshot wounds the umbilicus was filled with blood. When this was cleaned away an additional gunshot wound was found within the umbilicus (Fig. 8-17).

Wounds in the head on which there is a thick growth of hair are not easily seen. Careful search must be made and for proper examination of the wounds the pathologist should not hesitate to shave the hair. Reflection of the scalp and opening of the cranium will reveal the bullet injury if the missile has entered the cranium.

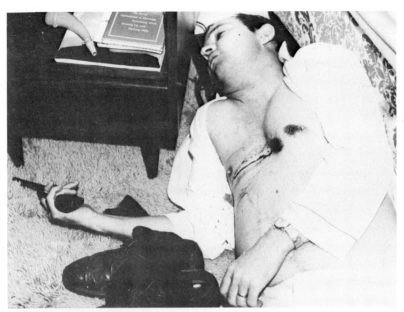

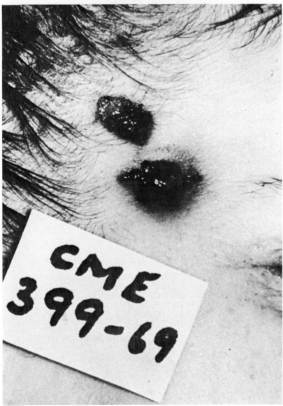

Fig. 8–15. *Top,* Two suicidal gunshot wounds of the chest. *Bottom,* Two suicidal gunshot wounds of the temple. (Reproduced with the permission of the Journal of Forensic Medicine. From Fatteh, A.: Homicide or suicide? J. Forensic Med., *122:* 18, 1971.)

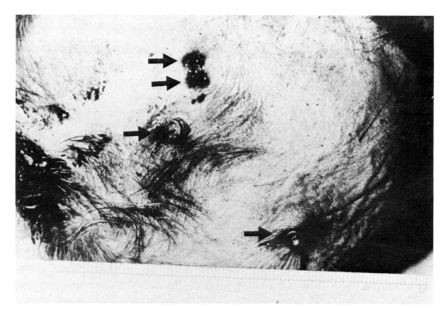

Fig. 8–16. Four suicidal gunshot wounds of the head. (Courtesy of Hobart Wood, M.D.)

The possibility of wounds in concealed sites should always be kept in mind.

Wounds in the mouth are not uncommon, most of these wounds being suicidal. A case of homicidal gunshot wound in the mouth has been reported.[8] In this case a woman was teasing her husband by putting her tongue out, when he placed the muzzle of a rifle against her tongue and shot her (Fig. 8-18). In another instance a sheriff's deputy was shot in the mouth by a man who was being arrested. Wounds in the mouth are difficult to examine especially if rigor has set in with the mouth closed. No effort should be spared, however, to explore such wounds. A mouth gag serves a useful purpose in such circumstances.

A wound in the nostril or one in the ear (Fig. 8-19) may escape detection if due care is not exercised at postmortem examination. A wound in the eye or in any of the body orifices, such as the rectum or vagina, may not be obvious. Therefore, the examiner must always look for bullet holes in the body orifices, axillae, perineum and back before and after the body is cleaned.

Unusual features of gunshot wounds may create difficulties in interpretation. The injury may not have the appearances of a gunshot wound if the missile passes through an object such as glass or if the bullet strikes the body after it has ricocheted. Fragments of bullets also cause unusual

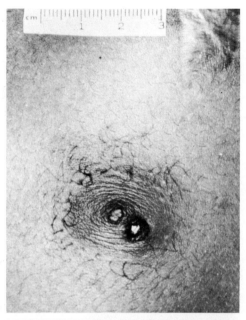

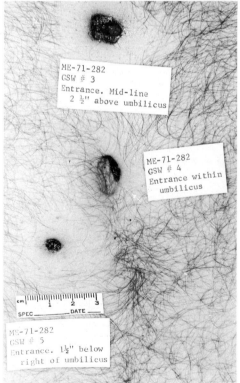

ME-71-282
GSW # 3
Entrance. Mid-line
2 ½" above umbilicus

ME-71-282
GSW # 4
Entrance within
umbilicus

ME-71-282
GSW # 5
Entrance. 1½" below
right of umbilicus

Fig. 8–17. *Top,* A gunshot wound of the chest. *Bottom,* multiple gunshot wounds, one in the umbilicus.

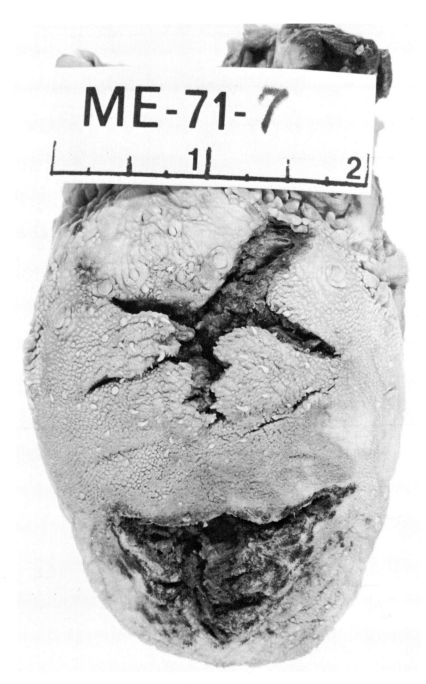

Fig. 8–18. A homicidal gunshot wound of the mouth. (Reproduced with the permission of S. S. Kind, Editor, Journal of The Forensic Science Society. From Fatteh, A.: Homicidal gunshot wound of mouth. J. Forensic Sci. Soc., *12*:347, 1972.)

injuries. Bullet grazes caused by glancing missiles sometimes resemble abrasions or lacerations (Fig. 8-20). A gunshot wound may be associated with other perforating injuries caused by fragments of the decedent's bones and these should be properly identified.

ARTEFACTS IN DEATHS FROM GUNSHOT WOUNDS

Occasionally, artefacts add to the difficulty of interpreting gunshot wounds. A victim of gunshot wounds may have been hospitalized for a period of time. During his hospitalization he may "sustain" additional "pseudogunshot wounds." Drainage holes in the chest or abdomen, such as the embalmer's trocar holes have also sometimes created problems (Fig. 8-21). Perhaps a more complicated situation is created by surgical altera- tion or suturing of gunshot wounds. A classical example of this is what may be termed the Kennedy phenomenon; surgical alteration of the gun- shot wound on the neck of President John F. Kennedy, the difficulty in the evaluation of that wound and the subsequent controversies about whether it was an entrance or an exit wound are well-known.

In decomposed bodies gunshot wounds are greatly modified. In one case of multiple wounds, a wound was twice the size of the others because in- testinal loops had protruded through it.

In the investigation of the cases of gunshot wounds, the finding of unex- pected bullets in the body is always a puzzle and may lead to false deduc- tions. Here is an example of an "old" bullet in the body:

> In the case of a severely burned body, x-rays showed a bullet in the pos- terior wall of the chest. This x-ray finding immediately raised suspicions of murder. However, when the bullet was localized and removed, it was found to be well wrapped with dense fibrous tissue.

In another case a "new" bullet formed an artefact:

> A man shot himself at the right temple and the bullet was recovered from the brain. There was, however, another bullet in the stomach. The scene in- vestigation showed a row of beer cans in the man's back yard, used as tar- gets. Part of the beer in the cans that had bullet holes had been consumed. It is surmised that the man drank beer from each can he shot successfully and "drank" a bullet with the beer.

X-ray Examination. It is advisable to x-ray the body of the victim of a gunshot wound prior to autopsy if facilities are available. Anterior and lateral films of the general area in which the bullet is suspected to be lodged save a considerable amount of the pathologist's time and effort in the search of the missile. In addition to the principal purpose of localizing

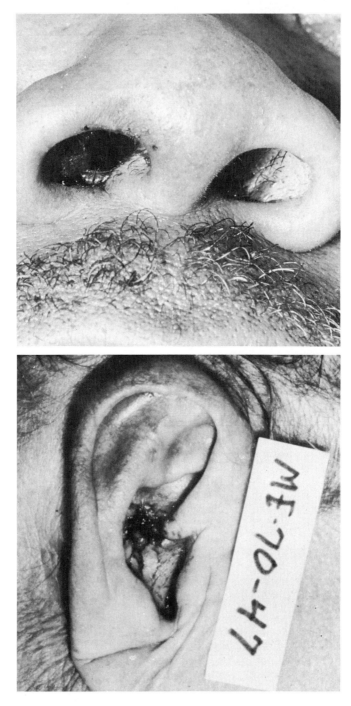

Fig. 8–19. (*Opposite*) *Top,* A homicidal gunshot wound in the nostril. (See Color Plate.) *Bottom,* A gunshot wound in the ear. (Courtesy of Page Hudson, M.D.)

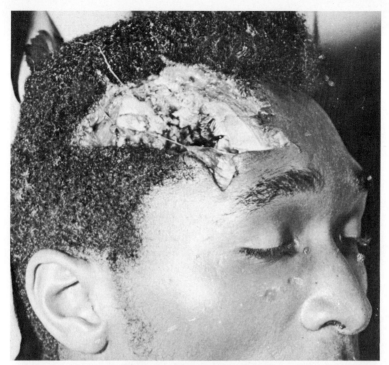

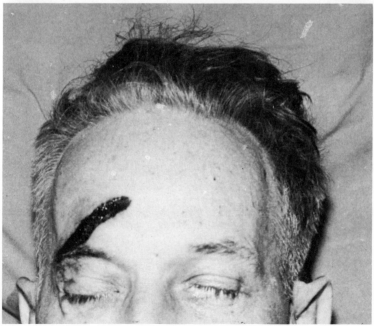

Fig. 8–20. (*Opposite*) *Top,* A gunshot wound caused by a bullet that first passed through a glass window. *Bottom,* A gunshot wound (caused by a glancing missile) resembling a laceration.

125

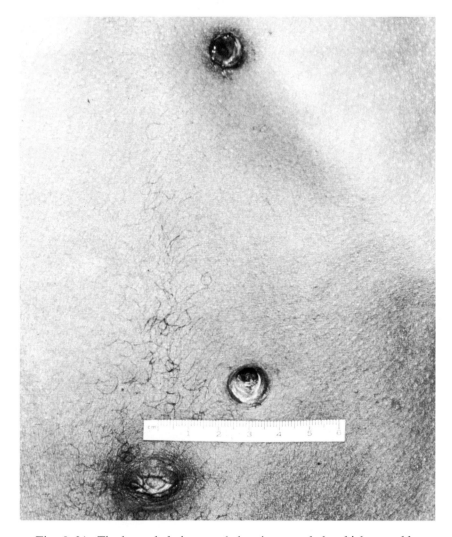

Fig. 8–21. The lower hole is an embalmer's trocar hole which resembles
the gunshot wound above.

the missiles, x-rays also help determine the number of bullets in the body,
evaluate the direction and angle of fire, estimate the distance of fire,[12]
assess the depth of the wounds and determine the type of firearm.

Occasionally x-rays reveal unexpected information. In a case of shooting, x-rays revealed not only shotgun pellets but also a small caliber missile. In another instance, shotgun pellets of different sizes were discovered
by radiologic examination. Bullet embolization is rare[4, 5] but if it does

occur the task of retrieval of the embolized bullet is extremely difficult without the help of x-rays (Fig. 8-22).

One of the other important values of x-rays is that they form a permanent record for use in the courts.

Test Firing. Sometimes the circumstances of shooting are not clear enough to indicate the precise manner of death. Conflicting stories may make the issue cloudy and the idiosyncracies of the gun in question may not be known.

To determine whether the suspected weapon was used and to find the range of fire, test firing may be necessary. If such an investigation is desired the help of the police may be sought.

Examination for Gunpowder. The so-called "Paraffin Test" for the detection of nitrates and nitrites in the gunpowder left on the hand of the person firing the gun, on the clothes and on the skin around the gunshot wounds is being used in many places. The method of testing is simple. A paraffin glove is prepared by placing layers of melted paraffin on the victim's hand or by soaking a piece of gauze with melted paraffin and while still melted wrapping it around the hand. After the paraffin is solidified the glove is removed and treated with diphenylamine or diphenylbenzidine reagent. The spots where nitrates, nitrites or other oxidizing agents are present will show blue discoloration. However, this test has limited value and, in fact, a critical study by Cowan and Purdon[3] indicates that it is useless and should be abandoned.

Histological Examination of Gunshot Wounds. Microscopic examination can help differentiate entrance gunshot wounds from exit wounds. Entrance wounds may show abrading of the skin, elongation and flattening of epidermal cells from the burning of the skin, as well as the presence of gunpowder particles in the epidermis, dermis and deeper tissues. Coagulation necrosis of the tissues, and swelling and vacuolization of the basal cells may also be seen.[1] The sections of exit wounds will not show these features. A special histological technique for forensic ballistics has been described by Rolfe and his colleagues.[15]

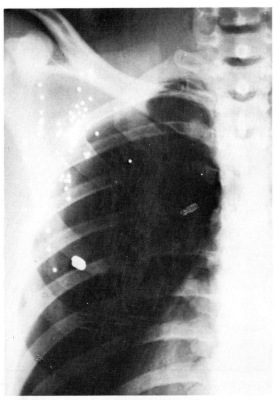

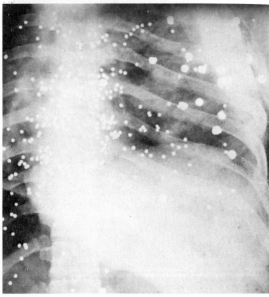

Fig. 8–22. *Top,* This chest x-ray shows shotgun pellets as well as a small caliber missile. (Courtesy of Harry L. Taylor, M.D.) *Bottom,* This chest x-ray shows pellets of two sizes. (Courtesy of Page Hudson, M.D.)

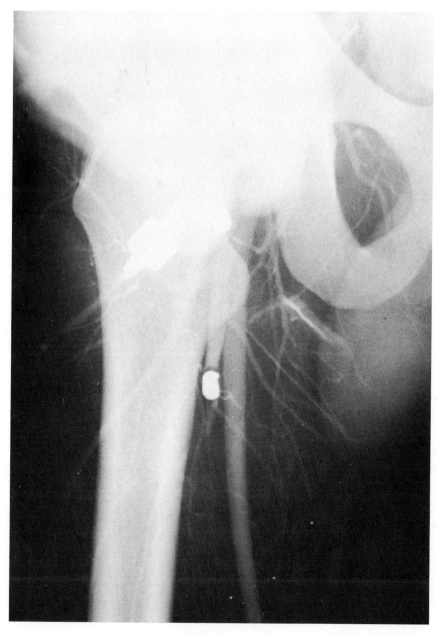

Fig. 8–22 (continued). An embolized bullet in the profunda femoris artery. (Reproduced with the permission of the Journal of Forensic Medicine. From Fatteh, A., Shah, Z. A., and Mann, G. T.: Bullet embolus of right profunda femoris artery. J. Forensic Med., *4:*139, 1968.)

REFERENCES

1. Adelson, L.: A microscopic study of dermal wounds. Am. J. Clin. Pathol., *35:*393, 1961.
2. Canfield, T. M.: Suicidal gunshot wounds of the abdomen. J. Forensic Sci., *14:*445, 1969.
3. Cowan, M. E., and Purdon, P. L.: A study of the "paraffin test". J. Forensic Sci., *12:*19, 1967.
4. DiMaio, V. J. M., and DiMaio, D. J.: Bullet embolization—six cases and a review of the literature. J. Forensic Sci., *17:*394, 1972.
5. Fatteh, A., Shah, Z. A., and Mann, G. T.: Bullet embolus of right profunda femoris artery. J. Forensic Med., *4:*139, 1968.
6. Fatteh, A., and Troxler, D.: The gun and its victims. A study of 1024 firearm fatalities in North Carolina during 1970. North Carolina Med. J., *32:*489, 1971.
7. Fatteh, A.: Murder or suicide? J. Forensic Med., *18:*122, 1971.
8. Fatteh, A.: Homicidal gunshot wound of mouth. J. Forensic Sci. Soc., *12:*347, 1972.
9. Fatteh, A.: Artefacts in forensic pathology. *In* Wecht, C. (ed.): Legal Medicine Annual 1972. New York, Appleton-Century-Crofts, 1972.
10. Fatteh, A., and Hayes, W.: Unpublished observations, 1972.
11. Guerin, P. F.: Shotgun wounds, J. Forensic Sci., *5:*294, 1960.
12. Krishnan, S. S., and Nichol, R. C.: Identification of bullet holes by neutron activation analysis and auto radiography. J. Forensic Sci., *13:*519, 1968.
13. Lyle, H.: Gunshot wounds. J. Forensic Sci., *6:*255, 1961.
14. Mason, M. F., Rose, E., and Alexander, F.: Four non-lethal head wounds resulting from improper revolver ammunition: report of case. J. Forensic Sci., *12:*205, 1967.
15. Rolfe, H. C., Curle, D., and Simmons, D.: A Histological technique for forensic ballistics. J. Forensic Med., *18:*47, 1971.
16. Wood, H.: Personal communication, 1972.

9

Asphyxial Deaths

Death caused as a result of obstruction to breathing forms the substance of this chapter. The forms of mechanical interference which disturb the mechanics of breathing (e.g., hanging, strangulation, smothering, choking, traumatic asphyxia) are grouped together. Death from cerebral anoxia resulting from mechanical obstruction of the neck arteries (e.g., manual strangulation and hanging, and vagal inhibition due to pressure on the neck) is also included here.

SCENE INVESTIGATION

The study of the circumstances of an asphyxial death and the findings at the scene of death can contribute considerably to the overall value of the investigation. Many questions may remain unanswered if the scene of death is not visited. In determining the questions concerning the cause, manner and time of death, the scene examination can be invaluable. Of particular importance is the opportunity to collect materials of value in the reconstruction of the case.

Cause of Death

In the majority of deaths from asphyxia the cause of death is obvious. Nevertheless, there are times when diligent effort is required at the scene of death to find the cause of the fatality. In most cases asphyxial changes are obvious at the autopsy, but in some the changes may be minimal or totally absent. No asphyxial changes may be found in the body of a baby dying of smothering or accidental strangulation in the crib (cot), in an adult dying of suffocation by being covered with sand or coal dust or in a victim of plastic bag asphyxia. In all such cases the investigator will have to rely heavily on the findings of the scene examination. The conclusion of death from vagal inhibition can be drawn in a case in which the autopsy is negative only with the full knowledge that can be best acquired at the scene of death. Additional findings at the scene such as disarray of the

131

furniture and of the decendent's clothing, evidence of robbery and indications of sexual assault may lend corroborative evidence to the suspicions of asphyxial death.

Manner of Death

The scene investigation frequently provides immediate clues to the question of the manner of death (Fig. 9-1). An asphyxial death may be natural, as from aspiration of vomitus during an epileptic seizure, or it may be accidental, homicidal or suicidal. The scene investigation reveals differentiating features and these are discussed at appropriate places in this chapter. In some instances it may be nearly impossible to draw any conclusions regarding the manner of death without visiting the scene or securing accurate details of the scene of death.

Time of Death

The scene visit provides the earliest opportunity to examine the body and the earlier it is examined after death the more reliable is the estimation of time of death. The condition of the body, rigor, livor and especially the rectal temperature readings provide more dependable estimates of the time of death during the first few hours after death. Therefore, if homicide is suspected, one of the important purposes of a scene investigation is the recording of the rectal temperature to determine the time of death. Belated efforts to make the estimates in the autopsy room will be less accurate.

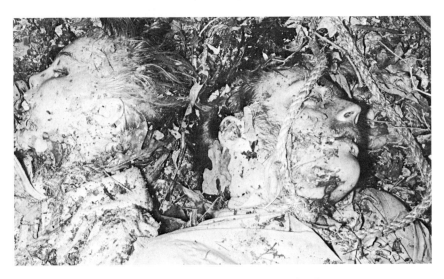

Fig. 9–1. A double murder. Strangulation by rope.

Collection of Evidence

A pathologist at the scene of death can do much more than just determine the cause and manner of death. In any medicolegal investigation the preservation of evidence and collection of articles that are likely to be important in the interpretation of the findings and in the reconstruction of the case are vital.

If a person is found strangled or hanging, the nature of the ligature knot frequently gives a clue to the manner of death. Sometimes thoughtless cutting of the ligature destroys the pattern of the knot or knots and the interpretation of the case is rendered more difficult. The medical investigator can prevent such a disturbance of evidence at the scene. To release the body, the ligature should always be cut away from the knots. Such a precaution allows the pathologist to make a detailed examination of the ligature in situ in the autopsy room and draw more reliable conclusions.

Trace evidence left by the assailant on the body of a victim of asphyxia should be carefully collected at the scene. Foreign hairs, fibers of clothing and blood spots can later help identify the assailant. Such pieces of evidence, if not collected at the scene, can easily be displaced or lost during the transportation of the body. A victim struggling to defend himself always attempts to use the hands unless they are tied. Sometimes telltale evidence may be found on the hands and under the nails of the victim. Nail scrapings may reveal the assailant's body tissue such as epidermis, and blood, in addition to fibers of clothing. If it is decided not to collect the materials from the hands and fingers at the scene, the hands should be wrapped in plastic bags to prevent such loss of vital information.

Frequently the motive for strangulation of a woman is sexual assault. Therefore, while investigating the death of a woman, if there is the remotest possibility of rape, vaginal secretions should be collected and examined for spermatozoa. There is always a better chance of identifying sperm from the material collected during the early hours after death than from the material collected at a delayed autopsy. The method of examination for the detection of sperm is described in Chapter 22.

GENERAL AUTOPSY FINDINGS

The general postmortem appearance in an asphyxial death is due either to the obstruction of the air passages or to the compression of the neck vessels leading to obstruction to the return of venous blood to the heart, and cerebral anoxia. Most of the outstanding features of asphyxia can be seen on external examination. Internal examination reveals additional features especially in the neck. Examination of the neck organs is the most important component of an autopsy on a case of asphyxia. Neck organs therefore, should be exposed and examined in the method described in Chapter 2. In a case of an asphyxial death, the general changes commonly seen are petechial hemorrhages, congestion, pulmonary edema and cyanosis.

Petechial Hemorrhages

Punctate hemorrhages of capillary origin are a constant feature of most asphyxial deaths. In death resulting from the compression of the neck vessels or of the air passages, the diagnosis of asphyxia should be questioned if such hemorrhages are absent. The mechanism of causation of these hemorrhages is either raised intracapillary pressure or increased capillary permeability due to anoxia. Petechial hemorrhages are commonly seen in the skin, conjunctivae, epiglottis, subglottic region, pleural and pericardial surfaces and in the surfaces of the internal organs.

In the skin, petechial hemorrhages are prominent wherever there is marked capillary congestion. They appear as a scatter of red spots most easily detected in the skin of the eyelids (Fig. 9-2) and forehead. Many hemorrhages may be seen in the scalp. A collection of these spots may also be seen in the skin just above the ligature mark. In a light-skinned person these are easily visible, but a careful examination with a magnifying glass may be necessary to detect them in a person with dark skin.

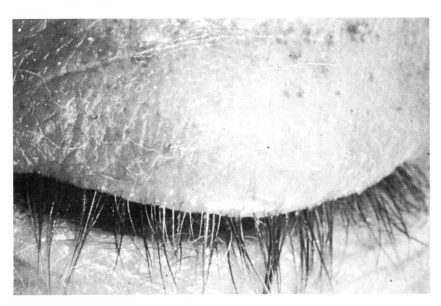

Fig. 9–2. Petechial hemorrhages in the skin of the eyelid. (See Color Plate.)

Petechiae are most easily detected in the conjunctivae where they are most commonly found because the capillaries are loosely supported (Fig. 9-3). They are present both in the palpebral conjunctiva as well as in the bulbar conjunctiva.

On internal examination, one may see a widespread distribution of petechial hemorrhages. They should be looked for in the larnyx, especially in the subglottic region in all asphyxial deaths. Petechial hemorrhages are as constant a finding in the subglottic region as in the conjunctivae, yet this fact does not appear to be amply stressed in textbooks. Punctuate or confluent hemorrhages may also be present in the submucosa of the epiglottis. The undersurface of the scalp and the skin of the forehead are other sites where petechiae are commonly present. The presence of these spots in the surface of the thymus, in the epicardium and in the pleural and pericardial surfaces are not difficult to detect. Careful search may, however, be required to find them in the mucosa of the intestines, under the renal capsules, in the renal pelvis, in the peritoneal lining and in the subarachnoid space on the surface of the brain. Cut surfaces of the internal organs (e.g., brain or thymus) may reveal minute hemorrhages in asphyxial deaths.

The presence of petechial hemorrhages at the sites described above does not necessarily mean that the death was from asphyxia. This fact should be borne in mind while interperting the significance of petechial hemorrhages, because they are frequently associated with many other conditions. For instance, in sudden death from coronary artery disease, the finding of petechiae in the conjunctivae in the skin of the eyelids is not uncommon. Other organic disorders that may be associated with hemorrhages are meningococcemia, blood dyscrasias and bacterial endocarditis. In fact, any natural disease that can cause extreme congestion will produce petechiae. Aspiration of regurgitated material may also be accompanied by petechiae.

Occasionally, positional hemorrhages appear postmortem; after death gravitational accumulation of blood in dependent parts may cause petechial hemorrhages. These, if present in the conjunctivae and larynx, may mislead the examiner. The knowledge of the circumstances of death and the consideration of the possibility of artefactual production of hemorrhages after death can help make a correct interpretation.

It must also be stressed that in some asphyxial deaths there may not be any petechial hemorrhages. In death from drowning, for instance, petechial hemorrhages are rarely seen. According to Polson[11] they "are frequently absent in hanging, especially when the body is completely or almost completely suspended." In death from suffocation by plastic bag, no petechial hemorrhages may be seen at all the sites described above.[2]

A 75-year-old man who has been depressed was found dead in bed at his home. He had committed suicide with a plastic bag wrapped around his head and face and tied around the neck. Autopsy revealed no petechial

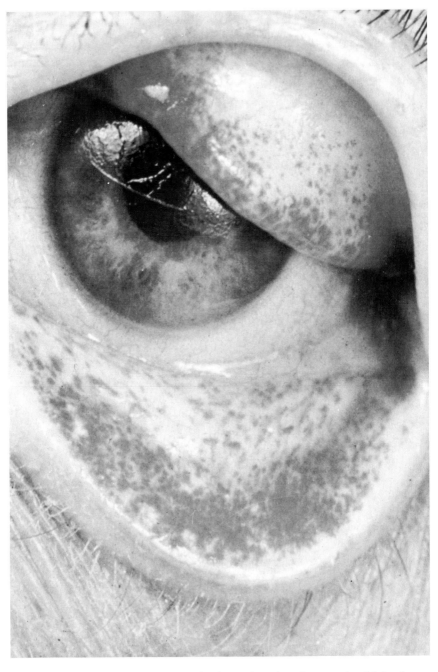

Fig. 9–3. Petechial hemorrhages in the conjunctivae in an asphyxial death. (See Color Plate.)

hemorrhages in the skin or conjunctivae. A few petechiae were present in the subglottic region. No significant natural disease or injury was found.

Congestion

In every asphyxial death there is some degree of congestion of the tissues. This may be visible in the skin of the face above the ligature, the face appearing purple and slightly swollen. Congestion of the blood vessels in the eyes is obvious and in the nasal septum or eardrums it may be so intense that hemorrhages may be caused from rupture of the engorged vessels. Of particular significance is congestion of the skin just above the ligature mark, for this indicates that the ligature was applied when the person was alive. On internal examination, the visceral organs, particularly the lungs, show congestion. Pulmonary hemorrhages also may be caused by rupture of the intensely congested capillaries. Associated with pulmonary congestion, there is usually dilatation of the right chambers of the heart.

The finding of congestion is just an additional postmortem finding in support of other evidence of asphyxia. Because congestion of the type seen in asphyxial deaths can be caused by a variety of conditions, it should be carefully interpreted.

Pulmonary Edema

No great significance can be attached to the presence of pulmonary edema in making the diagnosis of asphyxia, since it is also a common finding in deaths from poisoning, organic disease or trauma. The edema is usually caused by rapid heart failure and its presence indicates struggle for survival for a time.

Cyanosis

Although cyanosis is commonly observed in asphyxial deaths, this too is a nonspecific finding, since it is also observed in a variety of other types of death. If present, it is reflected as bluish lips and nails. The intensity of cyanosis may alter after death; it may disappear from nondependent parts of the body, or conversely, decomposition of the cyanotic areas may accentuate its effect.

STRANGULATION

Strangulation can be defined as asphyxia caused by the constriction of the neck with a ligature when the body is not suspended. Manual strangulation is compression of the neck with the hands.

Strangulation with a ligature may be accidental, suicidal or homicidal. Manual strangulation is often homicidal and rarely suicidal.

Ligature Strangulation

While investigating a death from ligature strangulation the following aspects should be studied: the scene, the ligature, the knot, the ligature mark, the injuries, the signs of asphyxia.

The importance of the *scene* investigation has already been stressed and the precautions to be taken to preserve the evidence noted.

The *ligatures* frequently used are stockings, scarves, neckties, jute ropes, cotton string, electric and telephone cord. Occasionally the victim's clothing or necklace may be used. If an unusual type of ligature is used, the identification of the source of the ligature may afford a vital clue to the crime. If the ligature suspected to have been used is found away from the body, it may be positively identified with the detection of fragments of the decedent's epidermis on it. Additional help may be obtained from a comparison of the pattern of the ligature with the ligature mark on the neck.

In a case of strangulation, the *knot* should be carefully examined before it is undone. Occasionally, the nature of the knot may help determine whether the death was homicidal or suicidal. The presence of two or more tight knots, for instance, should arouse strong suspicion of foul play. If it is desired to preserve the knot, the ligature should be cut away from the knot at the time of postmortem examination and the cut ends identified by wrapping them with labels using gummed tape.

Certain features of the *ligature mark* help differentiate strangulation from hanging. In strangulation cases, the mark on the neck is usually lower than in hanging cases. The strangulation mark, most often, is horizontal, encircling the neck once or more than once. On the other hand, the mark in suicides by hanging is higher, almost always above the thyroid cartilage, and turns upward producing an inverted *V* shaped mark on the side on which ligature reaches the point of suspension. In either type of case, the decedent's clothing may interrupt the mark. In a case of homicidal strangulation, the decedent's fingers may cause an interruption in the mark. If a rough ligature such as jute rope is used it leaves a distinct groove showing the imprints of the strands and of the knot (Fig. 9-4). Soft ligatures may not leave any identifiable external mark. In a majority of strangulation cases the mark is in the form of a groove with a parchmented pale brown base and in some cases petechial hemorrhages may be present in the groove. The lower margin of the mark is usually pale, whereas the upper margin reveals some degree of congestion or the presence of petechial hemorrhages.

External and internal examination of the body will reveal *injuries* which

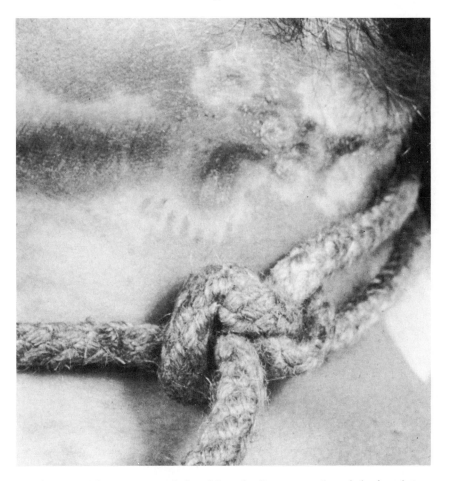

Fig. 9–4. Ligature strangulation. Note the ligature mark and the imprint of the ligature knot.

can throw light on the mode of strangulation. In a homicidal strangulation if there is struggle and the victim is thrown on the back, the body may show such external injuries as abrasions around the elbows and on the shoulder blades as well as bruises at the back of the head. The ligature mark may be associated with abrasions of the skin of the neck and bruising of the subcutaneous tissues. The thyroid cartilage may be fractured and in rare instances the hyoid bone may be broken. If there is a sexual assault, evidence of injuries to the external genitals, tears of the hymen and contusions and lacerations of the vagina may be seen.

The general changes seen in asphyxial deaths are invariably also seen in the cases of strangulation.

Manual Strangulation

Manual strangulation is the more common form of strangulation. A case of manual strangulation must be presumed to be homicidal unless the contrary is proved. The pattern of this form of asphyxia is more or less constant. The victims are usually children or women, and if a woman is manually strangled the motive is frequently sexual assault. In most instances death results from obstruction of the airway; rarely does vagal inhibition cause death.

External appearances vary considerably, depending on the degree of the force used. In some, the evidence of strangulation is clear. In others, the injuries on the neck may be so faint that they can be easily missed if care is not exercised. In dark-skinned individuals, the bruising of the skin of the neck may be missed if the neck is covered with clothing, if the lighting is inadequate or if the neck is not examined. If the investigation is not approached with an open mind, miscarriage of justice may result.

> A middle-aged woman was found dead in bed at her home. Examination of the body at the place of death revealed no suspicious circumstances and no marks of violence. There was no history of medical ailment. An autopsy was performed to determine the cause of death. On external examination the only injury seen was a small, faint bruise on the neck. Internal examination showed massive contusions of the neck structures and a fracture of the hyoid bone.

> In another case, an 84-year-old woman was found dead at home dressed in underclothes. After "examining" the body at the scene, the medical examiner considered the death natural. He sent the body to the autopsy room where he was to draw blood for a routine check for alcohol. While the body was in the postmortem room, a senior forensic pathologist noticed obvious injuries on the neck (Fig. 9-5). The autopsy revealed clear evidence of manual strangulation and it resulted in the arrest and conviction of the assailant.

In manual strangulation, the *external injuries* on the neck are of two types—abrasions caused by fingernails and bruises caused by finger pads. Abrasions caused by fingernails are sometimes the characteristic crescent shape of the curvature of the assailant's fingernails. In a majority of the cases, however, the nail injuries are indefinite scratches or grazes associated with slight contusion of the margins of the injuries. Occasionally, the nails cause distinct small purplish or bluish bruises, the bruise being a little larger than the area of the tip of the finger causing it. The sites of the injuries caused by the nails and the finger pads depend on whether one or two hands were used by the assailant and whether the assailant was right- or left-handed. If only one hand was used by a right-handed assailant from the front of the victim, the thumb would cause abrasion and contusion of the skin in the region of the upper end of the right side of the neck. The

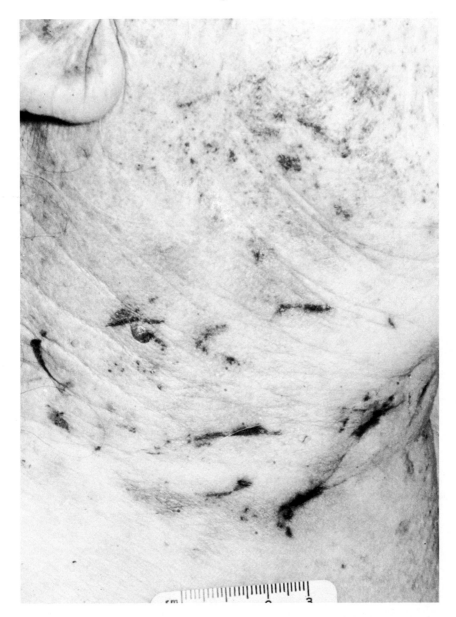

Fig. 9–5. Abrasions, contusions and lacerations on the neck in a case of manual strangulation. (Courtesy of Page Hudson, M.D.)

assailant's four fingers would cause corresponding injuries down the left side of the neck beginning approximately at the tip of the hyoid bone. If two hands were used from the front of the victim, the thumbs would cause injuries in the midline and the fingers on either side of the neck. With a two-handed grip from the back, the fingers would cause damage in the front and the thumbs in the posterior aspects of the victim's neck. The significance of fingernail abrasions has been well discussed by Shapiro and his associates.[12]

Careful note of injuries on other parts of the body and of the signs of asphyxia should be made. Injuries caused during struggle also may be present such as abrasions and contusions on the face, arms, back and, in female victims, on the breasts. With sexual assault, injuries to the genital organs may be present. Injuries may be due to intercourse or to attempts by the assailant to introduce a foreign object into the vagina. In the following example such injuries were present:

> A 67-year-old obese woman who lived alone was found dead on her apartment floor fully dressed. She was known to have had heart trouble. Examination of the body at the scene of death revealed nothing spectacular until the body was turned to examine the back. There was a pool of blood under the buttocks. Her underpants were torn and pulled down. At autopsy a one-inch long laceration in the vagina was found to be the source of the hemorrhage. Faint bruises were seen on the neck and dissection of the neck structures showed extensive contusions of the soft tissues and fractures of the thyroid cartilage.

On *internal examination,* as a rule there is marked bruising of the soft tissues of the neck. Fresh hemorrhages will be obvious in the subcutaneous tissues, fascia and the muscles. The strap muscles, especially the sternomastoids, may show laceration in addition to contusions. Bruising of the soft tissues is pronounced on the front of the neck, whereas hemorrhages are minimal in the back tissues. Fractures of the hyoid bone and thyroid cartilage are common but by no means always present in the cases of manual strangulation. They are seen with a greater frequency in the elderly, in whom calcification of these structures predisposes them to easier fracturing. In younger persons these structures are elastic and not easily broken. The superior horn of the thyroid cartilage is the most vulnerable part. With grips higher up in the neck the horns of the hyoid bone fracture. Fractures of the hyoid bone, thyroid cartilage and the cricoid cartilage indicate considerable pressure on these structures. At the autopsy the best guide to the detection of any of these fractures is the presence of recent hemorrhage in the soft tissues around the sites of the fractures.

While examining the neck structures, antemorten injuries should be carefully evaluated. Artefactual postmorten hemorrhages can mislead the pathologist.[3, 4] Therefore, each structure should be dissected individually and in situ photographs of the injuries taken as the tissues are removed layer by layer.

Other internal injuries in the cases of manual strangulation may be bruising of the tongue, pharnyx, larynx and the salivary glands. Injury to the trachea is rare.

Changes common to asphyxial deaths are also present in cases of manual strangulation.

Accidental Strangulation

Death from accidental strangulation can occur in a variety of ways. It is important to correctly determine the manner of death, since an attempt may be made to conceal a homicide by making it look like an accident, or the defense of accident may be raised during a trial for homicide by strangulation.

Accidental strangulations are not uncommon in infants. The body of a child may slide between the side bars of a crib (cot) and the neck may be compressed by one of the bars should the head not pass between them. Occasionally, an infant is strangled with a string attached to a toy tied to the crib. Strangulation can also occur with the tightening of the umbilical cord around the neck of the fetus in utero.

In adults, accidental strangulation may occur while the person is under the influence of drugs or alcohol. Asphyxiation may result from the necktie or if the intoxicated person rests the neck against a bar or other hard object. In industry, belts, ropes or parts of clothing may be caught in the rollers or other parts of the moving machinery and cause accidental strangulation.

Suicidal Strangulation

This is an uncommon event and can cause considerable difficulty in determining the manner of death. All the facts of the case including the background of the victim should be considered with the autopsy findings. The nature of the ligature knot and the general scene assist in formulating the conclusions. The suicide may pass the ligature around the neck several times and then tie the free ends with a single knot. Some suicides pass the ligature around the neck and tighten it by twisting a stick or rod tied to it or passed under it. The victim may also pass a ligature around the neck and pull it with a hand. In order to do this the ligature may be passed around the hand once or twice. These variations have been described in detail by Polson.[11] The materials used by the suicides also vary—ropes, scarves, clothing fabric, rubber tubes, electric and telephone cords. The ligature mark in the cases of self-strangulation is horizontal and not rising on one side of the neck, as in hanging. Invariably the ligature is tied around the upper half of the neck at about the level of the larynx. Scattered reports of suicidal strangulation can be found in the literature.[13] For information on a series of 26 cases of suicidal strangulation, the reader is referred to the works of Wiedmann and Spengler.[17] Suicide by manual strangulation is considered impossible.

Strangulation and Vagal Inhibition

An attempt at squeezing the neck or strangling may result in sudden death from reflex cardiac arrest. Such a death reveals no evidence of asphyxia and there are no injuries of the neck tissues. With the history of some pressure on the neck and negative autopsy, the possibility of vagal inhibition should be strongly considered. Such a situation raises an important medicolegal question of whether the death is accidental or homicidal. In a case cited by Polson,[11] a man, while dancing, squeezed the neck of his partner either playfully or erotically. The woman went limp and suddenly died. The man was charged with murder but acquitted. In another instance, a man squeezed his wife's neck while they were having sex relations. She died instantly. The husband was acquitted of her murder.

HANGING

Hanging is death from asphyxia caused by constriction of the neck as a result of suspension of the body with a ligature.

In hanging, death usually results from the obstruction of the air passages as well as of the arteries and veins. The airway obstruction depends on the degree of suspension and the type of ligature. Obstruction of the vessels on both sides occurs if the ligature passes completely around the neck at least once. Occasionally, the vessels on the side of the neck along which the ligature rises are only partially obstructed. In judicial hangings, if there is a drop, fracture of the spine and injury to the spinal cord occur and cause death.

A majority of the deaths from hanging are suicidal.[9] However, in recent years there has been an increase in accidental hangings in persons involved in auto-erotic activities. The increase perhaps is not real but merely a reflection of proper recognition of these deaths as being accidental.

Suicidal Hanging

The important aspects of a case of hanging are the scene of the death, ligature, external appearance and internal injuries.

The *scene* may reveal features of suicide-privacy, suicide note and so on. Relatives or friends of the decedent at the scene may provide background information such as marital, social or financial problems; history of depression and of previous suicide attempts. At the scene it is possible to study various details about the type of ligature, point of suspension, the platform used to gain height to hang without touching the ground and so on.

The *ligatures* commonly used by suicides are strings, ropes and portions of clothing. The victim in Figure 9-6 used rubber hose. In a jail the commonly used ligature is a belt, since nothing else is available. The ligature is usually applied in a simple loop. Some victims may be found with multiple ligature turns around the neck. The ligature is invariably above the level of thyroid cartilage and the knot, most frequently, is on one side of the neck. When the ligature rises on one side of the neck to the point of suspension, the head is turned slightly away from the rising part of the ligature. This causes maximal pressure of the ligature on the side opposite the rising part of the ligature or the knot.

External appearances in a case of suicidal hanging are significantly different from those seen in strangulation. The ligature mark is high in the neck, invariably above the thyroid cartilage. The mark has a light-brown parchmented base and pale margins. The ligature groove is deepest at the site of maximal pressure, usually opposite the knot or the rising parts of the mark. The margins or the base of the groove may reveal the pattern of the material used. The arms of the ligature rising to the point of suspension impart an inverted *V*-shaped mark and the arms of the mark taper off at their highest points. The above features of the mark and the absence of any obvious vital changes often give an erroneous impression that the mark was caused after death. As in strangulation, a soft ligature may not leave any mark at all.

Other external appearances in a hanging case are pallor of the face,

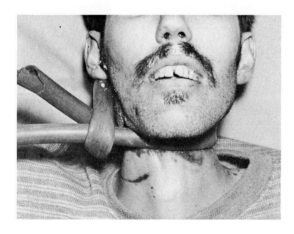

Fig. 9–6. A suicidal hanging by means of a rubber hose.

excessive salivation, and in males evidence of discharge of prostatic secretions. The mouth is partially open and the swollen tongue frequently pro-
trudes between the lips.

The important negative finding in some cases, is the absence of petechial
hemorrhages in the skin and conjunctivae.

Internal injuries are strikingly absent. Immediately beneath the ligature
mark the skin is pale, and bruising of the subcutaneous tissues is rarely
seen. With a gradual hanging, injuries to the soft tissues are minimal. If,
however, there is a rapid jerk or if there is a drop of the body, bruising of
the tissues and laceration of the sternomastoid muscles may be present.
Due to the pull of the tissues, the muscles may be torn and the cartoid
arteries injured.

The cartilaginous and bony structures also seldom show injuries. According to Smith and Fiddes[15] the "hyoid bone is practically never injured"
in hanging. Ganapathi[7] studied 152 cases of suicidal hanging by carefully
removing the hyoid bone in each case and x-raying it. In none of his cases
was the hyoid bone found to be fractured. Injuries of the thyroid cartilage
and the larynx are also not common. The likelihood of the injuries of the
bony and cartilaginous structures is greater in elderly persons in whom
these structures are calcified. Fracture of the spine with damage to the
spinal cord and medulla sometimes occurs in the subjects of judicial hanging.

Accidental Hanging

One of the most interesting groups of cases in medicolegal practice
is that of death from auto-erotic activity. These are cases of hanging, occurring during the course of abnormal sexual practices. The principal consideration in the investigation of a death from sexual asphyxia is the proper
certification of the manner of death. Most of the cases are typical and easy
to identify. A pathologist who sees a case once, or is made aware of the
general features of such cases, is unlikely to have any difficulty in interpreting the cause and manner of death because certain aspects are common to most of these cases.

Hanging resulting from the activities of sexual deviation almost always
involves males in the age group of 15 to 25 years. The body of the victim
is either nude or partially dressed, with the genital organs exposed (Fig.
1-1). The man or the boy may be attired in female garments; a brassiere
with false pads, female underpants and even sanitary pads are frequently
used. An important characteristic finding is the presence of some sort of
fabric, such as a scarf, handkerchief or towel, interposed between the skin
and the rope. Photographs of nude females and obscene literature are frequently found at the scene. Some of the minor variations include tying of

the body in an unusual fashion, bandaging of the genitalia and fastening of the wrists. Some use mirrors to observe their own activities and they may be found at the scene of death.

This deviation is not well understood. It may be just an unusual method of masturbation. Males involved in such activities usually reveal a background of "normal" sexual life and no psychiatric illness. They choose a site such as a bedroom, bathroom, attic or wooded area for secrecy. There may be evidence on the neck of previous episodes of similar activity such as old scars or grooves. Repetition of such activity indicates that the purpose of the ligature is not to commit suicide.[6] The purpose of placing fabric between the skin and the rope is to prevent ligature marks on the neck.

A degree of asphyxia causes sexual stimulation. However, when the man or boy is in a state of orgasm and the asphyxiation is accentuated, he loses control over the circumstances and is hanged. This, therefore, is an accidental death and the medical examiner or pathologist should not hesitate to label such a death as accidental. Proper recognition of these cases is important for various reasons.[10] The case may be treated as a murder with unnecessary waste of investigational time and effort. If it is misinterpreted as a suicide, the family faces its stigma and is deprived of the benefits of a double indemnity insurance policy the decedent may have had.

Though accidental asphyxiation during aberrant sexual activity in the male is common, such a death in females is extremely rare. Henry,[8] who found no instances of sexual asphyxiation in females in the forensic literature, has reported an "authentic" case of a female victim.

> A 19-year-old white female was found dead in her bedroom, hanging from the hinge of a closet door. She was dressed in the attire of an Oriental "harem girl." A towel was wound round her head and a window sash-cord was wound around the body in a complicated fashion. The cord was passed around the breasts in a "figure of eight" fashion and then down between the labia majora. A blindfold and mouth gag made from a housecoat belt was passed across the eyes, behind the neck, then back across the mouth and again to the back of the neck (Fig. 9-7).
>
> An "underground" magazine and a paperback Alfred Hitchcock book found at the scene explained the fantasy. The center fold-out of the magazine showed a bizarre dance involving a clock. A nude male figure was bound to the hour arm of the clock and a nude female figure was bound to the minute hand. A verse on the fold-out showed how the two clock hands would move and the two figures would perform the sex act at the stroke of the hour. The paperback contained a story (which had been read so many times the papers were loose) about an Oriental harem. In the story the harem master provided girls to his lord and after the girls were "used" they were "stored" by hanging them around the walls on hooks.

Sexual deviation may take other forms. The victims may inhale coal gas, anesthetic gases or other gases such as carbon tetrachloride. Some merely

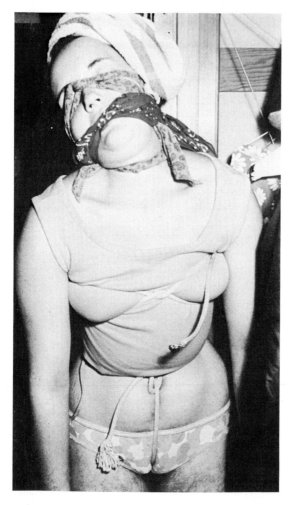

Fig. 9–7. A "sex" hanging in a female. (Courtesy of R. C. Henry, M.D.)

suffocate themselves in plastic bags which they use to produce asphyxia and consequent sexual stimulation.

Accidental hangings may occur under circumstances similar to those causing accidental strangulation; these have already been noted.

Homicidal Hanging

This is extremely rare. Only a few cases are recorded in the literature. An adult may be able to kill an infant or an intoxicated individual this way. During the investigation of a death at the place the body is found hanging, the possibility of a staged suicide after the victim is killed should be borne in mind. A thorough autopsy will settle the issue satisfactorily.

SUFFOCATION

Suffocation is asphyxia caused by all means other than constriction of the neck by hands or ligature. Various forms of asphyxia from suffocation are smothering, choking, overlaying and traumatic.

Suffocation may be accidental and homicidal but rarely suicidal.

In all forms of suffocation the general asphyxial changes are pronounced. The exceptions are noted in the following discussion.

Smothering

In smothering, the obstruction of the nose and mouth causes asphyxia.

Accidental smothering is possible in infants during the first few weeks after birth. This may occur if the infant's face is buried in a soft pollow or if heavy bedclothes and plastic materials cover the face. Before the diagnosis of smothering is given in such cases, the possibility of natural death must be ruled out. In adults, accidental smothering may occur during perverse sexual activity, during an epileptic seizure or when the person is under the influence of drink or drugs. In the following instance from England death was ruled at the coroner's inquest as from "misadventure."

> A 25-year-old healthy unmarried man living a happy life and having no obvious sexual disturbances, was found dead in his bedroom. He was lying face down. A thin polythene bag held in position by motorcycle goggles covered the face. The man was dressed in motorcycle-overalls and had on a new helmet and Wellington Boots. He also wore polythene gloves which were covered by motorcycle gloves. The motorcycle suit and the helmet had been acquired recently. The autopsy showed signs of asphyxia.[5]

It has been pointed out earlier that in some cases of suffocation the use of a plastic bag, typical asphyxial changes may not be seen. Accidental smothering occasionally may occur at work from being covered with sand, coal dust and grain. Such accidents involving middle-aged or elderly persons with some history of medical problems, and showing total absence of typical autopsy findings of asphyxia, can create diagnostic challenges.

> A middle-aged man was working at a sand quarry when he apparently slid down a height and was completely covered with sand. The autopsy revealed a moderately severe degree of coronary artery disease. There were no petechial hemorrhages in the skin or conjunctivae. A little sand was found in the pharynx, larynx and the trachea. Death was considered accidental.

The investigation of a case of *homicidal smothering* can be extremely difficult. Though the autopsy may reveal signs of asphyxia, there may not be any corroborative medical evidence to prove that death was the outcome of foul play.

Infanticide can easily be committed by smothering. If a soft object such as a pillow is placed on the face to obstruct breathing, the existence of the signs of asphyxia alone may not help to establish the commission of crime. An adult in poor health or one who is incapacitated from the effects of drugs or drink can similarly be killed.

Occasionally, the assailant uses his hands to suffocate the victim. Pressure on the nose and the mouth may be associated with asphyxial changes and localized injuries. There may be abrasions on the face caused by the assailant's nails. The nose may be broken and the lips and gums show bruising and laceration (Fig. 9-8). If there was a struggle, other parts of the body may show injuries.

Suicide by smothering is rare. Reported cases indicate that they occur mainly in prisoners and mental patients. Taylor[16] has described an unusual suicide by smothering.

> A man was found dead lying on his face in a prison cell. His nostrils and mouth were stuffed with pieces of cloth held in position by a handkerchief which was tied around his mouth.

Choking

This is a form of asphyxia in which the obstructing material is within the air passages—the larynx, trachea or bronchi. Choking is mainly accidental. Accidents in children follow the inhalation of candies, chewing gum, buttons and so on.[1] The elderly may choke on food or partial dentures. (Fig. 9-9). Cases of choking on food are described in Chapter 18. One of the commonest forms of choking is the inhalation of regurgitated material. A finding of aspirated material in the air passages should be cautiously interperted for this could merely be a result of terminal aspiration and not a true cause of death.[4]

Overlaying

A death may be caused by overlaying when an infant sleeps with a parent. The accident is more likely if the parent is intoxicated. In a case of homicidal suffocation the defense of death from overlaying may be advanced.

Traumatic Asphyxia

Compression of the chest by a heavy weight causes traumatic asphyxia. The most common cause of traumatic asphyxia in day-to-day practice of Forensic Pathology is the running over of a victim by an automobile. Mass

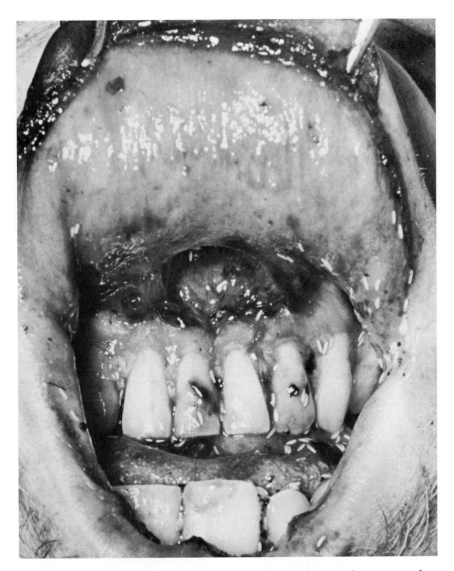

Fig. 9–8. Bruising and laceration of the lips and gums in a case of smothering.

casualties from traumatic asphyxia occur in human stampedes,[14] in coal mines and in building collapse.

Autopsy appearances in the cases of traumatic asphyxia are fairly typical. The head, neck and upper part of the chest are a dark purple color due to intense cyanosis. This hue is frequently associated with hemorrhages in the skin of the eyelids and in the conjunctivae. Confluent hemorrhages

Asphyxial Deaths

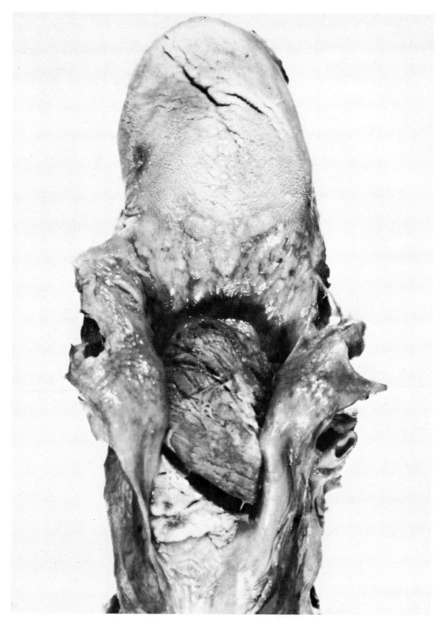

Fig. 9–9. Choking on food. A large piece of unchewed meat plugged the larynx.

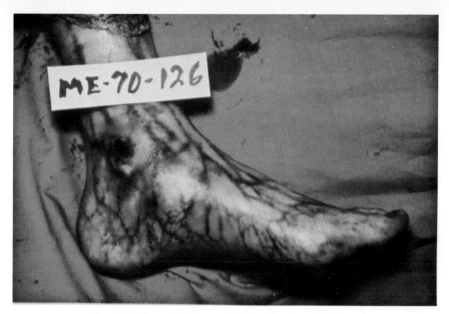

Fig. 3-2. Distended foot veins in a decomposing body.

Fig. 3-4. Skin slippage in a decomposing body.

Fig. 6-2. A patterned bruise caused by a tire.

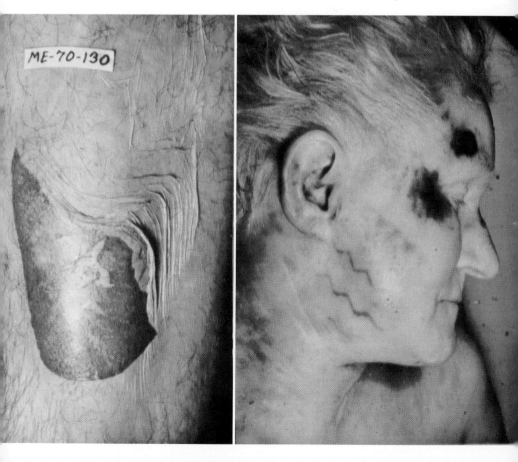

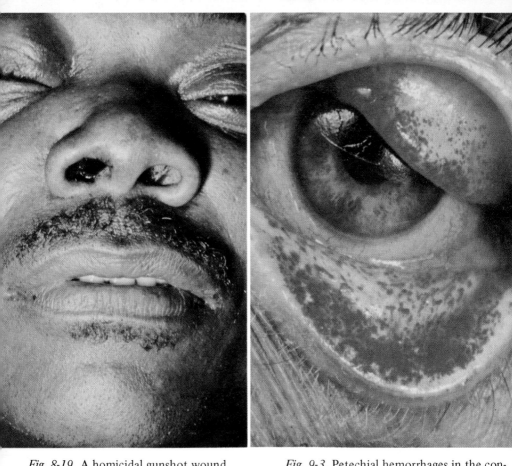

Fig. 8-19. A homicidal gunshot wound in the nostril.

Fig. 9-3. Petechial hemorrhages in the conjunctivae in an asphyxial death.

Fig. 9-2. Petechial hemorrhages in the skin of the eyelid.

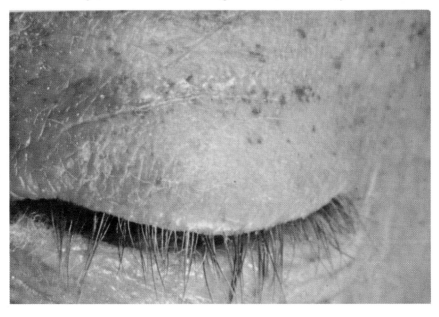

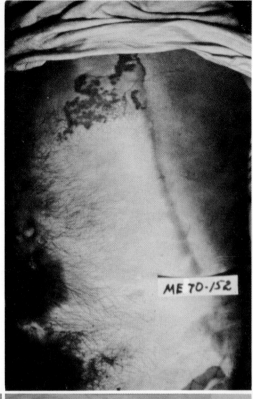

Fig. 11-1. (Top) The line of vital reaction at the junction of burned and unburned areas of the skin. This reaction is indicative of antemortem origin of burns.

Fig. 11-5. (Bottom Left) An extradural hemorrhage caused by burns after death.

Fig. 11-6. (Bottom Right) A typical electrical burn.

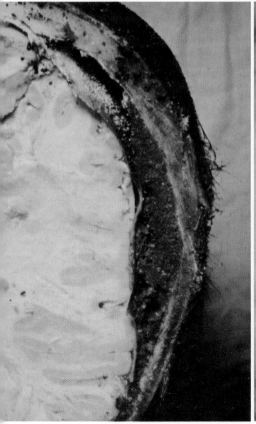

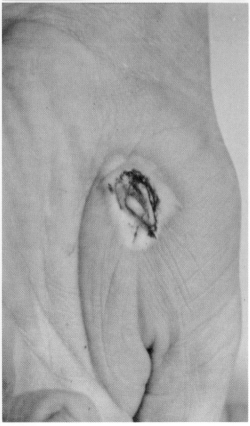

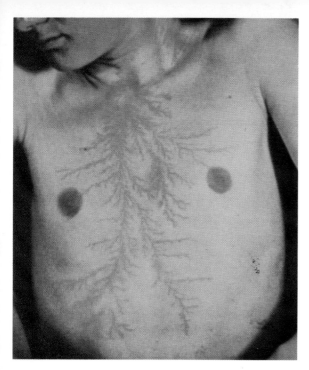

Fig. 11-8. (Top) Lightning stroke. Arborescent markings of the skin.

Fig. 17-5. (Bottom) A pseudo-strangulation mark on the neck was caused by a shirt collar.

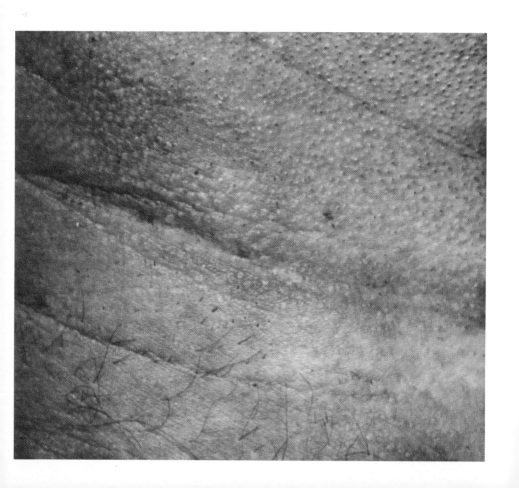

are often present in the skin on the neck and on the chest. The chest below the level of purple coloration is pale, although there is generalized cyanosis, more marked in the upper extremities.

REFERENCES

1. Blumberg, J. M., and Johnston, E. H.: The forensic pathologist and the unsuspected foreign body. J. Forensic Sci., *8:*231, 1963.
2. Camps, F. E., and Hunt, A. C.: Plastic-bag suicide. Brit. Med. J., *1:*378, 1962.
3. Camps, F. E., and Hunt, A. C.: Pressure on the neck. J. Forensic Med., *6:*116, 1959.
4. Fatteh, A.: Artefacts in forensic pathology. *In* Wecht, C. (ed.): Legal Medicine Annual, 1972. Appleton-Century-Crofts, New York, 1972.
5. Fatteh, A.: Plastic bag fatality. Brit. Med. J., *1:*875, 1962.
6. Ford, R.: Death by hanging of adolescent and young adult males. J. Forensic Sci., *2:*171, 1957.
7. Ganapathi, M. N.: Personal communication, 1967.
8. Henry, R. C.: "Sex" hangings in the female. Medico-Legal Bull. No. 214, Office of the Chief Medical Examiner, Richmond, 1971.
9. Luke, J. L.: Asphyxial deaths by hanging in New York City, 1964–1965. J. Forensic Sci., *12:*359, 1967.
10. Mann, G. T.: Accidental strangulation during perverse sexual activity. J. Forensic Sci., *5:*169, 1960.
11. Polson, C. J.: The Essentials of Forensic Medicine. Springfield (Ill.), Charles C Thomas, 1965.
12. Shapiro, H. A., Gluckman, J. and Gordon, I.: The significance of finger nail abrasions of the skin. J. Forensic Med., *9:*17, 1962.
13. Simpson, C. K.: Strangling-Murder or Suicide. Int. Crim. Pol. Rev., *138:*137, 1960.
14. Simpson, C. K.: Mass asphyxia. Lancet. *2:*309, 1943.
15. Smith, Sir S. and Fiddes, F. S.: Forensic Medicine. ed. 10. London, J. & A. Churchill, 1955.
16. Taylor, A. S.: Principles and Practice of Medical Jurisprudence, ed. 11, vol. 1, p. 468. Smith, S. and Simpson, K. (eds.). London, J. & A. Churchill, 1956.
17. Wiedmann, W., and Spengler, H.: Der Selbstmord durch Erdrosseln und Seine Unterscheidung vom Mord. Arch. Criminol., *117:*29, 75, 145, 1956.

10

The Diagnosis of Drowning

Death from drowning is common. In Eastern and Far Eastern countries drowning is one of the popular methods of committing suicide. In the Western world death from drowning is predominantly accidental. Homicide by drowning is distinctly rare in adults, but infanticide by drowning is not uncommon.

If the circumstances of death are known, the diagnosis of drowning will not present any difficulty. However, when a body is found in water and no circumstantial details are available of how it got there, the case may pose a difficult problem. In some cases, the diagnosis of drowning cannot be established for lack of definite signs; hence one has to draw conclusions on the basis of the exclusion of other causes of death. In such situations every detail of the case must be considered with an open mind.

When a dead body is found in water, the investigating pathologist is expected to answer the following common questions:

1. Did death occur prior to entry in the water? If so, what was the cause of death?
2. Did drowning cause death? If so, was it fresh water or salt water drowning?
3. Were there any antemortem injuries? If so, did they play any part in the death?
4. Was there any natural disease or any evidence of poisoning? If so, did the finding contribute to death in any way?
5. What was the manner of death?

A careful investigation of the circumstances of death, examination of the scene and a thorough postmorten examination of the body provide answers to these questions. If the body is decomposed, the medical investigator will have the additional responsibility of establishing the identity of the decedent.

INVESTIGATION OF CIRCUMSTANCES OF DEATH AND EXAMINATION OF THE SCENE

Fatalities from drowning occur in seas, rivers, lakes, swimming pools, ditches, puddles, and even in bathtubs or toilets.

Accidental drowning deaths, involving all ages, can result from boating and bathing accidents (e.g., falls because of old age, disease or intoxication and accidents involving children who cannot swim take many lives). In most of the accidents, the circumstances are clear.

If the accident is not witnessed, findings at the scene of death may give an indication of the nature of death. A person falling into the water accidentally may be fully dressed. Those unclothed or with only a swim suit on are also likely to be victims of accident. Trivial injuries on the body may be present especially on the arms caused by a fall or an attempt to grasp an object. These should be properly identified as accidental in origin. If the body is recovered from navigable waters, extensive trauma may be present from being hit by a moving vessel or its moving parts (especially propellers) and from being bitten by marine life. At the scene of death, marks of slipping should be looked for.

A fatal accident in the bathtub is frequently associated with an epileptic attack, an episode of acute coronary insufficiency and alcohol or drug intoxication. In such a death also minor injuries from a fall may be present. The body should be examined for injection marks and electrical burns. Past medical history of the decedent must be reviewed.

The scene investigation may reveal distinct evidence of *suicide.* The person intending to commit suicide may remove some of his clothes before he enters the water. He would remove a hat, overcoat and gloves, for instance, before he jumps into the water; these articles are usually found neatly piled up at the scene. Background information or the finding of a suicide note would confirm the intent. A suicide may tie his hands or feet to make sure that he does not survive with a last moment change of mind, and occasionally victims tie heavy weights around the body to ensure drowning. With such findings, however, the possibility of homicide must be ruled out before rendering the verdict of suicide. Suicide by jumping into the water from a bridge is not uncommon. In the absence of any clues at the scene, the personal history of the decedent will help establish the manner of death. Suicide in the bathtub is rare but when it does occur the features indicating the intent are usually obvious. Death can occur in just a few inches of water.

An attempt may be made to conceal a *crime* by dropping a dead body into the water. In such cases and in cases of infanticide in which the body is disposed of in water, only a thorough autopsy can detect the true cause of death, provided, of course, that the body is not decomposed. Obvious contusions and significant antemortem injuries must arouse suspicion of foul play. Unless the circumstances of death in a case of drowning are clear enough to point to the precise cause and manner of death, an autopsy is indicated. If the circumstances of death are bizarre and if the facts of death are simply not known, nothing short of a complete postmortem examination will provide answers to important questions:

The body of a teenage girl was found washed up on a beach. The body was fully clothed lying face up. A considerable amount of foam was present in the mouth and nose. A few scratches were present on the face. A routine autopsy revealed a gunshot wound in the back of the head. The principal cause of death was drowning. The presence of the gunshot wound led to extensive investigation and arrest of the girl's boyfriend who confessed to shooting her.

While dealing with a dead body in a bathtub the possibility of homicide must be excluded. The presence of needle puncture marks may give an idea about the manner of death (Regina vs. Barlow, Leads Assizes, England, 1957).

Personal effects on the body should be left undisturbed at the scene of death, since these may prove valuable in establishing the identity of the decedent. Before leaving the scene of death, a sample of the water in which the decedent was found should be collected so that a comparison may be made of diatoms in the body with those in the water.

EXTERNAL EXAMINATION

None of the external appearances on the body is diagnostic of drowning. There may be signs, however, that lend support to such a diagnosis. Changes in bodies found in water are of two types—those caused by contact with water and those caused by inhalation of water.

By merely being in water the body will be cold and wet. In a floating body, livor is pronounced in the head, neck and chest areas, since these parts are lower in the water. Livor is usually pink. The skin of the palms and soles becomes sodden, bleached and wrinkled. Gooseflesh or cutis anserina is frequently present.

Vital signs associated with inhalation of water during life should be considered as true signs in support of the diagnosis of drowning. One of the most important of these signs is the presence of persistent tenacious foam in the mouth and nostrils (Fig. 10-1). Although foaming can occur in any condition causing pulmonary edema, in drowning it is usually seen in large quantities. If decomposition has set in or if resuscitative measures have been applied, no foam may be present. The other vital phenomenon is the instantaneous rigor usually affecting the hands which show objects such as grass blades or sand tightly grasped. This, however, is an uncommon event. Although drowning is an asphyxial death, petechial hemorrhages are rarely seen in the skin or the conjunctivae.

In addition to the above signs, other findings of note may be present. Injuries of varying degree may be obvious. In persons jumping into water from a height, serious injuries are not uncommon. Fatalities associated

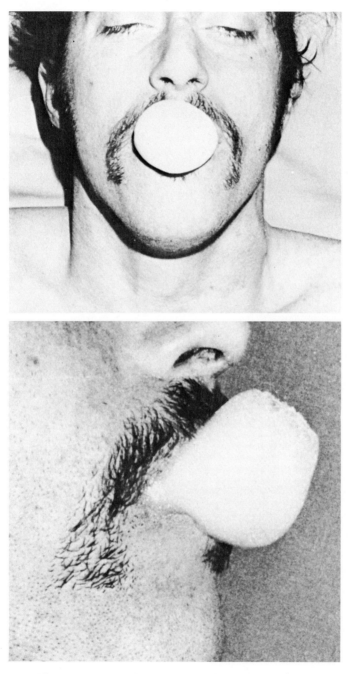

Fig. 10–1. Drowning. Persistent foam at the mouth.

with diving into swimming pools or jumping from high bridges frequently show injuries. A study of 169 suicides by jumping from the Golden Gate Bridge showed fractured ribs in 85.2 percent of the cases, lacerated lungs in 76 percent and ruptured livers in 53.8 percent of the cases, brain injury occurred in 62 of the 169 cases.[11] It is important to determine whether the injuries are antemortem or postmortem. The significance of antemortem trauma should be carefully assessed to exclude the possibility of homicide.

INTERNAL EXAMINATION

In a body recently recovered from drowning and without any putrefactive changes, perhaps the best guide to the diagnosis of drowning is the appearance of the lungs. Changes in the lungs are usually characteristic and it should be possible not only to make the diagnosis of drowning but also to differentiate saltwater drowning from freshwater drowning. Features that help differentiate the two have not been adequately explained in any of the textbooks.

The lungs in a victim of *freshwater drowning* are large or ballooned but light in weight, and their anterior margins usually overlap in the front of the heart. The lungs are pale pink in color and appear uniformly emphysematous. When they are removed from the chest, they retain their normal shape and tend to maintain an uncollapsed status. When the lungs are sectioned, a crepitus of a kind that is heard while cutting dry emphysematous lungs is easily appreciated. After sectioning, each portion of the lung retains its normal presectioning shape and tends to stand erect. When the cut tissue is compressed between the thumb and the fingers a little froth is squeezed out, and there is no fluid in the tissue unless there is edema. Thus, *the lungs are dry in the cases of freshwater drowning.*

In contrast, in the case of *saltwater drowning* the lungs are large or ballooned but heavy, sometimes weighing over 2000 grams. Because they are voluminous, their anterior margins overlap in the front of the mediastinum. The lungs are purplish or bluish in color with glistening surface. They are soggy and jelly-like in consistency and pit on pressure. When they are removed from the body and placed on a cutting surface, they do not retain their normal shape but tend to flatten out. While sectioning, no crepitus is heard and even without compressing the tissue copious amounts of fluid pour out of the tissue. The sectioned portions do not retain their shape and when squeezed the tissue is found to be filled with fluid in most areas of the lungs. *Thus in the cases of saltwater drowning the lungs are wet and soggy.*

Of course, with the onset of decomposition these changes in the lungs in saltwater and freshwater drowning begin to become obscured. With advanced putrefaction, none of the above signs will be present. The longer the delay in recovering the body after drowning, the poorer are the chances of discerning the evidence of drowning.

The other postmortem finding that supports the diagnosis of drowning is the presence of froth in the air passages. There may also be fluid, grass, weeds or sand in the upper respiratory tract.

A drowning person usually swallows water during the struggle for survival and some amount of water may be found in the stomach.

Inhalation of water causes obstruction of the pulmonary circulation. This results in dilation of the right side of the heart and the great veins.

Hemorrhages are present in the middle ear in about 60 percent of drowning cases. The correlation of this finding with the circumstances of drowning indicates that the hemorrhages result more often when the victim struggles to survive. Similar hemorrhages are also frequently seen in other types of asphyxial deaths.

In addition to the evaluation of the internal injuries, the role of any natural disease condition in the collapse or death of the person found in water should be properly assessed. Adequate microscopic and toxicologic studies must be made. Sections of the lungs from drowning cases show evidence of acute emphysema with rupture of many of the alveoli. The analyses for alcohol should be done routinely. Analyses for drugs that the decedent was known to be using also should be a part of the investigation especially in a bathtub death and in suicide.

OBSCURE CASES

It is possible that there will be no anatomical findings in the body of a drowning victim. If the autopsy is negative, it is most likely that one of the following three factors will explain the lack of positive evidence:

1. Decomposition obscuring the signs of drowning
2. Death from vagal stimulation
3. Death due to laryngeal spasm

Decomposition of the body is a major and frequent obstacle to the diagnosis of drowning. The air passages and lungs are among some of the organs that decompose early. Putrefactive changes affecting the respiratory system rapidly render the findings in cases of drowning equivocal. This makes the consideration of the circumstances of death mandatory.

If death occurs from *vagal stimulation* causing cardiac inhibition, the examination of the body may reveal none of the signs of drowning. When no changes indicative of drowning are present the evidence of trauma, natural disease or intoxication should be searched for. Only after all other possibilities are excluded should the likelihood of cardiac inhibition be considered to explain death. Vagal stimulation may result from a sudden inrush of water in the larynx and nasopharynx or from a blow on the abdomen with a fall into water in a horizontal position. Vagal stimulation is usually associated with instantaneous limping of the body and unconsciousness. These observations lend support to the conclusion of vagal inhibition as a cause of death.

The entry of water into the larynx may cause *laryngeal spasm*. In rare instances the degree and duration of spasm may be such that death results from mechanical asphyxia. Signs of asphyxia such as cyanosis and petechial hemorrhages are present in such cases but there are no signs of drowning, since no water enters the air passages. Other causes of death must be excluded before the diagnosis of laryngeal spasm is given. It must be remembered that no spasm of the larynx is present in dead bodies and the diagnosis has to be based on the circumstantial evidence and exclusion of other explanations of death.

DROWNING IN SKIN AND SCUBA DIVING

It is estimated that in the United States there are approximately eight million skin divers and one million scuba divers (*Time,* Nov. 19, 1965). This sport entails the risk of death; in 1965 there were 26 deaths from drowning from skin diving and 60 from scuba diving in the U.S.[22] Serious accidents are caused by equipment failure, environmental factors or human factors (e.g., exhaustion, panic, preexisting disease) and improper use of equipment.

The signs, symptoms and pathological changes are caused by rapid decompression. The most frequent signs and symptoms of decompression sickness, in order of frequency, are: localized pain, numbness or paresthesiae, muscular weakness, skin rash, dizziness or vertigo, nausea or vomiting, visual disturbances and dyspnea ("chokes").[15]

Fatalities in divers occur from one or more of the pathological findings of air embolism, mediastinal emphysema, subcutaneous emphysema and pneumothorax. As a result of panic, the diver voluntarily holds his breath and this leads to trapping of air in the lungs. Supersaturation of nitrogen during ascent causes it to change from liquid form to gas form. Excessive pressure within the lungs produces tears within the lung tissue and air bubbles enter the blood circulation. In most instances death results from cerebral air embolism.

Any time a diver surfaces unconscious or becomes comatose immediately after surfacing, the most likely cause is air embolism.[21] If death occurs, the signs of air embolism, pneumothorax and emphysema of subcutaneous tissues and mediastinum must be looked for.

SPECIAL INVESTIGATIONS IN DROWNING CASES

In the absence of decomposition it is possible to make the diagnosis of drowning with some degree of certainty. However, when the postmortem findings in a case are equivocal, additional investigations are required. Some of the approaches currently in use are outlined in brief.

Detection of Diatoms

Diatoms are unicellular plants with cell walls made of silica. They are found in all types of salt and fresh water.[11] Diatoms and other plankton elements enter the lungs when a drowning person inhales water (Fig. 10-2). The first approach to making the diagnosis of drowning by the detection of diatoms in the lung tissue was advanced by Revenstorf.[14] Later, Corin and Stockis[1] demonstrated that microscopic particles such as lycopodium, yeast and starch penetrate the lung capillaries and travel from them to the left side of the heart. In view of the works of Mueller and Gorgs,[9] it is now generally accepted that in the case of drowning in water rich in diatoms, a small number of these planktons enter the blood circulation. Some forensic pathologists consider the finding of diatoms in blood and in major internal organs as pathognomonic evidence for the diagnosis of death by drowning. Since diatoms are also found in air and in the tissues of nondrowning individuals,[17] it is important to detect the diatoms in the tissues from a dead body and compare them with the diatoms in the water in which the individual drowned. The finding of similar diatoms in the water and in the body tissues can be regarded as reliable evidence in favor of the diagnosis of drowning.

The significance of the demonstration of diatoms in the cases of drowning has been discussed by several investigators.[7, 10, 19] Details of the methods for the detection of diatoms in bone marrow and in various organs have been described by Thomas and his colleagues[20] and by Porawski.[12] The two methods widely used for the detection of diatoms are: incineration of the material in an electric oven and then dissolving the ashes with nitric acid, and direct digestion of the material with nitric acid and sulphuric acid. A new method which has advantages over other methods is described in Chapter 22. The method makes use of a filtering apparatus with a millipore filter membrane.

Chloride, Sodium, Potassium, Magnesium and Hemoglobin Studies

In 1921 Gettler declared that the determination of chloride in the blood from the heart chambers is a good test for drowning.[6] Many investigators have expressed divergent views on the validity of chloride studies in the

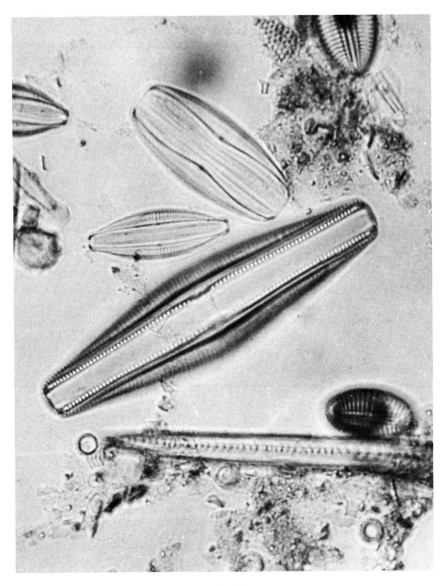

Fig. 10–2. Diatoms.

diagnosis of drowning. Moritz reviewed the subject in 1944 and expressed the view that the differences of chlorides in samples of blood from the right and left ventricles are of diagnostic value only if the analyses are made soon after death. He stated that a difference of 17mEq/L or more of chloride in freshwater drowning can be regarded as presumptive of drowning. A recent study indicates that in freshwater drowning the serum chloride level in blood from the left side of the heart is lower than the chloride level in blood from the right side of the heart.[4] Despite the conclusions of various investigators,[3, 8] in practice, chloride estimations give widely varying results. The diagnosis of drowning cannot and should not be made merely on the basis of chloride studies.

When fresh water enters the lungs, the plasma sodium falls and the potassium rises; with inhalation of seawater plasma sodium rises considerably and the potassium slightly.[18] In freshwater drowning, the serum sodium concentration in blood from the left ventricle is lower than that in blood from the right ventricle.[4] Too much reliance should not be placed on the soduim and potassium studies, since postmortem diffusion of fluid can alter the true levels.

Moritz has stressed the importance of magnesium determination in seawater drowning.[8]

It is recognized that when fresh water is inhaled, it passes from the alveoli into the capillaries leading to hemodilution and hemolysis. On the other hand, inhalation of seawater causes hemoconcentration and hypovolemia. In most cases, postmortem changes affect the reliability of such observations.

Plasma Specific Gravity

A study by Durlacher and his colleagues[2] indicates that in all cases of drowning the specific gravity of plasma from the left side of the heart is less than that of the plasma in the right side of the heart. These investigators found that the reverse was the case in the control cases of nondrowning deaths. They suggest that the determination of the difference of specific gravity of plasma from the two sides of the heart is more reliable than the chloride studies for the diagnosis of drowning.

Further studies of 80 drowning deaths and 80 control cases[5] indicate that the plasma specific gravity determinations can help conclude that a particular death was *not* caused by drowning.

Electron Microscopic Studies

In drowning, movements of fluid occur in both directions at the blood-air barrier. The inhalation of freshwater and seawater with different salinity and the passage of water across the alveolar-capillary junction can be expected to cause morphologic changes. Such changes, even if present, cannot be detected by light microscopy. Therefore, Reidbord and Spitz[13] made an ultramicroscopic investigation. They studied ultrastructural alterations in rat lungs. The study revealed clear morphologic differences in the lungs of rats drowned in saltwater and freshwater and in control cases. Logically, similar observations can be expected in human lungs. This field of investigation has, however, remained unexplored for obvious reasons. If the material is not examined shortly after death, postmortem changes make the task of interpreting the changes extremely difficult.

CONCLUSION

No forensic pathologist would deny the fact that there is not one pathognomonic autopsy finding indicative of the diagnosis of drowning. The best chance of making the diagnosis of drowning is when the body is not affected by putrefaction. In every case the diagnosis of drowning should be made by the evaluation of the findings suggestive of drowning, the circumstantial details and the exclusion of other causes of death.

REFERENCES

1. Corin, G., and Stockis, E.: Le diagnostic medico-legal de l'asphyxie par submersion. Bull. Acad. R. Med. Belg., *23:*42, 1909.
2. Durlacher, S. K., Freimuth, H. C., and Swan, H. E.: Blood changes in man following death due to drowning. Arch. Path., 56:454, 1953.
3. Fisher, I. L.: Chloride determination of heart blood; its use for the identification of death caused by drowning. J. Forensic Med., *14:*108, 1967.
4. Foroughi, E.: Serum changes in drowning. J. Forensic Sci., *16:*269, 1971.
5. Freimuth, H. C., and Swan, H. E.: Plasma specific gravity changes in sudden deaths. Arch. Path., *59:*214, 1955.
6. Gettler, A. O.: A method for the determination of death by drowning. JAMA, *77:*1650, 1921.
7. Koseki, T.: Fundamental examinations of experimental materials and control animals on the diagnosis of death from drowning by the diatom method. Acta Med. Biol., *15:*207, 1968.
8. Moritz, A. R.: Chemical methods for the determination of death by drowning. Physiol. Rev., *24:*70, 1944.
9. Mueller, B., and Gorgs, D.: Studien uber das Eindringen von corpuscularen Wasserbestandteilen aus den Lungenalveolen in den Kreislauf wahrend des entrinkungsvorganges. Dtsh Z. Gerichl. Med., *39:*715, 1949.
10. Neidhart, D. A., and Greendyke, R. M.: The significance of diatom demonstration in the diagnosis of death by drowning. Am. J. Clin. Path., *48:*377, 1967.
11. Patrick, R., and Reimer, C. W.: The diatoms of the United States. Monographs of the Academy of Natural Sciences of Philadelphia, No. 13, May 10, 1966.
12. Porawski, R.: Investigations on the occurrence of diatoms in organs in death from various causes. J. Forensic Med., *13:*134, 1966.
13. Reidbord, H. E., and Spitz, W. U.: Ultrastructural alterations in rat lungs. Arch. Path., *81:*103, 1966.

14. Revenstorf: Der Nachweis der aspirierten Ertrankungsflussigkeit als Kriterium des Todes durch Ertrinken. Vjschr gerichtl. Med., *27:*274, 1904.
15. Rivera, J. C.: Decompression sickness among divers: an analysis of 935 cases. Milit. Med., *314,* 1964.
16. Snyder, R. G., and Snow, C. C.: Fatal injuries resulting from extreme water impact. Aerosp. Med., *38:*779, 1967.
17. Spitz, W. U., and Schneider, V.: The significance of diatoms in the diagnosis of drowning. J. Forensic Sci., *9:*11, 1964.
18. Swann, H. G., and Spafford, N. R.: Body salt and water changes during fresh and sea water drowning. Tex. Rep. Biol. Med., *9:*365, 1951.
19. Thomas, F., Hecke, W. V., and Timperman, J.: The medico-legal diagnosis of death by drowning. J. Forensic Sci., *8:*1, 1963.
20. Thomas, F., Hecke, W. V., and Timperman, J.: The detection of diatoms in the bone marrow as evidence of death by drowning. J. Forensic Med., *8:*142, 1961.
21. U.S. Navy Department: U.S. Navy Diving Manual, U.S. Government Printing Office, Washington, D.C., 1963.
22. Webster, D. P.: Skin and scuba diving fatalities in the United States. Public Health Rep., *81:*703, 1966.

11

Deaths from Burns, Electrocution, Lightning

BURNS

Burns may result from dry heat, moist heat (scalds), chemicals or electrical charge. When death results from the effects of burns, most jurisdictions require that the case be investigated by the coroner or medical examiner. The pathologist is frequently asked to perform an autopsy to aid in the investigation.

The medicolegal investigation of a death from burns should be aimed at answering the following questions.

1. Was the person alive before the fire started?
2. Did the burns cause death?
3. If death was from causes other than burns, did the burns contribute to death?
4. Were there any natural diseases or injuries that could have caused death or contributed to it?
5. Were the burns sustained accidentally or did the person commit suicide?
6. Was death a result of crime?
7. Was there any attempt to conceal crime?
8. What was the cause of the onset of fire?
9. What was the source of fire?
10. What evidence was found to identify the decendent?

Occasionally, with multiple fatalities, one may be asked who died first in order to determine the rights of survivorship.

Circumstances of Death

The majority of deaths from burns are results of *accidents*. These accidents involve all ages, but more commonly the aged and the children. Accidents from clothing catching fire are common. In houses, such accidents result from inadequately guarded fires or from kitchen stoves. Epileptic attacks or episodes of angina can cause accidents leading to fire. The habit of smoking in bed, unfortunately, is common and frequently leads to fatal accidents. A person under the influence of alcohol or drugs, or one falling asleep may drop a lighted cigarette on the bedclothes.

> An elderly gentleman who had a habit of smoking in bed was found dead in a smoke-filled room. He had sustained minor burns on his right hand. The mattress was still smoldering when the room was broken open after the smell of smoke was detected. An ash tray on a side table was filled with cigarette stumps and some cigarette ash was found on the floor. Autopsy revealed no significant disease. The blood alcohol level was 230 mg. percent. The cause of death was carbon monoxide poisoning from smoke inhalation; the carboxyhemoglobin level was 69 percent.

A fire thus caused may involve a whole house or a building, resulting in multiple fatalities. Multiple fatalities from burns may also result from plane crashes or automobile accidents. In industry burns may be caused by explosions from flammable liquids and by flashes from furnaces.

Suicide by burning is almost unheard of in the Western world but in Asian countries it does occur. In India there was a custom which allowed a widow to cremate herself in the funeral pyre of her dead husband; this is now prohibited. For want of any other means, some suicides saturate their clothes with kerosene and set themselves on fire. To express protests of political nature, suicide by burning, self-immolation, is occasionally committed.

Murder by burning is rare. While investigating a death with bizarre circumstances, the possibility of crime should be considered, since a criminal may set fire to an abode to kill the occupant. Often an attempt is made to conceal crime by destroying the body of a victim in a fire. Burns may obscure evidence of wounding or strangling, but a careful postmortem examination may reveal evidence of crime in some cases.

Examination of the scene may reveal information regarding the cause of fire and may also indicate the site of origin of the fire. The overall study of the circumstances of death at the scene may yield information concerning the manner of death.

From the scene of death, all personal effects such as keys, watchband, belt buckle, buttons, cuff links and pieces of unburned clothing should be collected. These can be helpful in establishing the identity of the decedent.

Autopsy Findings

The autopsy will provide answers to some of the questions listed above. No case of fatality from burns can be investigated adequately without a complete postmortem examination. In some instances, because of extensive burns and charring of the remains, the material may appear most unpromising from the investigation point of view. Even in such cases, the autopsy should not be dispensed with, because a proper examination may yield valuable, even unexpected information.

Burns may be one of four degrees: reddening (first degree), blistering (second degree), scorching (third degree) and charring (fourth degree). The external examination will reveal the degree and extent of the burns. The heat may cause drying of the skin with scorching (brownish discoloration of skin) and this may be associated with splitting of the skin. Such a split may resemble an antemortem injury. This artefact and others are discussed below. Heat causes contracture of the tissues and this becomes obvious in the extremities which show flexing at the larger joints. The pugilistic attitude with flexion of elbows, knees and thighs is frequently seen in severely burned bodies. With charring of the body, breaking of the bones may mimic fractures. If a person dies from inhalation of smoke there may not be any burns.

In some instances the smell of gasoline or other flammable substance on the clothing or on the body indicates the use of such a substance to set fire.

How Does an Autopsy Help?

First of all, in many instances the *identity* of the body needs to be established. Without an autopsy, this is often impossible. The following check list will help in identification.

1. Note personal details and if possible estimate height and weight.
2. Record identifying stigmata such as scars, tattoos.
3. Retain unburned pieces of clothing and all personal effects.
4. Collect samples of unburned hair.
5. Record presence of natural diseases.
6. Make dental examination and if possible take fingerprints.
7. Do radiographic examination.
8. Determine decedent's blood group.

The question of *whether the person was alive or dead prior to the onset of fire* is important. The presence or absence of the following findings will greatly aid in determining the answer to this question: pink livor, vital reaction at the margins of the burns, soot in the air passages, carboxyhemoglobin in the blood.

Pink livor. In most burn cases, the color of livor is ill-defined. If large areas of the body are unburned, livor may be visible in the dependent unburned areas. In cases where the person dies from carbon monoxide poisoning from smoke inhalation, the livor, if visible, will be pinkish in color. This should lead to the suspicion of carboxyhemoglobin in the blood and to confirmation by chemical analysis.

Vital reaction. Burns caused after death do not show any vital reaction at their margins. The presence of a zone of vital reaction indicates that the burns were sustained during life. Such a zone of reaction is a distinctly pinkish red line at the junction of burned and unburned areas (Fig. 11-1). It is, however, not always identifiable. If the line of vital reaction is not

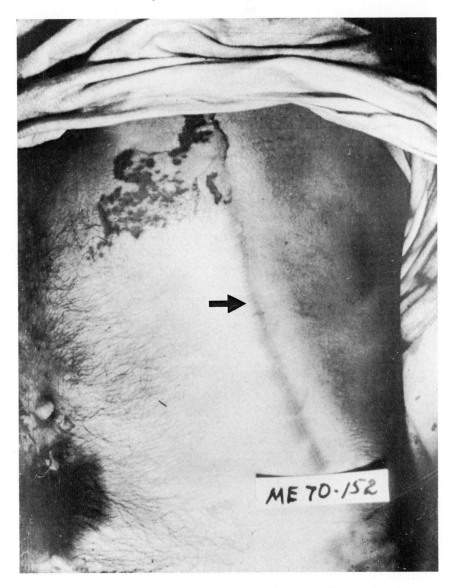

Fig. 11–1. The line of vital reaction at the junction of burned and unburned areas of the skin. This reaction is indicative of antemortem origin of burns. (See Color Plate.)

well defined and is not seen grossly, microscopic examination of the skin bordering the burn is necessary. This will reveal congestion of the area with hemorrhages and leukocytic infiltration. Specialized techniques have been used to differentiate antemortem burns from those sustained after death. Malik[5] studied the presence of enzymes—alkaline phosphatase, acid phosphatase, leucine amino peptidase and nonspecific esterase—in burns and concluded that an increase in the enzyme reaction in the periphery of an antemortem burn was a definite indication of its vital origin, because no such increase in the enzyme reaction was observed in the burns caused after death. He also found that enzyme reactions appeared earlier than the conventional histologic changes.

If blisters on the body are caused by burns, the examination of the fluid within the blisters may help differentiate antemortem from post-mortem burns. In case of burns sustained during life, the blisters contain fluid rich in protein; blisters formed after death contain scanty albumin.

Soot in the air passages. The presence or absence of carbon particles in the larynx, trachea and bronchi should always be checked for. If black soot is present in the air passages, it indicates that the victim had inhaled smoke and was alive when the fire started. The absence of soot in the air passages merely indicates that the person had not inhaled smoke. Fatalities can occur from burns without the inhalation of smoke as would happen if the victim runs in the open and the smoke arising from the clothing blows away. Death occurring indoors invariably shows black soot in the trachea and the main bronchi (Fig. 11-2). Occasionally, the carbon particles are deep in the smaller bronchi. The soot is mixed with mucus and sticks to the mucosa lining the air passages.

In an attempt to prevent inhalation, the victim may cough loose the soot from the larynx and posterior pharynx and it may be swallowed. At autopsy carbon with mucus may be found in the esophagus and stomach.

Carboxyhemoglobin in blood. Smoke contains carbon monoxide. If a person is alive during a fire he inhales smoke, particularly in closed spaces. Persons who die in fires after inhaling smoke have elevated levels of car-boxyhemoglobin in the blood. In most instances it is possible to conclude from the raised carboxyhemoglobin in the blood that the person was alive when the fire started. Therefore, a sample of blood must always be taken during an autopsy on a burned body to determine the level of carboxyhe-moglobin. If the analysis shows the level to be above 8 to 10 percent of carboxyhemoglobin, it can be assumed that the person had inhaled smoke and was alive before the fire started. A negative result (i.e., carboxyhe-moglobin saturation of less than 8 percent) should not be regarded as a proof of death prior to the onset of fire. If death occurs outdoors, no smoke may be inhaled and the victim's blood may not show any carboxyhemo-globin. Also, if death is caused by flash fire there may not be any car-

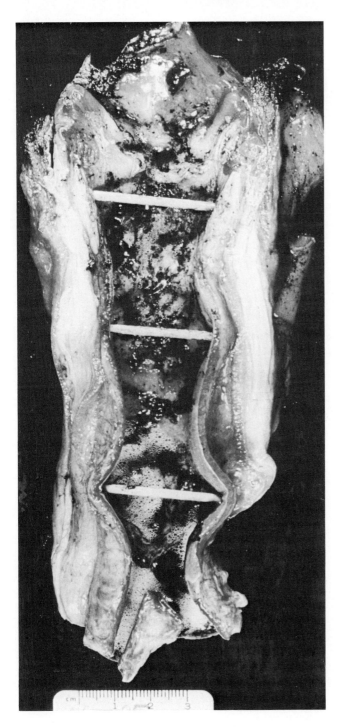

Fig. 11–2. Soot in the trachea indicates inhalation of smoke.

boxyhemoglobin in the blood.[2, 4] Hirsch and Adelson, who described five cases of flash fire with no carboxyhemoglobin, postulate that the intense flash of heat "can cause impregnable laryngospasm or immediate respiratory arrest" preventing the inhalation of the products of combustion. Similarly, an explosion associated with the onset of a fire can kill a person rapidly and no carboxyhemoglobin may be found in the victim's blood.[11]

The autopsy will, of course, help determine *the cause and the manner of death.* Apart from the obvious purpose of excluding the possibility of crime, the determination of the true cause of death by autopsy will provide accurate data for vital records and more important, the information will be useful for the settlement of insurance claims. Once it is determined that the burns were caused while the person was alive, it is then necessary to establish whether the burns were the sole cause of death. At times there may be other factors contributing to death. The role of injuries from falling objects or the presence of significant diseases must be carefully evaluated. If it is not certain whether the burns were caused before or after death, a complete autopsy will settle the issue. A case such as the one described below may be certified improperly if an autopsy is not performed.

A man in his sixties who lived alone was found dead in his living room seated in a chair. Some of the furniture was gutted. The lower extremities of the man were charred and there was scorching of the upper part of the body. A whiskey bottle was found on a table near the body and ash trays contained several cigarette stumps. It was thought that smoking while being intoxicated probably had caused the fire and death from burns. At the autopsy no vital characteristics of the burns were seen on external examination. No soot was found in the air passages and his blood contained no carboxyhemoglobin or alcohol. The cause of death was coronary thrombosis.

The investigation and autopsy can yield valuable information that can determine the manner of death. If the victim had a life insurance policy with a double indemnity clause for accidental death, it is important to resolve the question of manner of death. Occasionally, a civil suit arises from a death; without a complete investigation, miscarriage of injustice can result.

A housewife who had always enjoyed good health was allegedly watching television in her living room. A few minutes after she was seen to carry a cup of coffee to the living room, the husband who was in another room noticed that the living room was full of smoke. In a few minutes the fire marshals were at the scene and the fire was extinguished within an hour. The woman was found dead lying on the floor with her head near the sofa and her feet toward the television set. Detailed investigation raised the possibility of fire having started from the television set, which was shattered. After preliminary investigation the body was buried without an autopsy. In view of lingering doubts as to whether she had died from natural causes, electrocution or burns related to explosion of the television set, the body was exhumed two weeks after burial.

Autopsy revealed total body burns. There was soot in the trachea and the larynx. The lungs were edematous. Apart from minimal atherosclerosis of the coronary arteries and an adenoma in each adrenal, no disease was seen. The blood alcohol concentration was 50 mg. per 100 ml. and the carbon monoxide saturation was 30 percent. On the basis of the autopsy findings and the examination of the television set, product liability suit against the manufacturer of the television set ensued on the contention that the explosion in the set caused the woman's death.

One of the most important objectives of an autopsy on a burned body is the exclusion of the possibility of foul play. Although murder by fire may be difficult to prove without strong circumstantial evidence, the autopsy may reveal evidence of killing by other means and destruction of the dead body by fire.

A middle-aged chronic alcoholic was found dead in a dilapidated abode which was often used by chronic alcoholics. His charred body was discovered after the fire which destroyed the abode was extinguished. The circumstances pointed to this being an accidental death. However, x-rays of the body prior to the postmortem examination revealed a bullet in the spine. Dissection for removal of the bullet showed recent hemorrhages along the tract of the missile.

On another occasion, severely burned bodies of a couple—husband and wife —were found in a burned house. Investigation indicated the possibility of murder-suicide. At the autopsy, a bullet was found in the brain of the woman and the point of entry of the bullet was in the back of the head. The autopsy on the man revealed two bullets in the head. Beveling of the skull indicated that one bullet had entered the cranium from the right side of the head and the other from the left. This was a double murder.

In view of cases such as those described above, the *need for radiological examination* of the body prior to the commencement of an autopsy cannot be overemphasized. In the following instance x-rays helped in the identification of the body. The case also illustrates various other interesting aspects of investigation.

One day parts of the body of a man were found in a burned automobile (Fig. 15-3 in Chapter 15). The automobile was a Pontiac with license plates that had been allocated to a Cadillac. In the car there were 24 bottles of "moonshine." The charred body consisted of the torso and several portions of bones. Except for a small portion of patterned underpants, all clothing was burned. With the body were a brass belt buckle with a name engraved on it, a wristwatch and a key ring with 12 keys. The head was missing with the level of separation at C2. This was also seen on x-rays which did not show any radioopaque objects in the body. There was some froth in the trachea and the main bronchi but no soot. The lungs were congested and edematous. No natural disease was found. There was some unburned, light brown hair in the pubic area. The decedent's blood type was B, blood alcohol level was 290 mg. per 100 ml. and the carboxyhemoglobin saturation was 15 percent.

The following day, a head and hand were found 3½ miles from where the charred body was found. The head and the hand were buried in a 2-foot deep hole on a farm (Fig. 11-3). Examination of the head showed a contact gunshot wound behind the left ear with an exit hole on the right side of the head. The head had been severed at the level of C2. The hair on the head and on the hand was light brown. Examination of the blood from the head showed alcohol concentration of 290 mg. per 100 ml., blood type B and negative carboxyhemoglobin.

The head was identified by visual identification of the face as being that of a 21-year-old man. The fingerprints from the hand and a scar on the wrist identified the hand as belonging to the same man. The circumstances and autopsy findings revealed several points that matched the charred remains with the head, leaving no doubt that all the remains were of one man. The personal effects found with the charred remains were identified as belonging

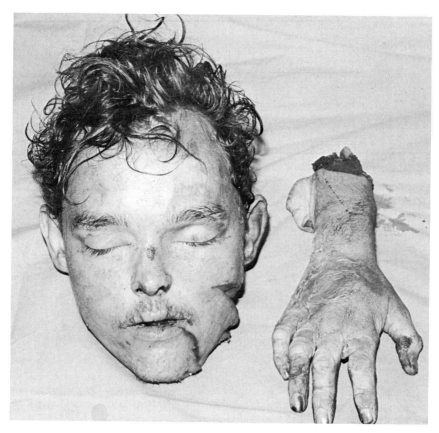

Fig. 11–3. Murder. The head and hand were removed before the rest of the body was burned in an automobile.

to a man who was later convicted of the murder of this man. The convict had attempted to fake his own death in order to collect insurance in the amount of $250,000.00.

Artefacts in Burned Bodies

The recognition of postmortem artefacts is important for the correct interpretation of the case. Therefore, a note on artefacts in burned bodies is added.

Postmortem artefacts in burned bodies can be many and varied. Heat ruptures may occur postmortem on any exposed part of the body and may resemble incised wounds or lacerations (Fig. 11-4). They can be easily differentiated from antemortem injuries by the absence of hemorrhage or vital reaction in the ruptures. Heat may cause rupture of the scalp or the skull. The famous case of R. vs. Rouse well illustrates these artefacts in the head.[10] In this case, heat had caused rupture of the victim's scalp which resembled a laceration, creating much confusion for a time. The victim's skull was shattered with herniation of the brain. To Sir Bernard Spilsbury, "that was due to bursting and splintering through the effects of heat, obviously."

In burned bodies, the occurrence of "heat hematoma" is a well-recognized artefact.[7] The condition, not due to antemortem trauma, is an

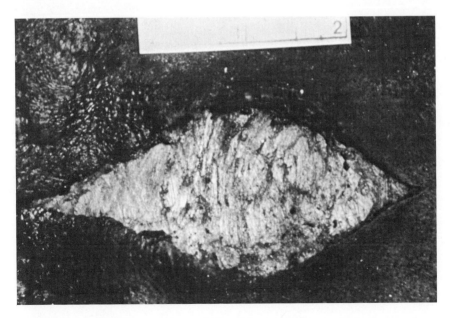

Fig. 11–4. This heat rupture of the skin resembles an incised wound.

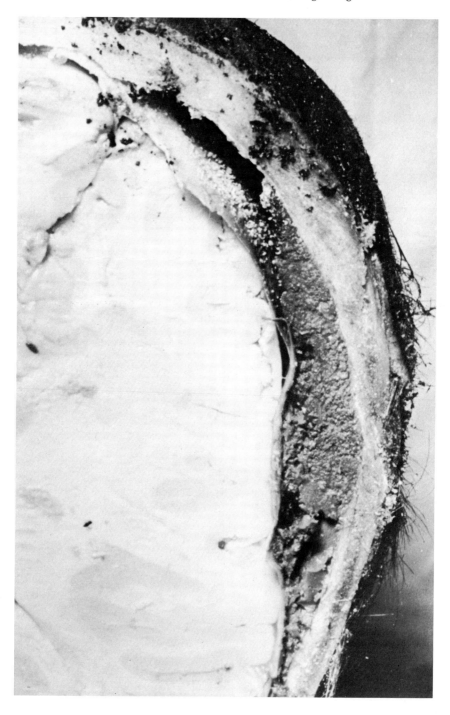

extradural hemorrhage of the extradural arteries, such as the middle meningeal artery, caused by burning and rupture after death. Distribution of the hemorrhage follows closely distribution of the charring of the outer table of the skull. The parietotemporal region is the most common site of such hemorrhages. The blood in the hematoma is a soft, friable clot of chocolate color or of a pink tint, if the victim's blood had a high concentration of carboxyhemoglobin. The clot presents a honeycomb appearance and is usually soft in the center. The thickness of the clot varies; in one case it was three fourths of an inch thick (Fig. 11-5). Such a hemorrhage should not be interpreted as evidence of antemortem trauma. In cases with history of head injury, careful evaluation should be made of such a finding.

Heat may also cause charring and fracturing of the vault of the skull. However, it is unlikely to cause fractures of the base of the skull. The finding of basal fractures must arouse strong suspicions of antemortem trauma and foul play.

Because the neck is relatively protected, it frequently escapes burns, particularly in clothed individuals. If the burned clothes are removed or fall off before the body comes to the autopsy table, the pathologist may see a deep unburned groove around the neck (caused by the collar) simulating a strangulation mark.

Droplets of fat are frequently observed in the pulmonary vessels of severely burned bodies.[6] These occur independently of antemortem injury and should not be confused with traumatically induced antemortem pulmonary fat embolism.

The toxicological artefacts encountered in burned bodies are included in Chapter 17.

ELECTROCUTION

A few facts concerning electrocution are worth noting.

The factors that play an important part in influencing the degree of severity of the effects of electrocution are:

1. *Amperage*: The intensity of the current (amperage) is an important factor. Currents above 100 amperes frequently prove fatal.
2. *Voltage:* The higher the voltage the more disastrous the effects. Voltages of alternating current as low as 50 can cause death.

Fig. 11–5. (*Opposite*) An extradural hemorrhage caused by burns after death. (See Color Plate.)

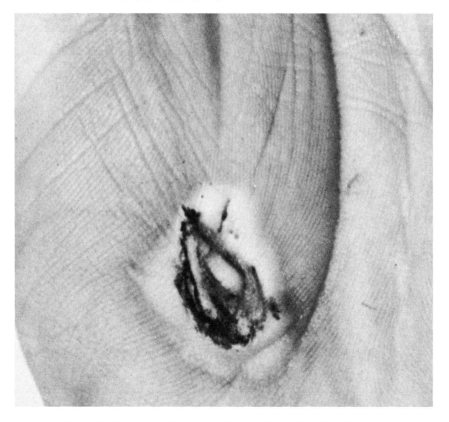

Fig. 11–6. A typical electrical burn. (See Color Plate.)

3. *Resistance:* Different body tissues offer different resistance. The skin of the palms and soles offers greater resistance than the skin elsewhere.
4. *Duration of contact:* Even a low voltage current with a prolonged contact is dangerous.

With electrocution, death usually results from ventricular fibrillation or respiratory failure.

Most deaths from electrocution are accidental. In homes, accidents result from contact with live electrical supply lines; the majority of the accidents being caused by defective equipment or negligence in the use of equipment. In industry, fatalities occasionally result from contact with live overhead cables or from handling of charged lamps, tools or switch gears.

Suicide by electrocution is rare. Polson has cited the work of Munck[7] who described four cases of suicide by electrocution and summarized reports of 29 cases published between 1885 and 1932.

Investigation of a Death

Careful investigation of death, particularly of a victim at work, is important because civil suits claiming damages for employer negligence might ensue is some cases. Occasionally, questions may be raised as to whether death was natural or was caused by injuries from a fall or by electrocution.

Most cases pose no investigative problems. Even if the death is not witnessed, examination of the place of death will reveal evidence indicating the possibility of electrocution. The decendent may be found grasping the object that electrocuted him. Occasionally, foam may be present in the mouth.

The important part of the investigation is the detection of the entrance electrical mark caused by contact with the live source of electricity. Search for an exit mark should also be made, but such marks may not be obvious in all cases. If electrocution is suspected, every part of the body must be carefully examined to locate the burn. Stiffened flexed fingers must be extended to look for marks on the hands and between the fingers. The feet may bear marks, especially exit marks. Ulcers and corns must be differentiated from electrical burns. An electrical burn on the head may not be obvious unless suspicious areas are shaved.

A *typical electric mark* consists of a round, oval or elongated crater. The floor of the crater is usually pale or a dark brown color. Around the depressed area there is a ridge of elevated skin. Immediately beyond the ridge there is a zone of whitish pale color which, in some cases, is surrounded by a zone of reddish vital reaction (Fig. 11-6). The conductor causing the mark may leave its shape and pattern in the injury (Fig. 11-7). Exit burns consist of small splits in the skin.

Microscopic examination of the electrical burn will show flattening of the epithelial cells. These flattened cells usually stain darker than the normal cells with hematoxylin and eosin stain. Microblisters and empty spaces also are seen frequently in the epidermis. Exit burns are also associated with empty spaces of varying sizes and shapes in the epidermis.

Adjutantis and Skalos[1] have described a test based on the detection of metallic deposits at the site of the electrical burn. If the importance of the case demands it, the existence of the burn can also be demonstrated with the detection of particles of the metal of the electrode by the technique of neutron activation analysis.

The general autopsy findings in a case of electrocution are usually non-

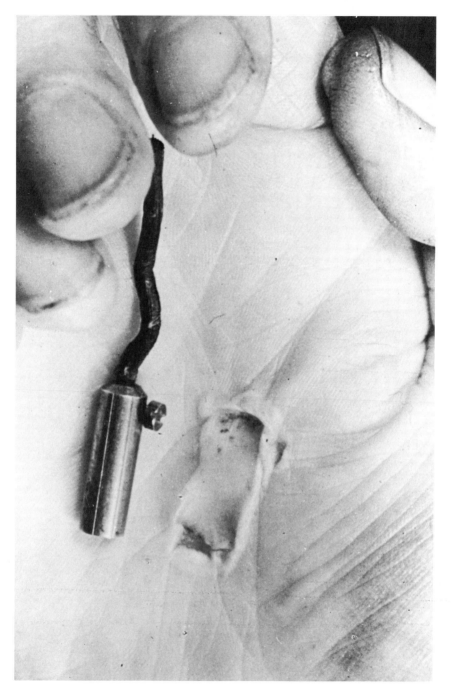

Fig. 11–7. Electrocution. An electric mark revealing the shape of the conductor.

specific. The visceral organs show generalized congestion. If the victim survives for a time, edema of the lungs with collection of foam in the air passages may be found. Details of changes in different organs are summarized in an exhaustive review of the subject of electropathology by Jaffe.[3] This review contains 137 good references. More recently Polson[8] has reviewed the subject.

LIGHTNING

In the diagnosis of death by lightning stroke, the history of storm and lightning is important. In the absence of such a history the cases can present reasons for suspicion.

At the scene of death there may be evidence of disruption of the ground, building and other objects caused by lightning.

The clothing on the body of the victim of a lightning stroke may show extensive tears with scorches or burns. The shoes and tight clothing may be burst open.

The body may, likewise, show extensive tears and splits in the skin, opening of body cavities and fractures of the bones. If there are any metallic objects on the body (e.g., belt buckles or buttons), these may be associated with corresponding burns on the skin. The lacerated exposed tissues are pale and bloodless and some may show the effect of heat. One of the most characteristic findings in a lightning death is the presence of arborescent markings on the skin (Fig. 11-8).

It must be remembered that not every case of lightning fatality presents such a picture. In some cases the changes may be minimal. Tears in the clothing and body injuries may be entirely absent.

The victim of a lightning stroke may be found in a isolated spot. This fact, together with the lack of a history of the lightning, disruption of clothing and bizarre body injuries would cause concern. Identification of electrical burns, especially the arborescent marks, lack of a definite pattern of injuries and the finding of magnetized metal objects (keys, wristwatch, belt buckles, buttons) would assist in making the diagnosis of death from lightning.

REFERENCES

1. Adjutantis, G., and Skalos, G.: The identification of the electrical burn. J. Forensic Med., *9:*101, 1962.
2. Hirsch, C. S., and Adelson, L.: Absence of carboxyhemoglobin in flash fire victims. JAMA, *210:*2279, 1969.

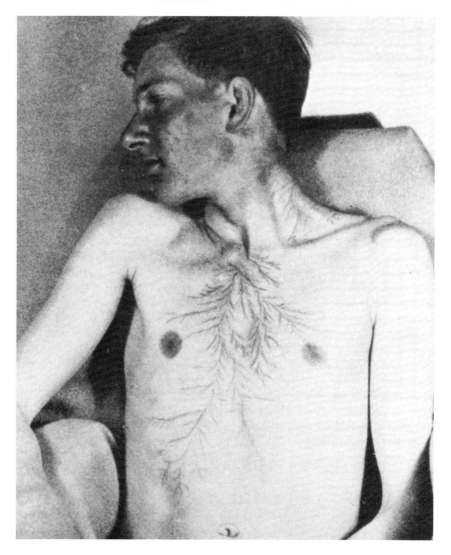

Fig. 11–8. Lightning stroke. Arborescent markings of the skin. (See Color Plate .)

3. Jaffe, R. H.: Electropathology—A review of the pathologic changes produced by electric currents. Arch. Path., *5:*837, 1928.
4. James, W. R. L.: Suicide by burning. Med. Sci. Law, *6:*48, 1966.
5. Malik, M. A. O.: Histochemical changes as evidence of the antemortem origin of skin burns. J. Forensic Sci., *15:*489, 1970.
6. Moritz, A. R.: Classical mistakes in forensic pathology. Am. J. Clin. Path., *26:*1383, 1956.

7. Munck, W.: Dtsch. Z. ges. gerichtl. Med., *23:*97, 1934. Cited by Polson, C. J.: The Essentials of Forensic Medicine. ed. 2. Springfield (Ill.), Charles C Thomas, 1965.
8. Polson, C. J.: Electrocution. Med. Leg. J., *27:*121, 1959.
9. Polson, C. J.: The Essentials of Forensic Medicine. ed. 2. Springfield (Ill.), Charles C Thomas, 1965.
10. R. v. Rouse: Trial of Alfred Arthur Rouse. *In* Normanton, H. (ed.): Notable British Trials Series. Edinburgh, Hodge, 1931.
11. Snyder, L.: Homicide Investigation. ed. 2. Springfield (Ill.), Charles C Thomas, 1967.

12

Deaths from Heatstroke and Hypothermia

HEATSTROKE

Deaths from heatstroke and hypothermia are unnatural deaths. Therefore, the investigation of such a fatality should be the responsibility of the medical examiner or the coroner. Medicolegal questions might arise if a person suffers fatal heatstroke while at work. These deaths are invariably accidental and the determination of the precise cause of death can be important in settling the questions related to insurance.

Heatstroke is an uncommon event but it carries high mortality. The principal factors in the initiation of heatstroke are high temperature, increased humidity, muscular activity and lack of acclimatization. Other factors of importance are old age, preexisting disease conditions, obesity, lack of air movement and unsuitable clothing. In sportsmen the use of "pep pills" may also be a factor.

Clinical Features. *Symptoms.* In the majority of cases the onset of symptoms is acute and without any warning signs. Sudden collapse and loss of consciousness is common. In some instances prodromal symptoms such as headache, dizziness, nausea, vomiting, weakness, faintness, staggering gait, purposeless movements, mental confusion, muscle cramps, restlessness, dryness of mouth and excessive thirst are experienced. The most serious of the manifestations are delirium, convulsions and coma.

Signs. The skin is hot, red and dry with absence of sweating. In most of the cases the rectal temperature is above 105°F. It could, however, range from 99° to 111°F. The pulse is rapid; usually the rate per minute is between 100 to 200. Respirations are rapid, deep and of the Kussmaul type. Fall in blood pressure is common but cases with normal blood pressure may be seen. Occasionally, other signs such as decerebrate rigidity, disturbances in muscle tone, pyramidal signs and tetany as well as hemorrhages in the skin and mucous membranes are seen.

Laboratory studies frequently reveal leukocytosis, moderate elevation of nonprotein nitrogen, reduced carbon-dioxide combining power, prolongation of prothrombin time, prolongation of clotting time, afibrinogenemia, increased capillary fragility, evidence of alkalosis and hypokalemia, albuminuria, hematuria and casts in the urine.

Death generally occurs within a week and almost two thirds of the victims of serious heat stroke die in the first 24 hours. Signs that indicate poor prognosis are coma, hypotension, azotemia, hyperkalemia (or hypokalemia) and body temperature of 106°F. or over.

Autopsy Findings. In heartstroke many of the organs are affected. A variable degree of some of the following pathological changes are seen in all cases of heatstroke.[5, 7]

Central nervous system. The increased weight of the brain, congestion and edema of leptomeninges with petechial hemorrhages, flattening of the convolutions, cellular changes with pyknotic nuclei, swollen dendrites and chromatolytic changes, dropping out and degeneration of neurons and diffuse proliferation of microglia are some of the changes seen in cerebral hemispheres. According to Malamud and his colleagues,[5] changes in the cerebellum are more striking, more consistent and more rapid in development than in any other part of the brain. These changes consist of edema of the Purkinje layer, and swelling, disintegration and reduction of the Purkinje cells. With survival of more than one day, complete degeneration of the Purkinje layer and gliosis are obvious. With prolonged survival, rarefaction of the granular layer occurs. In the hypothalamus, the center with heat regulatory role, no significant changes are seen other than edema of the nuclei.

Lungs. Frothy hemorrhagic fluid in the trachea and main bronchi, edema of the lung tissue, intense vascular congestion and widespread petechial hemorrhages are frequently seen in cases of heatstroke. Complicating pneumonia may be seen in some cases.

Heart. Dilation of right auricle, flabbiness of muscle, petechial or confluent subepicardial and subendocardial hemorrhages and histological evidence of degeneration of the myocardium are often seen.

Liver. Congestion of the liver and centrolobular necrosis are common in cases of prolonged survival.

Kidneys. They are usually congested, edematous and increased in weight. Hemoglobinuric nephrosis, uncommon in early cases, is common in cases of longer survival.

Adrenal glands. Pericapsular hemorrhages, engorgement of sinusoids and degeneration of cortex may be seen.

General changes. In many cases petechial and confluent hemorrhages are seen commonly in most of the organs.

The following case illustrates many of the features of heatstroke:

A 20-year-old man who had always enjoyed good health collapsed during football practice on a hot, humid day. On admission to the hospital, he was comatose, with the blood pressure of 70/0 mm. of Hg. and the body temperature of 108°F. The patient was oliguric, had episodes of cardiac arrythmia and showed petechial hemorrhages in the mucous membranes. Serum potassium was 1.9m Eq/L and blood studies revealed prolonged clotting time and decreased quantities of Factors V, VIII, IX and X and platelets. Blood urea nitrogen (BUN) fluctuated between 78 and 175 mg. %. The patient's stools were benzidine positive and the liver function tests indicated acute hepatic necrosis. Despite treatment to combat hyperthermia, control electrolytes and maintain blood pressure, the patient terminally developed massive gastrointestinal bleeding and atrial fibrillation and became hypotensive. Death occurred two weeks after admission.

At the autopsy, evidence was seen of diffuse intravascular coagulation with areas of infarction in the heart, lungs, spleen, liver, pancreas, stomach, colon, kidneys and skeletal muscle. In addition, the liver showed acute centrolobular necrosis and the kidneys revealed acute tubular necrosis. There were acute ulcers in the stomach and colon. Acute fungal peritonitis due to Candida organisms was found. There was also diffuse lobular pneumonia in all parts of both lungs. Culture studies indicated septicemia with two strains of Klebsiella.

HYPOTHERMIA

The state of hypothermia is said to exist when the body temperature falls below 95°F. Hypothermia can cause dangerous physiologic changes and even death. In winter months many people die from the effects of cold weather. A "sudden unexpected" death from possible hypothermia is a medicolegal problem and the determination of the exact cause of death can be significant. In the case of hypothermia, circumstantial evidence is immensely important. Fatal hypothermia is associated with certain pathological changes in the body that may escape the attention of the general pathologist. Therefore, a brief review of gross and microscopic alterations in hypothermia cases is presented in this chapter.

External Changes. In most cases of fatal hypothermia the body temperature is below 90°F. unless the body has been exposed to higher temperatures prior to autopsy. (In every case of suspected hypothermia, rectal temperature should be recorded at the start of the autopsy.) The skin is pale because of ischemia of the subcutaneous tissues and feels doughy. The presence of patchy erythema is common due to sludging of blood in the cutaneous blood vessels, a feature that can be verified by microscopic examination. Frequently the legs and feet are edematous and the skin on these parts may be shiny with areas of slippage of superficial epidermis.

Internal Changes. The following changes may be seen in the internal organs in the cases of hypothermia.

Gastrointestinal tract. Obvious changes caused by hypothermic states are commonly seen in the gastrointestinal tract. The esophagus frequently shows superficial sloughing of the mucosa. Occasionally, the changes are more pronounced. In Brennan's case[2] the esophagus showed extensive necrosis involving the mucosa and part of the submucosa with inflammatory reaction and edema. The stomach more or less constantly exhibits changes in the mucosa. In twelve consecutive cases this author has seen acute gastric ulcers. The changes are variable and range from multiple ecchymoses of altered blood to frank ulcers. The hemorrhages in the mucosa are blackish because of the altered blood, and the ulcers are superficial with hemorrhage in the base. If death is delayed, sloughing of the gastric mucosa is more pronounced. Similar changes may occur in the duodenum, but these are not as frequent as in the stomach. In the rest of the gastrointestinal tract submucosal hemorrhages are seen infrequently. In a case of hypothermia described by Mant,[6] an elderly woman who lived for five days after admission to the hospital had not only multiple gastric erosions but also a large perforated acute duodenal ulcer.

Pancreas. Fat necrosis along the pancreas is another more or less constant pathological change in hypothermia. This chnge is variable; in some, occasional patches of fat necrosis are seen while in others there is obvious nonhemorrhagic pancreatitis with fat necrosis along the entire organ. Occasionally, necrosis extends into the neighboring tissues. Necrosis can be easily verified by microscopic examination; therefore, many sections of the pancreas should be taken at autopsy for a histological examination.

Respiratory system. Changes in the respiratory system are nonspecific. Pulmonary congestion is nearly always seen and sometimes it is associated with intrapulmonary hemorrhage and edema. Hunter[3] noted gross and microscopic evidence of hyperemia, hemorrhage and edema in all of his ten cases. In his study nearly all vessels showed perivascular hemorrhages. In addition, some alveoli were filled with proteinous fluid mixed with trapped air and masses of erythrocytes and macrocytes. He stresses the constancy of these pulmonary changes as being the most striking pathological phenomenon in the cases of hypothermia. It has been suggested[4] that pulmonary edema results from altered capillary permeability or a decrease of the osmotic pressure of blood largely attributable to changes in protein concentrations.

Cardiovascular system. The heart is not significantly changed in a morphological sense. The right side of the heart is usually distended with blood, whereas the left side is empty. In most cases the blood is thick because of the marked and uniform increase in its viscosity and it is cold. In one case, a middle-aged woman was found dead in the woods covered with snow. The autopsy on her revealed all large blood vessels and the right side of the heart packed with ice caused by the freezing of the serum. In all cases of hypothermia the blood vessels of different sizes are enor-

mously distended, and frequently there is associated sludging of the erythrocytes and perivascular hemorrhages. Congestion of internal organs is due
to packing of blood cells in the capillaries.

Brain. The brain is usually unremarkable. Occasionally, one may see a
ring and ball appearance due to sludging of the erythrocytes and perivascular hemorrhages.

Adrenal glands. The adrenals may show a stress effect in the zona
fasciculata.

Associated Conditions. Healthy adults may succumb to cold, but it is the
elderly and infants who become victims of hypothermia more easily. The
presence of wasting diseases and certain other acute and chronic conditions
increases the susceptibility to cold. Conditions that deserve particular attention are myxedema, hypopituitarism, steatorrhea, rheumatoid arthritis,
anemia and malnutrition. Acute and chronic alcoholism as well as the use
of barbiturates accelerate the effects of cold. Hence, in suspected cases of
hypothermia, analyses for these chemicals should be made.

In conclusion, erythematous skin lesions, gastric erosions and fat necrosis along the pancreas, together with distended vessels with viscous
blood and congestion of organs, are some of the more helpful findings in
hypothermia cases. To substantiate this diagnosis, the circumstances of
death and the presence of associated pathological conditions should be
carefully evaluated. Because histological details of all organs are well preserved for long periods, the use of microscopic examinations should be
encouraged to help make the diagnosis of hypothermia.

REFERENCES

1. Austin, M. G., and Berry, J. W.: Observations on one hundred cases of
   heartstroke. JAMA, *161:*1525, 1956.
2. Brennan, J.: Case of extensive necrosis of the esophageal mucosa following
   hypothermia. J. Clin. Path., *20:*581, 1967.
3. Hunter, W.: Accidental hypothermia. Northwest Med., *67:*569, 1968.
4. Kreider, M. B.: Pathological effects of extreme cold. Medical Climatology,
   Elizabeth Licht, New Haven, 1964.
5. Malamud, N., Haymaker, W., and Custer, R. P.: Heatstroke—a clinicopathologic study of 125 fatal cases. Milit. Surg., *99:*397, 1946.
6. Mant, A. K.: Some observations in accidental hypothermia. Med. Sci. Law,
   *4:*44, 1964.
7. Romeo, J. A.: Heartstroke. Milit. Med., *131:*669, 1966.

13

Sudden, Unexpected Natural Deaths

Sudden death from a natural cause can be described as rapid termination of an acute or chronic disease. When the symptoms of disease are not experienced by the patient, or they are unknown to friends, relatives or the patient's physician and when such a disease proves fatal, death is termed "unexpected." Death is not necessarily "sudden" but when a person who had apparently been in good health is found dead, such a death is categorized as "sudden, unexpected death." Such cases fall within the jurisdiction of medical examiners and coroners, since the cause and manner of death are not known.

Investigation of a sudden, unexpected death is necessary for several reasons:

1. Determination of whether violence in any form played any part in the death is important.
2. Insurance claims or civil suits based on allegations that death resulted from accidental injury may arise.
3. The question of workmen's compensation may be raised if death occurs at work or if there is possibility of industrial disease or accident.[3]
4. The possibility of death from poisoning may exist.
5. The investigation may serve public health interest if a communicable or epidemic disease is detected.

From the medicolegal point of view the principal objective in the investigation of sudden, unexpected death is the determination of the manner of death. In some instances the study of the circumstances of death indicates that death was from natural causes. In some jurisdictions disposition of a case without an autopsy is permitted if there is no doubt in the investigator's mind that the death was natural. Conclusions without an autopsy, however, cannot always be accurate. There is always a possibility that a death presumed to be natural may be an unnatural one. Several investigations have pointed out the value of ascertaining the true cause of a sudden, unexpected death.[2, 4, 6] In a few cases the circumstances of death do not provide any clue to the cause and the manner of death. In such cases the investigation cannot be complete without a thorough postmortem examination of the body. The body of a person who has died suddenly and unexpectedly might bear injuries. If so, the significance of the injuries must be clearly determined.

The autopsy provides the cause of death from gross examination in a majority of natural deaths. In some cases histological studies are required. Of course, with the slightest suspicion of poisoning adequate toxicological studies must be performed.

CAUSES OF SUDDEN DEATH

Following is a systematic listing of pathological lesions causing sudden and unexpected natural death in adults. Pathological conditions involving infants and young children are discussed in Chapter 14.

Diseases of the Cardiovascular System

1. Coronary artery disease—narrowing and obliteration of the lumen of the coronary artery by atherosclerosis
2. Coronary atherosclerosis with coronary thrombosis, old or recent, with or without old or recent myocardial infarction
3. Coronary atherosclerosis with hemorrhage in the wall causing occlusion of the lumen
4. Coronary artery embolism (rare)
5. Occlusion of the ostium of the coronary artery associated with atherosclerosis or syphilitic aortitis
6. Rupture of the fresh myocardial infarct or aneurysm of the heart wall; delayed rupture
7. Myocarditis, acute, subacute or chronic
8. Bacterial endocarditis, acute or subacute
9. Cardiomyopathies: alcoholic myopathy, asymmetrical hypertrophy of the heart
10. Lesions of the conducting system: fibrosis, necrosis
11. Myocardial hypertrophy: hypertension, hyperthyroidism
12. Valvular lesions: aortic stenosis, aortic regurgitation, mitral stenosis, rupture of the chordae or leaflets, ball-valve thrombus
13. Pericarditis and constrictive pericarditis: septic, rheumatic, tuberculous, malignant
14. Lesions of aorta: rupture of a dissecting or an atheromatous aneurysm
15. Congenital lesions

Diseases of respiratory system

1. Acute infections: acute bronchitis, bronchopneumonia, lobar pneumonia, laryngitis
2. Pulmonary embolism with or without infarction
3. Status asthmaticus
4. Pneumothorax caused by rupture of emphysematous bleb
5. Chronic lesions: pulmonary tuberculosis, bronchogenic carcinoma, lung abscess, bronchiectasis
6. Sudden airway obstruction: laryngeal edema from infection, hemorrhage from pulmonary tuberculosis or carcinoma, prolapsing tumor mass
7. Cor pulmonale

Diseases of the Nervous System

1. Subarachnoid hemorrhage due to a ruptured berry aneurysm
2. Spontaneous intracerebral hemorrhage associated with atherosclerosis and hypertension
3. Pontine hemorrhage
4. Cerebellar hemorrhage
5. Hemorrhage in a brain tumor or abscess
6. Acute meningitis
7. Meningococcemia without gross meningitis
8. Acute, chronic encephalitis
9. Cerebral artery thrombosis and embolism with or without cerebral infarction
10. Carotid artery thrombosis
11. Status epilepticus

Diseases of the Alimentary System

1. Hemorrhage from esophageal varices, a gastric or duodenal ulcer or tumor
2. Acute peritonitis associated with ruptured viscera, intestinal obstruction, strangulated hernia
3. Mesenteric thrombosis with infarction of the bowel
4. Acute pancreatitis
5. Severe fatty metamorphosis of the liver
6. Spontaneous rupture of the spleen in infectious mononucleosis or malaria

Diseases of Urogenital System

1. Rupture of ectopic pregnancy, complications of abortion
2. Eclamptic toxemia of pregnancy
3. Acute pyelonephritis
4. Uremia associated with chronic renal disease

Miscellaneous

1. Diabetes mellitis: hypoglycemia, diabetic coma
2. Sickle cell crisis
3. Addison's disease
4. Pheochromocytoma
5. Hemorrhage from varicose ulcer of the leg
6. Hyperthyroidism
7. Blood dyscrasias

In medicolegal practice, coronary artery disease accounts for a majority of sudden, unexpected natural deaths. Severe narrowing of the coronary arteries without thrombosis or myocardial infarction is the commonest finding in such deaths. Fresh thrombotic lesions are seen in less than twenty-five percent of the cases. Although coronary artery disease is common in middle-aged and elderly persons, it is not uncommonly a cause of sudden death in young adults. In many of the cases symptoms of the disease are absent. In some the complaints of chest pain are discarded as being insignificant and no medical help is sought. Occasionally, even a careful medical checkup does not reveal any abnormality.

A 28-year-old truck driver was a potential kidney donor for his ailing brother. In order to determine his fitness as a donor an elaborate medical examination was made by a team of physicians. His electrocardiographic tracings were normal. After the examinations he was pronounced fit to donate the kidney and was asked to remain prepared for the operation. The day after he was so told, he collapsed and died at the wheel in his truck parked at his place of work. The autopsy on the man revealed severe coronary artery disease with a fresh thrombus in the descending branch of the left coronary artery.

In an apparently natural death, if the fatal lesions are not obvious on gross examination of the organs, it is advisable to retain the entire heart. Lesions such as myocarditis, fibrosis and necrosis of conducting tissue may otherwise escape detection. The narrowing of the valves must be carefully evaluated before the valve orifices are slit open.

Respiratory diseases usually present no problems. If the upper respiratory tract is not examined, lesions of the larynx may be missed. Occasionally, foci of bronchopneumonia are not obvious on gross examination; hence multiple sections of the lungs should be examined microscopically in such circumstances. The presence of air in the pleural cavities should be checked for when pneumothorax is suspected. In the absence of adequate history the interpretation of the cases of bronchial asthma may be rendered difficult.

Subarachnoid hemorrhage due to rupture of a berry aneurysm is not uncommonly found in deaths of young adults. Likewise, spontaneous intracerebral hemorrhage in the region of the basal ganglia caused by rupture of a lenticulostriate artery is common in middle-aged and elderly persons. Therefore, in a case of sudden, unexpected death the examination of the brain must not be omitted, even if an apparently satisfactory cause of death may be evident elsewhere. If a subarachnoid hemorrhage is suspected to have been caused by a ruptured aneurysm, it is best to dissect the cerebral arteries on a fresh unfixed brain. In a medicolegal case it is advisable to make at least one transverse cut at the level of basal ganglia to exclude or detect intracerebral hemorrhage before the brain is fixed. In one instance a pathologist studied sections of all organs which revealed nothing and obtained negative results of exhaustive toxicological studies only to find a massive intracerebral hemorrhage when he cut the brain one month after the autopsy.

TRAUMA AND DISEASE

In the investigation of a medicolegal case of sudden, unexpected death the vital objective, it has been pointed out, is the exclusion of an unnatural cause of death. The victim of a fatal heart attack may sustain serious injuries in a fall or a person may develop a fatal heart attack or cerebral hemorrhage during an altercation. If any injuries are found on examination of the body, the examiner must answer the following questions:

1. Did natural disease alone cause death?
2. Did natural disease contribute to death?
3. Did trauma alone cause death?
4. Did trauma contribute to death?

With the history of altercation or in the presence of trauma, the conditions that frequently pose problems of interpretation are coronary artery disease, hypertensive cardiomegaly, aortic aneurysm, spontaneous intracerebral hemorrhage and rupture of a berry aneurysm. If death occurs a certain time after the injury is sustained, the role of injury in the causation of death must be carefully evaluated. Commonly encountered cases of this nature are those with spinal fracture and hip fracture.

On rare occasions the pathologist may be asked to determine whether a certain stress or trauma caused the disease or precipitated death.

As far as the heart is concerned it is generally accepted that an excessive work load can make silent coronary artery disease symptomatic, accentuate the existing symptoms or even lead to heart failure. Death precipitated by stress or trauma usually occurs immediately after the episode of such extraneous factors. Sometimes in compensation cases it is claimed that a blow on the chest caused coronary thrombosis, heart failure and death. Impact on the chest may initiate arrhythmia or cause hemorrhage in the wall of the coronary artery. Severe body injury leading to shock may predispose to cardiac dysfunction in a person with a diseased heart.

Can a mechanical injury cause cancer? Before a sound case for a cause-and-effect connection between injury and cancer is presented certain criteria must be met—previous integrity of the part, substantial injury to the part, reasonable time interval for the development of growth, development of tumor at the site of injury and proof of the nature of the tumor by microscopy.

Trauma may lead to immediate or delayed infections which may prove fatal. This complication and other aspects of the relation of trauma to disease have been discussed in detail by Moritz[5] and Brahdy.[1]

REFERENCES

1. Brahdy, L.: Disease and Injury. Philadelphia, J. B. Lippincott, 1961.
2. Johnson, H. R. M.: The incidence of unnatural deaths which have been presumed to be natural in coroners' autopsies. Med. Sci. Law, *9:*102, 1969.
3. Lasky, I. I.: The importance of autopsies in workmen's compensation cardiac fatalities. J. Forensic Sci., *15:*507, 1970.
4. Marshall, T. K.: The value of the necropsy in ascertaining the true cause of a non-criminal death. J. Forensic Sci., *15:*28, 1970.
5. Moritz, A. R.: Pathology of Trauma. ed. 2. London, Kimpton, 1954.
6. Turkel, H. W.: Merits of the present coroner system. JAMA, *153:*1086, 1953.

14

Stillbirths and Infant Deaths

The principal objective in the investigation of the death of a newborn is to establish whether the child was born alive or was stillborn. If the pathologist is involved in the investigation, he must ascertain whether the death was entirely natural, a consequence of neglect or a result of a criminal act.

STILLBIRTH

In North Carolina, as in some other states, a fetal death (stillbirth) is not treated as a reportable death unless the fetus has reached 20 weeks of uterogestation. The investigation of stillbirths by a medical examiner is not required unless there is indication that death occurred by criminal act or default, or under suspicious, unusual or unnatural circumstances. In England a stillbirth is legally defined as an infant of 28 weeks' gestation or over who has been born dead. Before 28 weeks' gestation the infant is not considered legally viable.

Every year many bodies of newborn infants are discarded in paper bags, thrown in rivers or sewers or abandoned in suitcases. Some of these are stillbirths; others are victims of negligence, adandonment or crime. When a medical examiner, coroner or the police surgeon is called upon to investigate such a death, his duty is to answer the following questions:

1. Was the child stillborn or born alive?
2. What is the intrauterine or extrauterine age?
3. What is the cause of death? Is there any evidence of negligence or crime?

Stillbirth vs. Live Birth. On external examination, an unequivocal evidence of stillbirth is maceration of the fetus, an asceptic decomposition consisting of soft, sodden skin with vesications, and laxity of joints with abnormal movements.[6] On internal examination, in a stillbirth the lungs will be unaerated, purplish, firm, noncrepitant and liver-like. They will readily sink when placed in water. If the child has breathed, the lungs will be aerated, pinkish, spongy and crepitant, and will float buoyantly in

195

water. However, if decomposition has set in, the typical characteristics of the lungs disappear. Decomposed lungs of a stillborn may not only appear aerated, feel crepitant, but may also float in water. Therefore, in the presence of decomposition the opinion as to whether the child was live or dead should be guarded. In the absence of decomposition the lungs of the stillborn weigh around 500 grains each, but the lungs of the child born alive are almost twice as heavy because of the presence of circulating blood in them (Fodéré's static test). Artificial mouth-to-mouth respiration causes expansion of the lungs.

Age. The intrauterine age of the fetus—that is, the period of gestation— can be approximated from the centers of ossification of bones and the crown-heel length of the fetus. The information in Tables 4-3 and 4-1 will be of help in determining the age of the fetus. Various criteria for assessing the age of infants born alive are discussed in Chapter 4.

Cause of Death. If signs of live birth are present in a newborn the precise cause of death should be established by a meticulous autopsy. Various causes of death in infants are discussed in the following paragraphs.

NATURAL DEATHS OF INFANTS

In infants under 28 days of age immaturity and postnatal asphyxia are the leading causes of death. In those dying in hospitals the leading causes of death are pulmonary hyaline membranes, inflammatory lesions, intraventricular (cerebral) hemorrhages.[13] According to Robbins[10] the relative frequency of some of the causes of death in infants under one year of age is:

Respiratory Infections	24	percent
Postnatal Asphyxia	18	"
Immaturity	17	"
Congenital Malformations	14	"
Birth Injuries	9	"

The medical examiner, coroner or forensic pathologist, however, is not ordinarily involved in the investigation of hospital deaths. The medicolegist has jurisdiction over sudden, unexpected, unusual and unnatural infant deaths. The commonest type of sudden, unexpected death in infancy seen in medicolegal practice is what is called crib death syndrome or cot death. This entity deserves special discussion.

Crib Death Syndrome (Cot Death)

Sudden, unexpected death in infancy known as "crib death," "cot death" or "sudden death syndrome" can be defined as "a disorder characterized by the sudden death of an infant who had previously been well or affected with a mild illness such as coryza, cough, or a mild gastrointestinal upset which was in no way felt to be of sufficient severity to have caused his death."[7]

The etiology of crib deaths is not known. Various factors such as suffocation by bedclothes and pillows, status thymolymphaticus, bacterial infection, neurogenic shock, hypogammaglobulinemia, metabolic disorders and anaphylactic shock have been incriminated by a variety of workers. Hypersensitivity to cow's milk antigens as a possible cause of crib deaths was suggested by Parish, *et al.*[9] with the finding of increased levels of milk antibodies in cases of sudden infant deaths. Geertinger[4] has suggested that incomplete embryological development of the parathyroids may be a cause of crib deaths. The majority of researchers agree that the death is from interstitial pneumonitis, and the possibility that viral infection caused this type of pneumonitis is widely recognized.

Every year in the United States alone an estimated 25,000 infants die suddenly and unexpectedly. In most places the medical examiners or the coroners are required to investigate these cases because deaths are sudden, unexpected and unattended. Often there is no medical history. The purpose of the investigation from the medicolegal standpoint is essentially to rule out the possibility of crime or accident.

General Features. The group of cases falling in the category of "crib death syndrome" reveal the following general features:

1. Age—A great majority of deaths occur during the first six months of life with the peak of infant deaths being two to four months.[11]
2. Sex—Generally, it is felt that there is a preponderance of males in the incidence of crib deaths.
3. Race—Several studies reporting population analyses indicate that (in the U.S.) Negroes show 1.7 to 3.0 times greater incidence of sudden unexpected infant deaths than do Caucasians.[12]
4. Incidence by months—It is generally agreed that the majority of infant deaths occur in the colder months of fall, winter and spring.
5. Time of day—The majority of the deaths occur between 3:00 A.M. and 9:00 A.M.
6. Preceding symptoms—Over 40 percent of the infants are well and symptom-free before being found dead. About the same number show symptoms of respiratory infection such as "cold," "sniffles," and/or "cough". A small percentage show signs of gastrointestinal disturbance.
7. Other factors—Low socioeconomic status of the family, poor infant care, illegitimacy, prematurity, young parents, large families and twin pregnancies are some of the factors that influence the incidence of crib deaths.

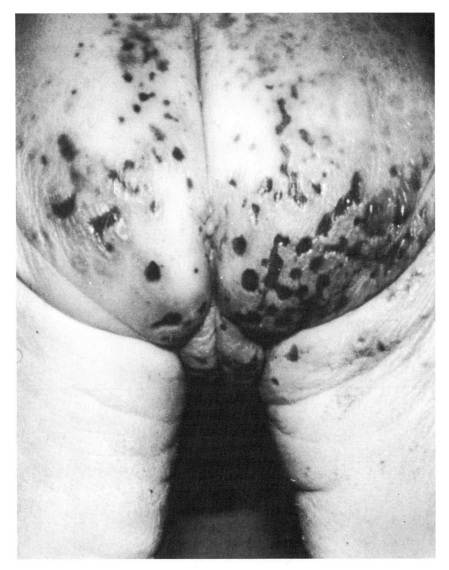

Fig. 14–1. Diaper rash (skin excoriation of buttocks) resembling abrasions.

Pathological Findings. In most (over 80 percent) of the cases of crib death syndrome the autopsy is, in a conventional sense, negative. The usual findings are increased weight of the lungs, patchy or uniform purplish discoloration of the surface of the lungs, slightly firm consistency of the discolored areas, congestion and slight edema of the tissue. Other visceral

organs do not show anything much more than congestion. Petechial hemorrhages may be seen in the surfaces of the lungs, heart and thymus gland.
Some children show evidence of prematurity and poor infant care such as
diaper rash (Fig. 14-1). Microscopically the lungs show congestion, patchy
endema and areas of alveolar collapse. The alveolar walls are thickened
with an infiltrate of lymphocytes, occasional neutrophils and monocytes
(Fig. 14-2). Occasional alveoli contain macrophages and alveolar lining
cells. Aspiration of the vomitus may be seen. Blood cultures are negative
and lung tissue cultures are either negative or reveal contaminants or
nonpathogens.

In some cases, of course, a well-defined pathological change is seen to
account for death. Conditions occasionally encountered are acute bronchopneumonia, acute tracheobronchitis, gastroenteritis, meningitis and congenital anomalies.

UNNATURAL DEATHS OF INFANTS

Laws concerning the killing of infants vary from country to country.
In England, the laws spell out special leniency to the mother killing her
child; the Infanticide Act provides that "where a woman by any wilful act
or omission causes the death of her child, being a child under the age of
twelve months, but at the time of the act or omission the balance of her
mind was disturbed by reason of her not having fully recovered from the
effects of giving birth to the child, or by reason of the effect of lactation
consequent upon the birth of the child," then she shall be guilty of infanticide. If guilty of this offense, in most instances, the woman is merely bound
over to be of good behavior. In the United States the person responsible
for the death of the infant is charged with murder; the imposing of lesser
charges in some instances however, is not uncommon.

Causes of death in infanticide or child murder seen in medicolegal practice include: blunt force (battered child syndrome), suffocation, strangulation, drowning, cutting and stabbing wounds, burns and scalds, poisoning.

Battered Child Syndrome

Child abuse has been aptly defined by Gil[3] as: "Non-accidental physical
attack or physical injury, including minimal as well as fatal injury, inflicted
upon children by persons caring for them." The victims are usually children
under the age of five. They are subjected to repeated trauma, most often
by one of the two parents. The method of inflicting injuries varies; the
parent may pull the scalp hair, hold the head and strike it against hard
objects, whip or kick the child or even inflict burns. The child may be

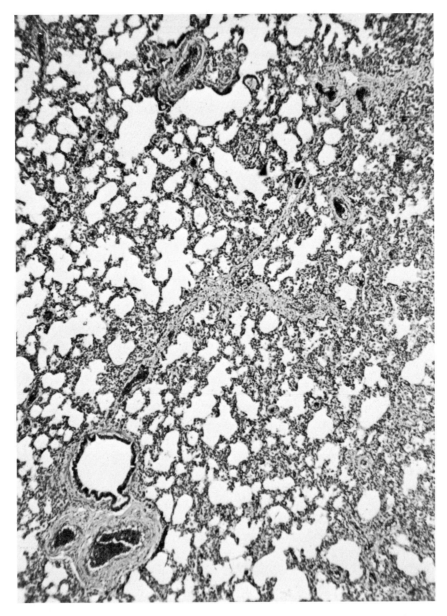

Fig. 14–2. Crib death syndrome. A section of lung showing thickening
of the alveolar walls (× 50).

starved or neglected. The child may be taken to hospital if the injuries are
not concealable. The parent usually alleges that the injuries were accidental. The parents frequently have mental, social, marital and economic
problems and regard the child as unwanted.

Tens of thousands of children are severely battered in the United States each year and many of them die from child abuse. Numerous papers and books have been written to document the history, incidence and social aspects of the battered child syndrome.[2, 5, 8] The pathologist should be aware of the method of investigation of this difficult group of cases.

Examination of the Scene. When a case of possible child abuse is reported and if the body is still at the scene of death, the pathologist must visit the scene to make a preautopsy investigation. The preliminary investigation should include detailed questioning of the persons responsible for the care of the infant, nearest relatives and neighbors. A social history of the parents and the past medical history of the deceased child must be carefully probed into, particularly previous hospital admissions. The person responsible for inflicting the injuries and causing death will, on questioning, probably come out with a variety of false explanations for the injuries. Statements to the effect that the child fell from the crib, was hit by an older sibling or was accidentally knocked while opening the door are not uncommon. The pathologist should proceed with an open mind and not fall into the trap of accepting such statements as true. The scene investigation should include notations about the general location of the home, the state of repair, degree of cleanliness, condition of heating and cooling appliances and so on. The examination of the body of the infant should include observations about general nutrition; stage of rigor, livor and decomposition; body temperature (record rectal temperature) and various injuries on the body. Every effort should be made to make an objective evaluation of the statements of the persons at home pretaining to the cause of injuries. Evidence of overturned furniture and other evidence indicating points of impact of the body with articles in the house should be noted. Whenever possible photographs of the scene should be taken.

Examination of the Body. The autopsy on the case of child abuse preferably should be performed by a competent forensic pathologist.

External examination. After the clothes are examined and removed and trace evidence collected, a thorough external examination should be made. General observations about the height, weight, state of nutrition, diaper rash and identifying features should be recorded. The body may bear evidence of recent and old trauma in the form of abrasions, bruises and fractures. The bruises and abrasions on the knees and elbows can be sustained in falls but those on other parts of the body should arouse suspicion of foul play (Fig. 14-3). General features of the injuries such as shape, color, location and pattern, together with precise measurements, should be recorded. Particular attention should be paid to the discoloration of bruises for this may indicate the time of infliction of injuries (see Chap. 6). On external examination the fractures of the skull, ribs and the long bones may be felt (Fig. 14-4). Photographs of the face and of all injuries should be made.

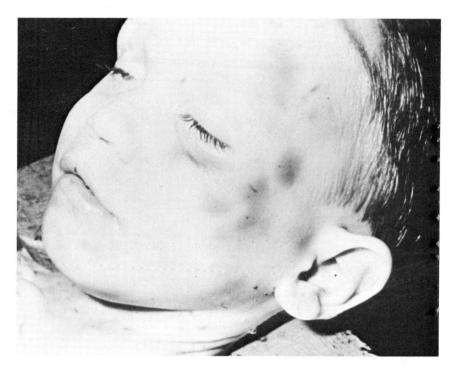

Fig. 14–3. Battered child syndrome. Multiple bruises should arouse suspicion of foul play.

Roentgenographic examination. The x-ray examination of the body must
always be a part of an autopsy on a case of battered child syndrome. As
a routine the entire body should be x-rayed. Fractures of skull and of the
distal parts of extremities may be missed if these areas are not x-rayed.
The x-rays will reveal recent and old fractures, may help in aging the
bony injuries and will serve a useful purpose in court (Fig. 14-5).
  Internal examination. All the internal injuries should be described in
detail and photographed. Reflection of the scalp will reveal old and recent
bruises that may not be visible on external examination. The pathologist
should incise various bruises for examination and should not hesitate to
excise the skin and scalp bearing injuries for histological examination.
  In the head there may be evidence of old injuries in the form of organizing subdural or subarachnoid hemorrhage, and brown-yellow areas of
cortical softening reflecting healing contusions. Recent injuries frequently
seen are fractures of the skull, fresh subdural and subarachnoid hemorrhage, and contusions and lacerations of the brain (Fig. 14-6). In the
chest, free blood may be present in the pleural cavities with recent trauma.
Multiple fractures of ribs, recent fractures and fractures showing variable
degrees of healing are commonly seen (Fig. 14-7). Recent fractures may
be associated with contusions of the lungs and heart. Blunt force on the

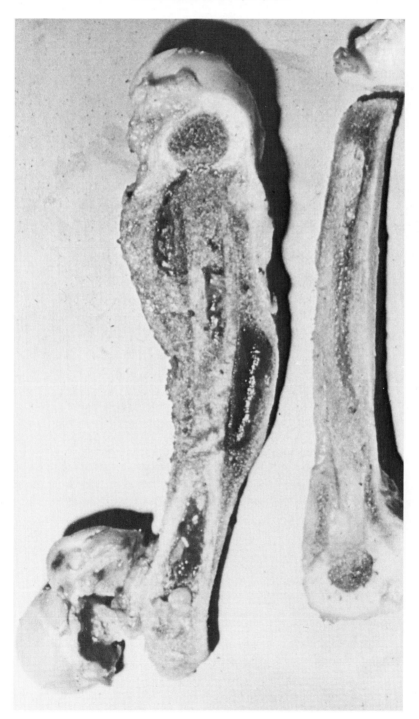

Fig. 14–4. Battered child syndrome. Healing fractures of the femur.

Stillbirths and Infant Deaths

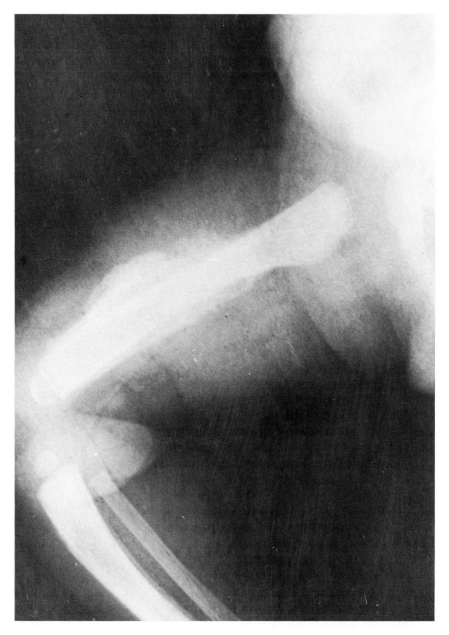

Fig. 14–5. Battered child syndrome. An x-ray of the thigh shows healing of a fracture of the femur.

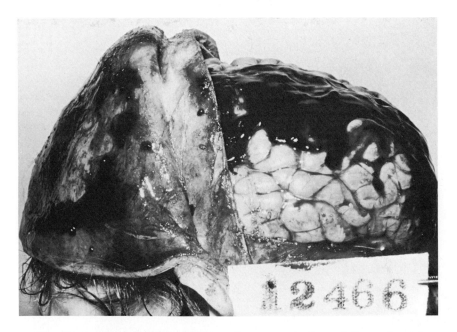

Fig. 14–6. Battered child syndrome. Recent contusions of the scalp and fresh subdural hematoma. (Courtesy of David K. Wiecking, M.D.)

abdomen may cause superficial and deep lacerations of the liver. Fatal laceration of the spleen may be seen.

Microscopic examination of various injuries is important in the case of battered child syndrome, since it will reveal the degree of healing and may assist in determining the time of infliction of injuries. Disparity in the changes in various injuries will point to the repetitious nature of the injuries. Therefore, areas bearing injuries, especially bruises, should be microscopically examined.

Suffocation, Strangulation, Drowning

Death from Suffocation. A newborn or an infant a few months old is likely to succumb without resistance if the mouth and the nose are obstructed by some means. Methods commonly used to obstruct breathing are placement of a soft pillow, bedclothes or hands over the face. Occasionally, death results from gagging when the infant's mouth is stuffed with some material.

These cases present two significant problems. First, airway obstruction may occur while the child is being fed at the breast or by overlaying of the

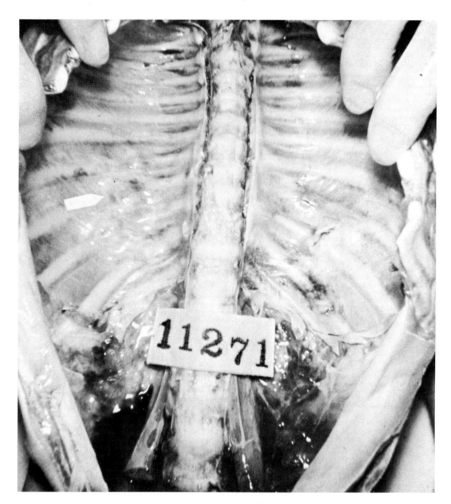

Fig. 14–7. Battered child syndrome. Healing fractures of ribs. (Courtesy of David K. Wiecking, M.D.)

sleeping mother. Occasionally a weak, sick infant may suffocate in a soft pillow. It may be difficult or even impossible to differentiate accidental suffocation from criminal killing if the circumstances are not clear.

The second major problem is created by the fact that the autopsy in these cases is frequently negative. Although such a death is an asphyxial one, changes such as petechial hemorrhages may be absent. Thus, it may not be possible to make the diagnosis of death from suffocation. The finding of bruising of lips and gums should arouse the suspicion of smothering.

Death from Strangulation. This usually presents little difficulty, since the ligature used (scarf, stocking or other material) is frequently in position on the neck or the ligature mark and the asphyxial changes (petechial hemorrhages in the skin, conjunctivae and larynx) are obvious. In considering the case of a newborn, the possibility of strangulation by the umbilical cord should be kept in mind for this would weigh heavily in favor of death being accidental. In the presence of advanced decomposition, the diagnosis of death from strangulation may be rendered extremely difficult because the ligature mark and the petechial hemorrhages may be obscured.

Death from Drowning. It is not uncommon to find bodies of newborn infants in toilet bowls. A pregnant woman in the second stage of labor may have a desire to defecate or urinate and go to the toilet. While she is on the toilet, precipitate delivery may cause the newborn to fall into the water and drown in the mixture of birth fluids and water. When blood, vaginal mucus and meconium are found in the air passages of the drowned newborn at the autopsy, no suspicion of foul play should be entertained if a consistent story of precipitate labor comes forth.

Cutting and Stabbing Wounds, Burns and Scalds, Poisoning

Death from Cutting and Stabbing Wounds. The use of cutting and stabbing instruments to kill infants is rare. When this type of killing is done the weapons used are those readily available in homes (e.g., scissors, kitchen knives and pen knives). Figure 7-3 illustrates a killing by knife.

Death from Burns and Scalds. Killing by fire is extremely rare. However, a maltreated child may be scalded, usually by hot water in a bathtub, probably because the defense of "accidental" scalds is easy to sustain.

Death from Poisoning. Other than by accidental overdosage, poisoning is not common in infants and children. A mother preparing to commit suicide may poison her child. Where coal gas is used for domestic purposes, poisoning by carbon monoxide is sometimes seen. On rare occasions narcotics and hypnotics are administered to children in lethal doses. Whenever poisoning is suspected, a thorough investigation must be carried out as outlined in Chapter 19.

REFERENCES

1. Caffey, J.: Multiple Fractures in the Long Bones of Infants Suffering from Chronic Subdural Hematoma. Am. J. Roentgen., *56:*163, 1946.
2. Fontana, V. J.: The Maltreated Child. Ed. 2. Springfield (Ill.), Charles C Thomas, 1971.
3. Gil, D. G.: Incidence of child abuse and demographic characteristics of persons involved. *In* Helfer, R. E., and Kempe, C. H. (eds.): The Battered Child. Chicago, University of Chicago Press, 1968.

4. Geertinger, P.: Cot deaths—associated with congenital anomalies of the parathyroids of infants. Experimental production of parathyroid abnormalities in the offsprings of rats. J. Forensic Med., *14:*46, 1967.
5. Helfer, R. E., and Kempe, C. H. (eds.): The Battered Child. Chicago, University of Chicago Press, 1968.
6. Mant, A. K.: Forensic Medicine—Observation and Interpretation. Chicago, Year Book Publishers, Inc., 1960.
7. Melton, J. W., Fatteh, A., and Mann, G. T.: Sudden and unexpected deaths in infancy. Va. Med. Mon., *95:*63, 1968.
8. Kempe, C. H., and Helfer, R. E. (eds.): Helping the Battered Child and His Family. Philadelphia, J. B. Lippincott, 1972.
9. Parish, W. E., Barrett, A. M., and Coombs, R. R. A.: Further investigations on the hypothesis that some cases of cot-death are due to a modified anaphylactic reaction to cow's milk. Int. Arch. Allergy, Appl. Immunol., *24:*215, 1964.
10. Robbins, S. L.: Pathology. ed. 3. Philadelphia, W. B. Saunders, 1967.
11. Valdes-Dapena, M.: Sudden and unexpected death in infants; the scope of our ignorance. Pediatr. Clin. North Am., *10:*693, 1963.
12. Valdes-Dapena, M.: Review article—Sudden and unexpected death in infancy: A review of the world literature 1954–1966. Pediatrics, *39:*123, 1967.
13. Valdes-Dapena, M., and Arey, J. B.: The causes of neonatal mortality: an analysis of 501 autopsies on newborn infants. J. Pediatr., *77:*366, 1970.

15

Transportation Fatalities

INVESTIGATION OF AUTOMOBILE ACCIDENTS

Vehicles of transportation are responsible for a great number of fatalities. In the United States alone automobiles kill over 50,000 people per year. Every vehicular death is a nucleus of a potential lawsuit or insurance claim. In view of this, every jurisdiction in the world requires that a medicolegal investigation of a transportation fatality be carried out. Many times the circumstances of the death demand that an autopsy of the decedent be a part of the investigation. Thus, a pathologist is frequently involved in the investigation and is required to answer several questions.

Ideally, investigation by a pathologist should include examination of the scene and performance of the autopsy.

Examination of the Scene

Every medicolegal investigation of a death should begin with the examination of the scene. Deaths resulting from automobile crashes should be no exception. As a part of the investigative team, whenever possible, a pathologist should visit the scene of death. There can be no substitute for the eyewitness study of the crash scene, for the eye sees much more at the spot than the mind can imagine at a distance. In addition to making the general survey at the scene of the fatality, the medical man should conduct a careful external examination of the body in order to render help in the exact reconstruction of the incident. Photographs should be an integral part of the scene investigation.

If the pathologist is unable to visit the scene, he should obtain as much information as possible from the investigators who were present. Sometimes the circumstances of the accident are clear and the cause of the crash obvious; at other times the pathologist may need to quiz the investigators carefully to get a clear idea of the happenings at the scene. In order to give a complete picture of the crash, investigators at the scene should be ready to provide the following information:

1. Time and date of accident.
2. Name(s) of decedent(s), whether driver, passenger or pedestrian.
3. Positions of victims (if more than one) and degree of injuries.
4. Brief background information about the decedent if suicide suspected.
5. Findings indicating suspicion of manslaughter or murder.
6. Make and position of vehicle and degree of damage.
7. Behavior of vehicle prior to crash.
8. Points of impacts and relative positions of vehicles (if more than one).
9. Estimated speed of vehicle and posted speed limit.
10. Condition of road.
11. Skid marks, brake marks.
12. Weather conditions (rain, fog) and lighting conditions.

Ordinarily the examination of the vehicle is made by appropriate investigators but the pathologist does not have to be involved in that part of the investigation. However, for the proper correlation of injuries sustained by the occupants and the impact points on the interior parts of the vehicle, it is sometimes necessary for the medical man to examine the vehicle. In lieu of this, the investigators concerned may be asked to look for items of evidential and correlative value such as fibers of clothing, human tissue and blood and hair at the possible points of impacts.

Police officers and other investigators make good notes of the findings of their investigations in most places in the United States and in Europe, and frequently record the scene with photographs. If it is not routine practice for them to take photographs, but if the gravity of the scene indicates, they should be requested to take photographs of the road, of the exterior and interior of the car at the points of occupant impact, and of the persons killed.[5] These pictures often are of invaluable help in the correlation of the various findings later. Police officers in many places also make drawings depicting various details of the crash. These give helpful information to the pathologist for his reconstruction of the crash.

The Autopsy

An autopsy on a transportation death is not always a simple matter of recording the gross injuries.[12] It involves careful consideration of various medical and legal questions and accurate correlation of the findings with these questions. No contemporary textbook of forensic pathology is complete without a discussion of the considerations of an autopsy on a vehicular death victim, since every pathologist has to deal with such a case.

The principal objectives of autopsies on vehicle-related deaths are:

1. Reconstruction of the crash to determine its cause.
2. Determination of the cause of death.
3. Determination of the manner of death (i.e., natural, accidental, suicidal, homicide).
4. Establishment of the identity of the decedent.
5. Identification of the driver and reconstruction of the positions of the victims prior to the accident.
6. Differentiation of injuries caused by being hit from those caused by being run over.
7. Identification of the automobile in the case of hit-and-run incidents.
8. Determination of the significance of previous injuries in a case of delayed death.
9. Documentation of the findings to aid legal processes.

There is no doubt that a pathologist can greatly aid in the investigation of a transportation vehicle fatality by providing answers to these vital questions that could otherwise remain unanswered if the autopsy were not performed.

Reconstruction of the Crash

A careful evaluation of all the aspects of the crash is essential for its accurate reconstruction. Details of the scene investigation form a vital part of this process. In the autopsy room the clothing should be inspected and meticulously described. All injuries on the external surface of the body—abrasions, bruises, lacerations and fractures—should be adequately described, drawn on body diagrams and photographed. A detailed analysis of even small and less serious injuries seen externally sometimes helps make an accurate reconstruction of the crash.[2, 13] The findings of the internal examination of the body may provide missing links.

Natural Death (at the Wheel) vs. Death from Injuries

Natural disease conditions can and do lead to accidents and cause the death of the driver while he is at the wheel. The most common cause of sudden, unexpected death is coronary artery disease. This condition causes disability of the driver while at the wheel more often than any other natural disease condition. A study by West[20] showed that 15 percent of the drivers who were dead within 15 minutes of an accident died from heart disease, mainly coronary artery disease. In general, chronic medical ailments are responsible for 15 to 25 percent of all crashes.[19]

When a person is found in a crashed vehicle, one of the most important questions to be resolved is whether he died from injuries sustained in the

crash or whether the death was natural. It is extremely important to determine this issue adequately, for a death insurance policy with a clause
for double indemnity for accidental death is bound to lead to an unsatisfactory situation or exhumation of the body if it is buried without a complete investigation. Only a complete autopsy can provide the right answer.
Mere absence of external injuries is no sound reason for doing away with
autopsy and pronouncing death natural. The conclusions could be wrong.

A 60-year-old man with a history of "angina" lost control of his car while
driving on a city street and gently crashed into a telephone pole. He was
found dead at the wheel. The only external injuries on the body were abrasions on the face and knees. The autopsy revealed no coronary artery disease and death was from hemothorax due to traumatic rupture of the
thoracic aorta associated with fractures of several ribs.

In another case, a middle-aged man who had always enjoyed good health
was driving along a road when the car swerved and crashed into a tree. He
was ejected from the car and was found dead with severe lacerations of the
face, fracture of the left clavicle and dislocation of the right ankle with skin
lacerations. At the autopsy, no significant internal injuries were seen. The
coronary arteries were severely atherosclerotic and the descending branch
of the left coronary artery contained a recent antemortem thrombus. This
explained the cause of the accident and of death.

In circumstances in which an acute illness causes the driver to lose control of the vehicle, commonly no major injuries are sustained by the driver,
the passengers or the pedestrian hit. A person suffering a heart attack
while driving is, more often than not, able to slow down or stop the vehicle in time to avoid collision.

In the case of pedestrians, cardiovascular or cerebrovascular disease,
poor vision, impaired hearing and reduced mobility may be some of the
factors leading to accidents. Also, a pedestrian lying in a street may be run
over after death. Positive determination of the cause of death and the evaluation of other factors is possible only with an autopsy.

Death may result a long time after the person sustains injuries in an
automobile accident. It then becomes important to determine whether the
death was entirely natural or directly or indirectly related to the remote
trauma. A common type of case is one in which a person sustains a fracture of the cervical spine and becomes quadriplegic. Such a person may
spend years immobilized in the hospital, with complications such as bed-
sores, bouts of pneumonia or urinary tract infections, and may eventually
succumb to one of these complications. Instances of survival for 20 to 30
years after the initial injury have been observed. If the autopsy findings,
evaluated in light of the history, indicate direct or indirect cause-and-effect
relationship between the injury and death, such a death cannot be considered natural and should be certified as a complication of the injury.

A death occurring suddenly sometime after even minor trauma should also be investigated carefully. The objective should be to establish or exclude the role of injury in the person's death. The following cases make the point.

An elderly woman pedestrian was hit from the back by a car. She sustained what appeared to be minor bruising of the right leg. Ten days later she was found dead in bed at home. Necropsy showed massive pulmonary embolism with thromboses of the veins of the right leg and extensive contusion of the calf muscles. The death was certified as accidental.

In another case a young man who was a front seat passenger in a car, sustained chest injuries during a collision. He was admitted to the hopsital and diagnosed to have two broken ribs on the left side. He was observed for two days and discharged since his general condition was good. A year later he suddenly collapsed while walking and died. The autopsy revealed a ruptured aneurysm of the left ventricle (Fig. 15-1). One of the fractured ribs had

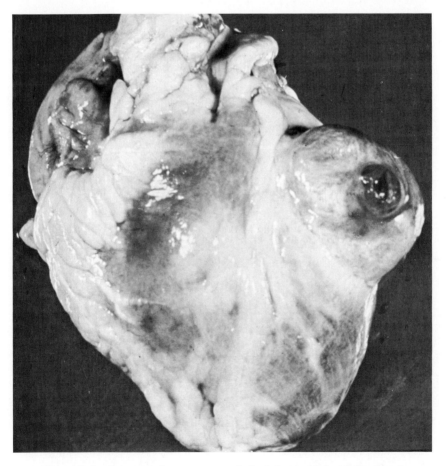

Fig. 15–1. A traumatic aneurysm of the left ventricle of the heart.

malunited and the broken end was directly in contact with the aneurysm. The coronary arteries were healthy and the aneurysm was considered to be traumatic in origin.

Thus, a pathologist is required to answer questions such as: (a) Did the natural condition lead to the accident; (b) did the injury or the natural disease cause death, and was death related to immediate or remote injuries? The answers may have far-reaching significance.

Homicide with the Automobile

The automobile is responsible for most accidental deaths. Occasionally it is used for criminal purposes. A crime may be committed with the help of a vehicle in the following four ways:

1. Premeditated murder by killing a pedestrian with an automobile: The investigation of such a situation is not a difficult problem if the killing is witnessed by others or the criminal makes a confession.

> After visiting a bar, two men were involved in an argument over a few cents. One of them told the other to wait on the street for a few minutes so that he could go home and get the money. The debtor got into his car, drove around the block and sped back at 60 mph. in a 25 mph. zone, running over the waiting man and killing him.

> On another occasion a man drove at another, forced him against a wall and crushed him with the automobile repeatedly until he died.

If the driver of the car leaves the scene and there are no signs of premeditation, such a killing may be easily classed as a hit-and-run death.

2. Hit and run: This is perhaps the most common crime with the automobile resulting in injury or death. The driver of the automobile "accidentally" kills or injures a person and leaves the scene to avoid blame. If death results some jurisdictions regard this as murder, others consider it manslaughter. Both offenses are grave; hence the investigation of such fatalities should be as thorough as possible.

The most important issue in the investigation of a hit-and-run fatality is the identification of the vehicle and the driver causing the death. A careful examination of the scene and of the body and collection of gross and trace evidence are essential. The materials that must be retained from a hit-and-run victim are: clothing, including shoes, blood, urine, hair from the victim's scalp and pubis, and dirt, grease, glass, oil and rust (if present) on the clothes and on the body.

The clothes may show a tire tread pattern that helps associate a suspected vehicle to the crime. In addition to the routine blood alcohol determination, the blood type of the decedent should always be determined. Examination of the blood on the vehicle may reveal the matching blood type. If any hair found on the vehicle matches hair of the victim by gross and microscopic examination and by neutron activation studies, identification of the criminal driver is more easily determined. Likewise, matching studies of other materials (e.g., dirt, grease, glass, paint, oil and rust) found on the victim and the vehicle in question can lead to the identification of the driver and the vehicle involved.

A less important issue to be resolved with respect to a hit-and-run death is whether the person was standing at the time he was hit or was run over while lying on the road. The pattern of injuries and other findings may help determine the position of the victim at the time of first vehicle contact.

Hit while standing. If the pedestrian is hit while standing, the impact on the left side of the body results in tearing of the left side of the trousers or stockings; abrasion, contusion, and laceration of the left leg; and fractures of the left tibia and fibula.[17] If the pedestrian is hit on the right side while crossing the road a converse picture results. Impacts from behind and in front result in injuries from secondary contact to the back of the head and forehead respectively, in addition to bilateral and sometimes symmetrical injuries to the lower extremities from primary impact with the automobile (Fig. 15-2).

Injuries from being run over. If a person is run over by a vehicle and dragged, there may be no impact injuries but the clothes are torn, avulsion (compression and tear abrasion) of skin is seen, especially in groin regions, and compression injuries of the internal organs are present. In addition, the body or clothing of the decedent may show oil spots and rust from the low parts of the automobile. The automobile, in turn, may show fibers from the decedent's clothing, as well as hair and blood on some of its low parts. The most convincing piece of evidence is the presence of tire treads on the decedent's clothing or on the body skin (Fig. 6-2). However, a vehicle may pass over a body without leaving any skin injuries.

When a person is believed to have been run over some additional questions must be answered: Was he first hurt and then run over? Was he dead before he was run over? Did running over kill him? If run over by two cars, which car killed him? Great caution should be exercised in answering these questions.

3. Accident faked to conceal crime: This is a rare event. A person may be killed by other means, the body placed in an automobile and pushed off the road to make the scene look like an accident. A high degree of suspicion is needed in dealing with such a possibility, in addition to careful evaluation of all the injuries and the cause of death. With the slightest suspicion of foul play the autopsy should include photographs and x-rays of the body.

4. Concealment of crime by burning a murder victim in a car: The following case history illustrates the various aspects of such a disposal of a dead body.

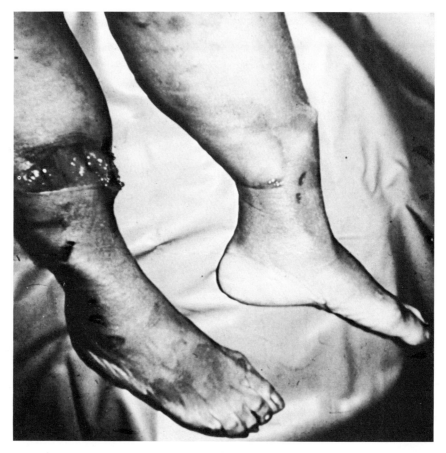

Fig. 15–2. Bilateral injuries from being hit from the back by the bumper of a car.

The torso of a 21-year-old white male was found severely charred in a burned Pontiac with license plates from a Cadillac (Fig. 15-3). Autopsy showed significant negative findings—absence of soot in the air passages and carboxyhemoglobin saturation of only 15 percent in the blood. The man had been shot to death, the hands and head cut off and the torso burned in the car (see pp. 173, 174).

Suicide with the Automobile

The interpretation of an automobile suicide is one of the most difficult tasks in the practice of forensic pathology. Unless the circumstances are clear, conclusions concerning the manner of death are hard to draw. The determination of the exact manner of death is often vital to the settlement

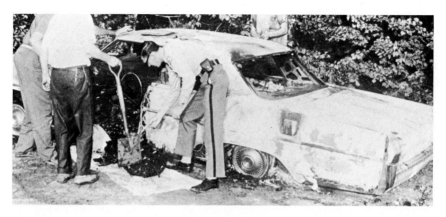

Fig. 15–3. An attempt was made to dispose of this body of a murder
victim by burning.

of insurance claims. The facts and findings that usually help identify suicide with an automobile are:

1. Previous suicide attempts, recent threats to commit suicide.
2. History of depression, recent as well as past, and evaluation of psychiatric data.
3. History of domestic quarrels, financial crises or other acute depres-
   sion-inducing circumstances.
4. Evidence of speeding.
5. Absence of evidence of braking.
6. Impact with a tree or bridge abutment usually at the dead center of
   the front of the vehicle.
7. Presence of a suicide note.

Lone occupancy of the car, presence of a slight to moderate amount of
alcohol in the blood of the victim and straightness of the road are factors
that are commonly observed.

A young man drove from home after a domestic argument with his wife,
saying as he left that he was going to kill himself. A few minutes later, at the
end of the straight section of a road he was found dead in the driver's seat.
The center of the front of his car was caved in due to impact with the bridge
pillar.

Driver Identification

If there is more than one occupant in the car that is involved in a crash
and the driver escapes with minor injuries, he may claim that he was not
a driver. Also, with multiple fatalities in a crash with ejection of the occupants of the car, it may not be clear who was driving. A pathologist may

be asked to render assistance in driver identification. Of all the investigators the pathologist is perhaps in a position to contribute the most in the problem of the identification of the driver. A helpful line of investigation is:

1. Detection of steering wheel imprint and/or injuries such as rib fractures, sternum with or without rupture of thoracic aorta and hemopneumothorax.
2. Finding of paint or glass from the door on the driver's side on the decedent's body or clothes.
3. Finding of cloth fibers, hair and tissue from the suspected driver on the driver panel, door or glass on the driver's side or on the steering wheel and column.
4. Search of the imprints of the brake or accelerator pedal designs on the sole of the driver's shoe.
5. Matching of the decedent's blood type with that of the blood on the driver panel, driver door and steering assembly.

The finding of injuries caused by the seat belt may also help in the identification of the driver. Seat belts can cause intestinal injuries (mesenteric and intestinal tears), spinal injuries, rupture of a pregnant uterus and rupture of a kidney, liver or spleen.[8, 11, 15]

Alcohol and Drugs

While performing an autopsy on a motor vehicle death, the possibility of alcohol and/or drugs playing a part in causing the accident and death always should be kept in mind.

It has been estimated that the consumption of alcohol by drivers and pedestrians leads to 25,000 deaths and a total of at least 800,000 crashes in the United States each year.[16] Alcohol is the largest single factor leading to fatal crashes and 1 to 4 percent of the drinking drivers are responsible for about 50 to 55 percent of all single-vehicle crashes.[3] Furthermore, it has been estimated that there are between 5 and 6 million chronic alcoholics in the United States and that about 80 percent of them drive automobiles.[1]

Psychoactive drugs are used by drivers and some crashes can be attributed to impairment from the effects of these drugs.[18] Long-distance drivers sometimes abuse amphetamine and this abuse may lead to an accident, as can the use of tranquilizers, depressants and marihuana. Antihistamines as well as other drugs taken therapeutically may affect driving safety, particularly in combination with alcohol.[7] Also, the possibility of carbon monoxide poisoning should not be forgotten.

With the exception of marihuana, the other drugs mentioned can be identified in the biological materials. Therefore, from the body of a traffic victim, a sample of blood and urine, if available, should always be obtained. Failing to get either of these specimens, a portion of the liver and of the brain should be retained. Details of the methods of collection of specimens are given in Chapters 1 and 19. The results of the toxicological analysis of the materials not only help explain the cause of the accident but also may be useful in the overall investigation of the case and the legal procedures that follow and the insurance claims that arise.

Conclusion

Investigation of an automobile death is frequently inadequately conducted by medical investigators partly because important questions are not anticipated at the time of investigation. There are many facets of the investigation and each one has far-reaching consequences. The importance of proper handling of an automobile fatality cannot be overstressed. The following components of investigation procedures should not be neglected.

1. Scene investigation with photographs.
2. Complete autopsy with recording of injuries by description, drawings and photographs.
3. Collection of evidence—clothing, paint traces, glass splinters, oil spots, rust, blood spots.
4. Follow-up studies—blood typing, analysis for carbon monoxide (if fire), alcohol (always), amphetamines (especially in truck drivers) and other drugs (if indicated).

The pathologist should expect to appear in court on at least some of these cases. Legal issues that require his testimony relate to

1. Double indemnity claims on accidental deaths.
2. Civil action for compensation for damages.
3. Criminal prosecution for murder or manslaughter.

Proper documentation of such cases is invaluable, since some of these cases may not go to court for several months or even years, and the memory of the facts may have faded completely. Record keeping is a vital part of the total investigation.

INVESTIGATION OF AIRCRAFT ACCIDENTS

The most important thing in the investigation of an aircraft accident is the preaccident organization. A pathologist in general practice and even a full-time forensic pathologist may never have to investigate an aircraft accident. On the other hand, one may be faced with the problem suddenly and unexpectedly. The need for planning and organization for such an eventuality cannot be overemphasized. The potential of the pathologist in the investigation of an aircraft accident is preeminent, since there are certain questions that cannot be answered by any other investigator.[9, 14]

The general objectives of the investigation of aircraft accidents are essentially the same as those for the investigation of automobile fatalities. In view of multiple fatalities, identification of the dead victims is a vital problem more often in aircraft accidents than in automobile accidents and identification of the pilot is an essential prerequisite to the detection of a pathological cause for the accident. (See Chaps. 4 and 5.) In this chapter, practical procedures for the pathologist to follow are outlined step by step. For greater detail the reader is referred to the publication of the Joint Committee on Aviation Pathology[6] and the United States Departments of Army, Navy and Air Force.[4] The three stages of investigation are:

1. Preaccident organization.
2. Scene investigation and autopsy.
3. Follow-up investigations.

Preaccident Organization. In order to be ready for an unanticipated disaster, a team consisting of the pathologist, Federal Aviation Agency investigators, local law enforcement agents, medical examiners (coroners or police surgeons), funeral directors and fire brigade and civil defense personnel should be formed to discuss and prepare plans for the handling of the accident. The team should prepare a list of supplies and the sources from which these can be obtained at short notice. Some of the important items that are needed at the time of investigation are body pouches, name tags, plastic bags, flashlights, photographic equipment and forms for recording findings of the investigation.

Scene Investigation and Autopsy. In case of an accident involving a small private airplane with no more than 3 or 4 fatalities, the investigation can be conducted almost in the same fashion as for the automobile crash. A well-coordinated team, however, should be implemented for the handling of a mass disaster with many casualties. The team of nonmedical investigators at the scene should do the following:

1. Seal off the area of disaster to prevent spectators and press reporters from interfering with the investigation.
2. Take photographs of the wreckage and bodies, before and after placing identifying numbers.
3. Examine the aircraft and its loose parts, including the seats, seat belts and surrounding structures.
4. Help the medical investigators to examine the bodies of the victims before they are moved.

The principal tasks of the pathologist begin when the bodies are removed from the scene for postmortem examinations. In order to be able to reconstruct the accident, the pathologist should first acquaint himself with its details and the type of aircraft. He should then systematically proceed as follows with each body:

1. Photograph the body, with and without clothes and take x-rays when indicated.
2. Describe clothing and personal effects in detail.
3. Obtain fingerprints or ask police to do it.
4. Make dental records or request a dentist to do it.
5. Note identifying features such as body build, height, weight, color of eyes, skin and hair, tattoos, scars, old fractures, bony deformities, absent organs surgically removed, and diseases.
6. Describe and photograph external injuries and burns and record them on body diagrams.
7. Make internal examination and record and photograph injuries.
8. Look for natural disease conditions and describe them in detail.
9. Retain tissues for histological studies and toxicological analyses and hair samples for identification.

For histological examination sections from all organs, skin and bone should be kept. For toxicological analyses the specimens of blood (50 to 100 ml.), urine (all available), liver (100 to 200 Gm.), brain (100 to 200 Gm.), one kidney, part of a lung and stomach contents should be kept. If none of these is available unburned skeletal muscle (200 to 300 Gm.) should be retained.

Before the bodies are released, if identity of the decedents is not established, relatives or friends should be invited to look at the bodies to make a personal recognition provided the features, especially facial, are recognizable.

Follow-up Investigations. Once the immediate tasks are completed, the pathologist can add up the information to reconstruct the mishap. Additional investigations to establish the identity of the decedent, cause of death, and cause of accident may be required. Records of the decedents' fingerprints and dental and medical records should be traced to determine identity. Relatives should be interviewed to obtain information about the body features, clothes and other personal effects.

Histological studies should be completed to confirm grossly seen diseases and to detect microscopic lesions such as myocarditis, myocardial fibrosis and so on. Despite careful examination conditions such as idiopathic epilepsy and hypoglycemia may not be detected.

Toxicological analyses should always be performed on the pilot, other crew members and if indicated on passengers. The analysis for *alcohol* should be done routinely. Some small plane crashes are caused by alcoholic intoxication. The use of tranquilizers, analeptics and narcotics may also cause accidents. The blood should also be tested as a routine for *carbon monoxide* intoxication, especially if there was a fire. The estimation of the concentration of lactic acid in the brain is considered to be helpful in recognizing hypoxia prior to death. It has been suggested that a concentration of over 200 mg. of lactic acid per 100 Gm. of gray matter of the brain is almost always from hypoxia due to low oxygen tension in the inspired air.[10] Such a concentration may also result from drowning or a state of shock for a short period of time prior to death.

REFERENCES

1. Campbell, H. E.: Traffic deaths go up again. JAMA, *201:*183, 1967.
2. Camps, F. E.: Reconstruction of accidents from examination of injuries. Med. Sci. Law, *3:*545, 1963.
3. Fatteh, A., Hudson, P., and McBay, A. J.: Highway homicides and suicides. North Carolina Med. J., *32:*184, 1971.
4. Government Printing Office: Autopsy Manual. Washington, Department of the Army Technical Manual TM 8-300, Department of the Navy Publication NAVMED P-5065, Department of the Air Force Manual AFM 160-19, 1960.
5. Huelke, D. F., and Gikas, P. W.: Investigations of fatal automobile accidents from the forensic point of view. J. Forensic Sci., *11:*474, 1966.
6. Joint Committee on Aviation Pathology: An Autopsy Guide for Aircraft Accident Fatalities. Washington, Armed Forces Institute of Pathology, 1957.
7. Landauer, A. A., and Milner, G.: Antihistamines, alone and together with alcohol, in relation to driving safety. J. Forensic Med., *18:*127, 1971.
8. LeMire, J. R., Earley, D. E., and Hawley, C.: Intra-abdominal injuries caused by automobile seat belts. JAMA, *201:*109, 1967.
9. Mason, J. K.: Aviation Accident Pathology. London, Butterworth, 1962.
10. Neiss, O. K., Lentz, E. C., Townsend, F. M., Davidson, W. H., and Chubb, R. M.: The role of the physician in the investigation of aircraft accidents. JAMA, *184:*115, 1963.
11. Porter, S. D., and Green, E. W.: Seat belt injuries. Arch. Surg., *96:*242, 1968.
12. Simpson, K.: Current studies in the pattern of traffic accidents. *In* Simpson, K. (ed.) Modern Trends in Forensic Medicine. London, Butterworth & Co., 1967.
13. Simpson, K.: The interpretation of surface pattern of vehicular injuries. Med. Sci. Law, *1:*420, 1961.
14. Stevens, P. J.: Fatal Civil Aircraft Accidents. Their Medical and Pathological Investigation. Baltimore, Williams & Wilkins, 1970.
15. Tourin, B., and Garrett, J. W.: A Report on Safety Belts to the California Legislature: Summary and Analysis of California Highway Patrol; Reports and Opinions on 54,348 Automobile Accidents, New York: Automotive Crash Injury Research of Cornell University, 1960.

16. U.S. Department of Transportation: Alcohol and highway safety—A report by the Secretary of the U.S. Department of Transportation to the Congress, Aug. 1968.
17. Voorde, M., and Vereecken, L.: An analysis of 285 legal autopsies in road accidents—reconstruction of the accident. Med. Sci. Law, *11:*187, 1971.
18. Waller, J. A.: Drugs and highway crashes. JAMA, *215:*1477, 1971.
19. Waller, J. A.: Medical impairment and highway crashes. JAMA, *208:*2293, 1969.
20. West, I., Nielsen, G. L., Gilmore, A. E., and Ryan, J. R.: Natural death at the wheel. JAMA, *205:*68, 1968.

16

Investigation of Deaths from Therapeutic Mishaps

OPERATIVE AND ANESTHETIC DEATHS

Medicolegal systems throughout the world require the investigation of deaths from operative and anesthetic mishaps. Such deaths are variously defined: In some jurisdictions they are deaths on the operating table; in others they are deaths before patients recover from the effects of anesthesia and anesthetics. In still other places they are all deaths within 24 hours after the operation. Whatever the definition, two facts should be clearly recognized: First, every operative or postoperative death does not spell negligence; second, every such death is not necessarily caused by the operation or anesthesia.

Investigation of a death from an operative or anesthetic mishap is not an easy task for the pathologist for several reasons: He has to attribute death, in some instances, to a mistake by a professional colleague, or he must rely on the information given to him by the defaulting parties. Furthermore, he has to draw important conclusions on many occasions from nonspecific autopsy findings. If the facts of the case are obvious enough to explain the death there is no difficulty. However, while dealing with borderline situations in which there is a question of professional negligence the objectivity of the pathologist may be shaken. He may tend to interpret the findings in favor of a colleague whose professional reputation may be at stake. Nevertheless, absolute impartiality must be maintained by the pathologist while investigating such deaths.

One or more factors may be involved in an unexpected death during or immediately after an operation. The pathologist should take into consideration the following aspects when faced with an investigation of an operative or anesthetic death.

1. History.
2. Condition requiring surgery.
3. Other preexisting conditions.
4. Preanesthesia medications.

5. Anesthetic agents and management of anesthesia.
6. Possibility of burn or explosion.
7. Bleeding and shock during and after the operation.
8. Incompatibilities of transfused blood.
9. Resuscitative measures.
10. Autopsy findings.
11. Toxicological analyses.

History. Before beginning an autopsy on any anesthetic or operative death, the pathologist should obtain full information about the facts surrounding the death. A thorough review of the hospital chart and discussions with the members of the operating room team and other involved personnel make the task of the interpretation of the findings easier. Extreme care should be exercised in obtaining the history from the persons involved. A sympathetic yet frank approach is more likely to result in the revelation of reliable facts than is terse questioning that is likely to antagonize the persons volunteering the information. Defensive postures and statements during history taking demand cautious interpretation.

Factual data should be carefully evaluated and should form a part of the autopsy report. Vital information (e.g., records of blood pressure readings on the chart and episodes of arrhythmias on the electrocardiograms) is readily found on the patient's chart. Such records are usually more reliable than oral statements. Experience indicates that in most instances the parties involved advance factual data and attempts to "cover up" the mistakes are rare. No doubt this is true because genuine errors are difficult to hide, and if there is no negligence there is no shame in explaining the facts. Only rarely is it necessary to interview independent observers and discard the information provided by members of the operating team.

Condition Requiring Surgery. Some conditions for which the operation is planned or performed are obviously high risk, and the team of the surgeon and anesthesiologist knowingly take a calculated risk. Resection of the aortic aneurysm and plastic repair can be considered a high-risk operation. These cases commonly come to the attention of a medical investigator. In some of these cases, while performing the operation even with due care, it becomes impossible to control the bleeding and the patient dies on the operating table. In many jurisdictions such cases are certified, quite justifiably, as natural deaths.

Occasionally, surgical errors cause death. For instance, the ligation of the ureter during abdominal surgery or ligation of the coronary artery while implanting a heart valve prosthesis are surgical mishaps. If death results from such an error it is classified as a therapeutic misadventure—in other words, an accident.

Other Preexisting Conditions. Preexisting conditions other than the one for which the patient is operated on should be adequately elucidated, since they may cause death under extra operative and anesthetic stress. These contraindications to operative procedures are not always easy to identify clinically, and even if they are identified their seriousness may not be appreciated. For example, symptomless coronary artery disease may prove fatal on the operating table because of accentuation of anoxia by the anesthetic agents. In elderly persons with brown atrophy of the heart, incipient heart failure may escape detection. Other conditions such as anemia, bronchitis, emphysema or interstitial pulmonary fibrosis, thyrotoxicosis, myxedema and hypertension, if present, may contribute to death. Proper assessment of such diseases helps to establish the degree of negligence if there was any.

It is the duty of the physicians in charge of the patient to exclude the contraindications before the administration of anesthesia and the performance of surgery. Even minor infections may create complications as in the following case [Butler vs. Layton, 164 N.E. 920 (Mass. 1929)].

> A doctor was found liable for damages in a suit by a patient who developed acute bronchitis after being given ether for a tonsillectomy. The patient was suffering from a severe cold on the day of the operation. The physician knew about the cold. It was established by expert testimony that the administration of ether caused the bronchitis.

Preanesthetic Medications. Errors in relation to preoperative medication are: giving a wrong medication, giving too much of a medication, or not giving any medication. Any of these errors can be a major factor in precipitating death. In a study of 1024 postoperative deaths, Phillips[20] indicated that "Errors in preoperative preparation and medication of the patient and the selection of the anesthetic agent accounted for about one fourth of the deaths." Therefore, the investigation of an anesthetic or operative death should include data on the name of the drug used for premedication, the quantity administered and the time of administration.

Anesthetic Agents. Anesthesia is the main cause of death in over 6 percent of postoperative deaths and a contributing factor in over 12 percent of such deaths.[20] Information about the anesthetic agent used, its quantity and the method of administration is vital. Note should also be made of the duration of time the patient remains under the anesthesia. Equally important is the information about the management of the anesthetic. In an excellent objective study of 1027 anesthesia-related deaths, Memery summarized the involvement of the anesthesiologist by saying "The primary fault of the anesthesiologist was improper management of the anesthetic and the secondary fault was improper management in the immediate postoperative period."[18] The Baltimore Study Committee[20] also concluded that "Faulty management of the anesthetic was the cause (of death) in around

50 percent of the cases." It becomes clear from these statements that adequate analysis of the facts about the management of the patient while under anesthesia is important. Gross errors such as inadvertent mixing of the anesthetic gases have occasionally resulted in deaths.

Possibility of Burn or Explosion. Deaths from anesthetic explosions are rare. However, Camps and Purchase[7] described two cases in which an explosion burst the bag and broke the bottles. At autopsy in one the esophagus was found to be bruised and the stomach torn to shreds; in another, the lungs showed blast injuries. In 1955, in a damage suit by a patient for injuries sustained by the explosion of anesthetic gas, the hospital was held liable. The explosion was caused by a spark of static electricity [Andrepont vs. Ochsner, 84 So. 2nd 63 (La., 1955)]. If death results from an anesthetic explosion, the pathologist's task is not difficult. Investigators should, however, take every care to establish the cause of the explosion.

Bleeding and Shock. In most operations bleeding is not a problem, since a continous replacement of blood is carried out as necessary. There are times when bleeding becomes uncontrollable, as in the operation for resection of an aortic aneurysm referred to above, and death results. In person with silent coronary artery disease, blood loss could lead to unexpected death. Blood loss and the consequent shock should be evaluated with other findings of the case.

Incompatibilities of Transfused Blood. General pathologists frequently have to investigate episodes of blood transfusion reactions and incompatibilities and are usually well aware of the method of investigation of such complications. Therefore, the discussion of this aspect of an operative death is omitted here, but a few comments are included with the discussion of iatrogenic diseases (p. 230).

Resuscitative Measures. Emergencies may arise either before, during or after an operation. Resuscitative measures can be instituted satisfactorily only if the equipment is readily available and there is someone with the patient who can render assistance. Failure to provide resuscitation is evident if care is exercised in ascertaining the details of the predeath moments.

Autopsy Findings. Where the circumstances and cause of death in an anesthetic or operative death are not clear, an autopsy is mandatory. Only a postmortem examination enables one to evaluate the nature of the disease or condition for which the operation was performed as well as the other conditions enumerated above. One may be able to detect an unsuspected cause of death (e.g., pulmonary, fat or air embolism or the evidence of asphyxia) from aspiration of regurgitated material. Such findings are not uncommon.[1] The findings of internal hemorrhage, peritonitis and retained swabs or instruments are of course obvious, but only if an autopsy is performed. The postmortem examination may also reveal the evidence of hypersensitivity reactions. Campbell[5] presented a fine review of autopsy findings in 195 cases in which death was associated with anesthesia.

No doubt there are some conditions that are not detected at autopsy. Vagal inhibition, fall in blood pressure, arrhythmias of the heart, spasm of the coronary arteries and spasm of the larynx do not leave traces at autopsy. Findings such as the impaction of the epiglottis into the larynx[4] and anoxial changes may not be easily detected at the postmortem table.

It is important to remember that anesthetic agents cause certain signs and symptoms and pathological changes. For instance, chloroform is hepatotoxic and sometimes produces ventricular fibrillation; ether leads to convulsions; cyclopropane and trichloroethylene cause cardiac irritability. These compounds cause anoxial changes, and microscopic examinations are necessary to detect them. The smell of the anesthetic agents used may be obvious during the course of autopsy.

Toxicological Analyses. From a case in which the anesthetic agent is suspected to be the cause of death, specimens should be retained for toxicological studies. In addition to routine specimens collected for poisoning cases, alveolar air should be collected with a needle and syringe by puncturing the lung before the chest is opened, and blood should be collected under oil.[6]

In some instances toxicological analyses render significant assistance in the overall interpretation of the case. The analyses help in (a) detecting and estimating the quantity of the drug mistakenly given, (b) estimating overdoses of premedications, and (c) estimating concentrations of anesthetic agents. The fatal concentrations of some of the anesthetic agents in blood are:[6]

	Percent (mg.)
Chloroform	40–60
Ethyl chloride	40
Ethyl ether	> 180
Trifluoroethylvinyl ether	50
Halothane	20
Divinyl oxide	68

LOCAL ANESTHETICS

Anesthetic agents for local anesthesia are administered as sprays and injections, and are commonly used for block infiltration and for spinal and epidural anesthesia. Despite extensive use of local anesthetics, their lethal potentialities are not sufficiently recognized. Deaths from local anesthetics usually occur from overdosages or from abnormal responses such as allergic reactions, hypersensitivity and idiosyncrasy. Overdose is, of course, by far the most common cause of fatalities from anesthetic agents.[14] Overdosages result from injections of excessive quantities, injections of concentrated solutions, accidental introduction of a drug into the blood stream or from topical application of excessive quantities of concentrated solutions to mucous membranes.[2] Factors that play an important role in influencing the toxicity of local anesthetics include: (a) the susceptibility of the patient, (b) the patient's general condition, (c) the rate of administration of the anesthetic agent and (d) the vascularity of the area injected. All these factors should be taken into consideration while investigating a death from the use of local anesthetic, and pertinent information with reference to these factors should be obtained *prior* to the autopsy.

Most local anesthetics are synthetic drugs, and in toxic quantities they act as central nervous system stimulants. The symptoms and signs of toxicity include nausea, vomiting, headache, excitement, muscular twitches and convulsions. Just prior to death there is a fall in blood pressure, shock, paralysis, areflexia and unconsciousness.

The purpose of an autopsy is to obtain additional evidence to establish or exclude the anesthetic agent as the cause of death. In most instances of death from overdose, the only change is that of anoxia. Hypersensitivity reactions may be obvious in some instances. A cause of death totally unrelated to the administration of the local anesthetic may be found with the gross and microscopic studies of the tissues. It may be possible to identify and quantitate the local anesthetic or its breakdown products in the biological materials. Therefore, blood, brain, liver and tissue from the site of injection should be routinely retained. Blanke[3] presented a review of the toxicological problems of local anesthetics in which he indicated that "Frequently, toxicological analysis of postmortem specimens is the only means by which the problem can be resolved."

THERAPEUTIC MISADVENTURE, IATROGENIC DISEASE

Almost every therapeutic drug on the market can cause death and every therapeutic procedure can prove fatal. In some of these deaths there may be an element of neglect on someone's part. Therefore, any death resulting from a therapeutic procedure or from the administration of a drug or drugs in which there is even a remote possibility of negligence should be investigated by the pathologist. The autopsy helps establish whether the death was, in fact, the outcome of the therapeutic misadventure or whether it was from a preexisting natural disease. In some cases the autopsy may not provide all the answers. It has been said that sometimes at autopsy "All that remains then is a catalogue of possibilities and suspicions and the Forsenic pathologist must bear in mind that almost any change found at autopsy, may, in fact, be referable to previous drug therapy."[13]

Mishaps can occur in different ways. In a thirteen-year study of fatalities from therapeutic misadventures, Gormsen (1960) found 60 cases. In this series, 20 deaths resulted from overdoses or wrong medications, 15 from administration of anesthesia, 10 from various therapeutic procedures, 9 from anaphylaxis and 6 from various diagnostic procedures.

Allergy, Anaphylaxis. The entity of anaphylaxis following an administration of certain drugs is well known. Deaths from anaphylaxis are rapid. The clinical features of allergy include skin rashes, urticaria, exfoliative dermatitis, necrotizing dermatitis, fever, asthma, conjunctivitis, arthralgia and capillary damage leading to purpura and hemorrhage. Blood studies may show eosinophilia, agranulocytosis, thrombocytopenia and hemolysis. With severe reactions there is shock, acute breathlessness and angio-edema.

The *autopsy findings* in the cases of anaphylactic death may include edema of the larynx, cyanosis, petechial hemorrhages in the surfaces of the lungs, heart and the thymus, dilatation of the heart, and edema of the lungs and brain. The reader is referred to an excellent study by Delage and Irey[9] in which clinicopathologic findings are discussed in 43 cases of anaphylactic death.

Among the drugs responsible for hypersensitivity reactions perhaps the most notorious is penicillin. Fatalities following injections of penicillin are not rare. Stajduhar[23] described deaths from anaphylactic shock due to injections of the combination of penicillin and streptomycin. Once the person becomes sensitized to penicillin, the sensitization lingers indefinitely and the person is always in danger of fatal reaction. Anaphylactic reaction to tetracycline has also been reported. Fellner and Baer[11] described a case in which the patient became dyspneic, dizzy and flushed, and developed tachycardia and generalized urticaria after the administration of tetracycline hydrochloride. Allergic reactions to aspirin, sometimes serious or fatal, occur in about 1 in 500 patients.[24] The usual manifestations are asthma, laryngeal edema and angioneurotic edema.

Overdoses. Acute poisoning due to massive overdoses of therapeutic agents and chronic poisoning due to repeated doses are discussed by Roche and Cotte.[21] Errors in prescribing, labeling and dispensing sometimes cause fatalities (Fig. 16–1). Johnson[15] discussed deaths from accidental therapeutic overdoses of adrenaline poisoning. He pointed out that such cases present difficulty in investigation, since the autopsy findings and the toxicological studies are negative because adrenaline decomposes rapidly and disappears from the tissues.

Complications of Transfusions. Mishaps following injections and trans-

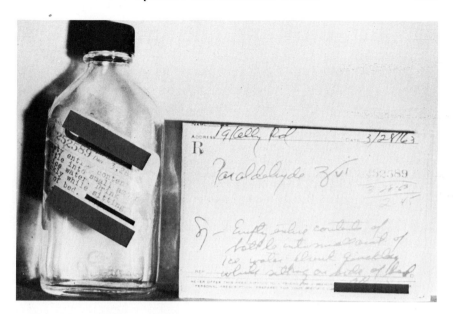

Fig. 16–1. An error in a prescription proved fatal. (Courtesy of Dr. Arthur J. McBay.)

fusion, such as entry of broken needles into the tissues or blood stream, frequently occur. Fatalities from injections of benzene, strophanthin and from air embolism during plasma transfusion have been described.[17] Serious or fatal complications of blood transfusion include episodes of bleeding as a manifestation of hemolytic reaction due to hypofibrinogenemia, hypothrombinemia and thrombocytopenia. Other complications of blood transfusion that may be found in fatal cases are hemosiderosis, viral hepatitis, hyperkalemia and hypocalcemia.

Complications of Diagnostic Procedures. Biopsy procedures and other diagnostic tests may be associated with fatal complications.

A 65-year-old woman was being examined for a gastric ulcer. A gastroscope was introduced to a length of 25 cm. with some difficulty. Thirty to 60 seconds later, however, the patient struggled to pull out the tube and became unconscious. Resuscitative measures failed to revive her. At the autopsy, three focal contusions of the mucosa of the proximal part of the esophagus, three ulcers of the gastric fundus, each 4 mm. long, and circumferential contusions of the larynx, trachea, right main bronchus and the bronchus to the right lower lobe were found. There was no significant disease condition in the body. Examination of the gastroscope revealed leakage of current within a portion of the instrument. Death was from low voltage current electrocution.[16]

Radiological procedures used for diagnostic purposes sometimes prove fatal. Accidents such as poisoning by barium enema, traumatic rupture of the rectum during the procedure of barium enema, and chemical peritonitis with the faulty use of barium enema have been described.[8]

Complications of Surgical Procedures. These have already been described briefly. Delayed complications which appear years or even decades after surgery should be interpreted in the right perspective. In the following instance the cause of death was a delayed, unexpected complication of a relatively safe surgical procedure.[10]

> A 65-year-old-woman sustained a fracture of the neck of the femur for which an open reduction and hip nailing were done. An abscess developed at the site of the fracture and one of the pins migrated inward through the head of the femur into the rectum (Fig. 16-2). She died from the effects of a large perirectal abscess despite removal of the pin.

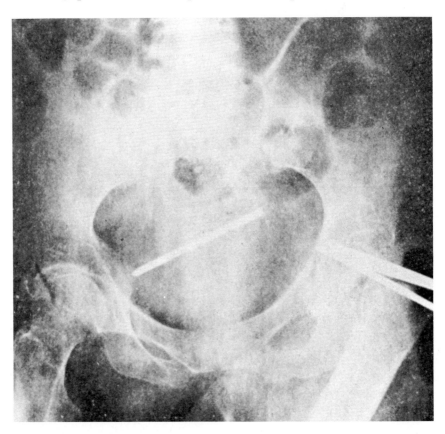

Fig. 16–2. Migration of a hip nail through the head of the femur into the rectum. (Reproduced with the permission of the editor, Military Medicine. From Fatteh, A.: Case for diagnosis. Milit. Med., *136*:291, 1971.)

Miscellaneous. Fetal and neonatal deaths in utero occur from adverse effects of drugs administered to the mother during pregnancy. Instances of fetal death from Dicumarol,* Diabenese,† Orinase,‡ Serpasil,§ iodides, synthetic vitamin K and thiazide diuretics when administered to pregnant women have been cited by Moser.[19]

There are numerous other iatrogenic diseases that may confront a pathologist with investigative problems. Details of these cannot be given in a text of this size. For additional reading the reader is referred to two excellent works on the subject. The book edited by Moser[19] is an encyclopedic manual dealing with almost every drug-related complication. Hundreds of references are included in this work. For pathologists the work of Spain[22] is recommended; in this the pathologic lesions of various iatrogenic conditions are described.

SUMMARY

When a death results from a therapeutic mishap several parties are involved—doctors, nurses, hospital, patient's kin and insurance companies. With an unexpected death the relatives of the decedent may believe that there was negligence on the part of the doctor and/or the hospital. The law demands that the professional personnel exercise due care and skill in their services to the patient. For these reasons every death from a therapeutic misadventure should be investigated by an independent medicolegal investigator. The most important part of the investigation of an operative, anesthetic or therapeutic death is a complete discussion of the case with all persons involved in the treatment of the patient. Some of the questions that the investigator is required to answer are:

1. What was the cause of death?
2. Was there any negligence on the part of the treating physician or other personnel of the hospital?
3. Was the error, if any, the sole cause of death?
4. How long would the person have lived if the therapeutic measures had not caused death?

Only the full knowledge of the circumstances of death and the autopsy findings will help answer these questions.

* Trademark, Wisconsin Alumni Research Foundation
† Trademark, Pfizer
‡ Trademark, Upjohn
§ Trademark, Ciba

REFERENCES

1. Adriani, J.: Selection of Anesthesia. Springfield (Ill.), Charles C Thomas, 1955.
2. Adriani, J.: Techniques and Procedures of Anesthesia. Springfield (Ill.), ed. 2. Charles C Thomas, 1956.
3. Blanke, R. V.: Toxicological problems of local anesthetics. J. Forensic Sci., *5:*539, 1960.
4. Caiger, G. H.: Role of epiglottis in anesthetic deaths. J. Forensic Med., *18:*78, 1971.
5. Campbell, J. E.: Deaths associated with anesthesia, Evaluation of 195 personally autopsied cases during a 30-month period. J. Forensic Sci., *5:*501, 1960.
6. Camps, F. E. (ed.): Gradwohl's Legal Medicine. ed. 2. Bristol, England, John Wright & Sons, 1968.
7. Camps, F. E., and Purchase, W. B.: Practical Forensic Medicine. London, Hutchinson, 1956.
8. Corby, C., and Camps, F. E.: Therapeutic accidents during the administration of barium enemas. J. Forensic Med., *7:*206, 1960.
9. Delage, C., and Irey, N.S.: Anaphylactic deaths: a clinicopathologic study of 43 cases. J. Forensic., *17:*525, 1972.
10. Fatteh, A.: Case for diagnosis. Milit. Med. *136:*291, 1971.
11. Fellner, M. J., and Baer, R. L.: Anaphylactic reaction to tetracycline in a penicillin—allergic patient. JAMA, *192:*997, 1965.
12. Gormsen, H.: On therapeutic misadventures in the last few years in Denmark. J. Forensic Med., *7:*179, 1960.
13. Goulding, R.: Mishaps of modern therapeutics—side-effects of drugs. *In* Simpson, K. (ed.): Modern Trends in Forensic Medicine. New York, Appleton-Century-Crofts, 1967.
14. Hirschfelder, A. D., and Bieter, R.: Local anesthetics. Physiol. Rev., *12:* 190, 1932.
15. Johnson, H. R. M.: Therapeutic accidents—adrenaline poisoning. J. Forensic Med., *7:*198, 1960.
16. Kazi, S. S., and Hlivko, T. J.: Iatrogenic disease—a constant hazard. Medico-Legal Bulletin No. 230, Office of the Chief Medical Examiner, Richmond, 1972.
17. Laves, W.: Therapeutic misadventures. J. Forensic Med., *7:*186, 1960.
18. Memery, H. N.: Anesthesia mortality in private practice: a ten-year study. JAMA, *194:*127, 1965.
19. Moser, R. H.: Diseases of Medical Progress: A Study of Iatrogenic Disease. Springfield (Ill.), Charles C Thomas, 1969.
20. Phillips, O. C.: The Baltimore Anesthesia Study committee, review of 1024 postoperative deaths. JAMA, *174:*2015, 1960.
21. Roche, L., and Cotte, L.: Therapeutic accidents from overdose of drugs. J. Forensic Med., *7:*190, 1960.
22. Spain, D. M.: The Complications of Modern Medical Practices. New York, Grune & Stratton, 1963.
23. Stajduhar, Z.: Fatal cases subsequent to application of antibiotics. J. Forensic Med., *9:*59, 1962.
24. Thomson, W. A. R.: Therapeutic poisoning. Med. Sci. Law, *5:*210, 1965.

17

Artefacts in Forensic Pathology

INTRODUCTION

In his Ward Burdick Award address at the thirty-fifth annual meeting of the American Society of Clinical Pathologists in Chicago, Alan R. Mortiz, comprehensively discussed "Classical Mistakes in Forensic Pathology."[11] His reflections touched upon, among other matters, the objectives of medicolegal autopsies, incomplete autopsies, misinterpretations of postmortem findings and mistakes in collection and presentation of evidence. The subject of artefacts has not been adequately discussed in the literature. Pathologists do sometimes misinterpret artefacts and draw wrong conclusions. A clear appreciation of what constitutes an artefact in a medicolegal autopsy perhaps will help reduce the number of mistakes. For this reason, a detailed discussion of various artefacts observed at autopsies on medicolegal cases is presented.

According to *Dorland's Illustrated Medical Dictionary,* an artefact is "Any artificial product; any structure or feature that is not natural, but has been altered by processing. The term is used in histology and microscopy for a tissue that has been mechanically altered from its natural state." For the purpose of the present discussion, this definition has been modified to be any change caused or a feature introduced into a body after death, that is likely to lead to misinterpretation of medicolegally significant antemortem findings, is considered to be an artefact. In other words, an artefact is a finding which is adventitious or physiologically unrelated to the natural state of the body or the tissues or the disease processes to which the body was subjected prior to death.

Artefacts can be broadly divided in two groups: those introduced during the period between death and the autopsy, and those introduced during autopsy. These are reviewed in this chapter. The artefacts encountered in the cases of gunshot wounds and burns are described in Chapters 8 and 11.

Artefacts Introduced Between Death and Autopsy

These artefacts are many and varied. For the purpose of simplification, they are classified into the following groups:

1. Agonal artefacts.
2. Resuscitation artefacts.
3. Embalming artefacts.
4. Interment and exhumation artefacts.
5. Artefacts due to handling of the body.
6. Artefacts related to rigor and livor.
7. Decomposition artefacts.
8. Toxicological artefacts.
9. Miscellaenous artefacts.

Agonal Artefacts. A common agonal artefact is regurgitation and aspiration of gastric contents. Frequently physicians give aspiration of gastric contents as a cause of death, often erroneously, when they see regurgitated material in the mouth and nose. Pathologists too may fall into the trap of misinterpreting the finding of aspirated material in the air passages. Regurgitation and aspiration occur, even in natural deaths, as a terminal event or from handling of the body or resuscitation, although it is often of no significance. In order to assess the incidence of aspiration of gastric contents in the larynx, trachea and the main bronchi, this author recorded observations on 210 medicolegal cases. The results showed that in cases with a distinct cause of death other than aspiration, the finding of aspiration of gastric contents was common; 23.5 percent of the cases showed evidence of aspiration.

Resuscitation Artefacts. A body subjected to resuscitative efforts may reveal injection marks, bruises and fractures. The injection marks are usually seen in the cardiac region or on the extremities. The intracardiac injection may be associated with bruising of the heart and collection of some blood in the pericardium. In cases of suspected drug abuse, recognition of the injection marks caused postmortem is, for obvious reasons, important. Also, many of the injection marks may be associated with postmortem bruises. A ringlike bruise is sometimes caused by a defibrillator applied to the chest.

Ribs, sometimes several, and even the sternum, are not uncommonly fractured during external cardiac massage. In the majority of cases these fractures can be indentified as postmortem if there is no hemorrhage at the fracture sites and no contusion of the intercostal muscles is present. Sometimes, however, recent hemorrhage may be present even in postmortem fractures. In such cases, confusion is avoided if the history regarding the resuscitative measures is carefully obtained. Evaluation of such fractures is of immense significance in deaths from violence, particularly in cases of beatings and battered babies. External cardiac massage, with or without fractures of the ribs or the sternum, is frequently associated with fat or bone marrow embolization. Hudson[8] made a controlled study of 1800 autopsy cases in which external cardiac massage had been applied at the time of death. He found marrow emboli in the lungs in 10 percent of the cases (Fig. 17-1), and fat emboli, with or without marrow, in 20 percent of the cases. In the control cases, such a finding was a rarity.

Rescue squads and hospitals employ positive pressure breathing apparatus (oxygenator) for resuscitation and this tends to leave the evidence of acute emphysema, occasionally with subpleural blebs, air in the medi-

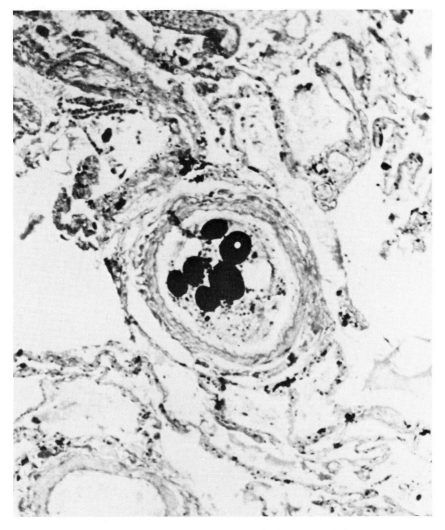

Fig. 17–1. A section of lung showing marrow embolus in an artery (postmortem embolization due to resuscitative measures). Osmic acid stain (× 250).

astinum and even tension pneumothorax. Resuscitative contusion of the soft tissues of the neck can raise suspicions of homicidal strangulation as in the following case:

> A 15-month-old child was brought to the emergency room of a hospital in a moribund state. The attending physicians attempted desperately to put a tube down the throat and had much difficulty doing so. Nevertheless, they persisted but the efforts were of no avail. At the autopsy marked contusion of the larynx and the surrounding soft tissues was seen (Fig. 17-2). The whole of the right lung was consolidated by pneumonia. The death was natural and the bruising of the neck tissues was artefactual.

Embalming Artefacts. In the United States, with rare exceptions, all bodies are embalmed before burial. The embalming may be arterial through

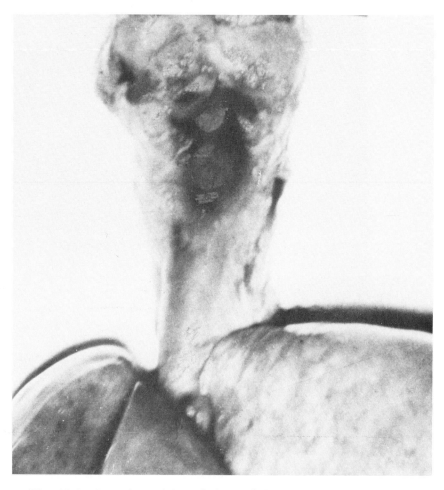

Fig. 17–2. Contusions of the soft tissue of the neck caused during efforts to introduce a rubber tube down the throat.

incisions at the sites of approachable arteries or with a trocar introduced through the abdominal wall. The embalmer may enlarge a homicidal stab wound to approach an artery or may introduce a trocar through a gunshot wound and modify its dimensions. In a case with multiple gunshot wounds, trocar holes may add to the difficulties (Fig. 17-3). In addition, the trocar may disturb the track of the weapon or the bullet, creating false tracks. Components of the embalming fluid often add to the worries of forensic toxicologists (see below).

Interment and Exhumation Artefacts. In bodies interred for some time and later exhumed, fungus growth is common at body orifices, eyes and sites of open injuries. When the fungus is removed, the underlying skin

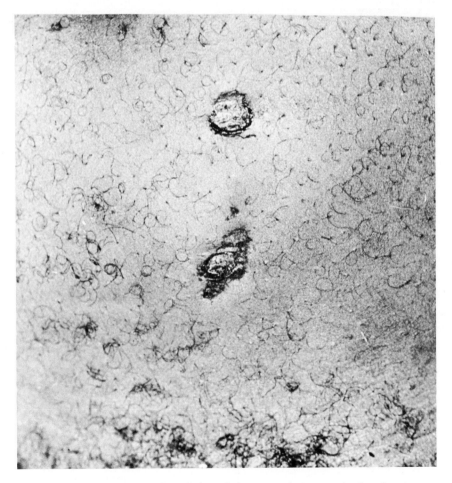

Fig. 17–3. Abdomen of a victim of three gunshot wounds showing two embalmer's trocar holes that were initially mistaken for gunshot wounds.

presents discoloration simulating bruising (see. Fig. 17-4). While performing an autopsy on an exhumed body, agonal artefacts and those due to resuscitation, embalming, handling of the body after death and to a previous autopsy should be borne in mind. The artefacts falling to the fate of the toxicologist and those due to decomposition are discussed elsewhere.

Artefacts Due to Handling of the Body. The artefact that stands out prominently, from the point of view of medicolegal significance, is fracture of the cervical spine. Rough handling of the body can and occasionally does result in such a fracture. In most cases the absence of significant hemorrhage helps to identify the fracture as postmortem in orgin. Slight hemorrhage at the fracture site, however, is not too uncommon. In a victim of a fall or other violence, a cervical spine fracture with some hemorrhage in the fracture line can create a puzzling situation.

Another postmortem injury that calls for care in interpretation is bruising in the region of the occiput. Robertson and Mansfield[14] noted the production of a postmortem "bruise" of the scalp, about an inch in diameter, from careless bumping of the head on a stretcher. In view of this instance, the possibility of a head injury during life should be excluded by collateral evidence whenever such a problem presents itself.

Artefacts Related to Rigor and Livor. *Rigor mortis.* In a case where estimation of the time of death is important, some reliance may be placed on the onset or state of rigor mortis. One of the commonest artefacts related to rigor mortis is the "breaking" of the rigor during the handling of the body. The onset or progress of rigor may be significantly affected by postmortem circumstances (e.g., extreme heat or cold) or antemortem conditions (e.g., extreme hyperthermia due to widespread infections). Rigor in a dead body may be erratic. To illustrate one extreme of this, two cases of antenatal rigor mortis, recorded by Paddock,[12] are cited. Rigor mortis may cause alterations in the heart that can lead to misinterpretations. As early as 1851 Maschka wrote: "The musculature of the heart affected by rigor mortis, and stiffened, may rather easily simulate concentric hypertrophy of that organ to the untrained postmortem examiner." Similarly, the presence of primary and secondary dilatation of the heart caused by rigor mortis, as discussed by Forster,[6] may create confusion.

Livor mortis. The color of the areas showing hypostasis is normally purplish. A characteristic "cherry" pink color is seen in the cases of carbon-monoxide poisoning. It must be noted, however, that pink hypostasis is a common finding in bodies exposed to cold temperatures in an open environment or in bodies refrigerated for some time. Localized areas of hypostasis may resemble bruises. There are, however, many definite points of distinction between the bruises and the localized areas of livor simulating bruises.[18]

Decomposition Artefacts. Changes caused by decomposition may be mis-

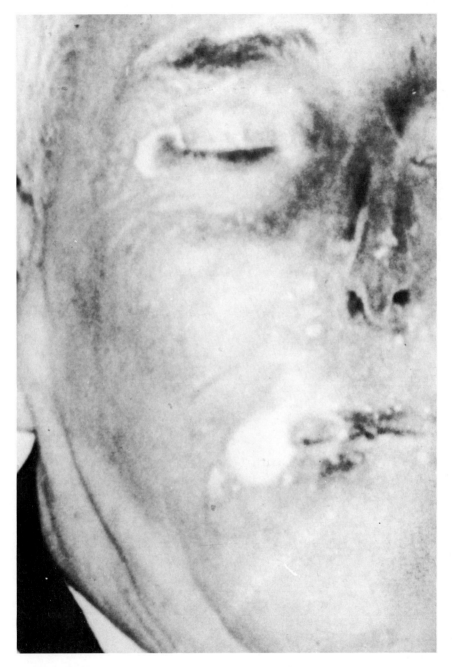

Fig. 17–4. The face of an exhumed body shows discoloration of the skin around the nose (caused by fungus), simulating antemortem burning.

takenly interpreted as pathological lesions. A statement made to this effect in 1882 by Schauenstein[15] in *Maschka's Handbook of Forensic Medicine* is valid even today. Decomposition of the body is responsible for perhaps the most common and the most significant of the artefacts. Advanced decomposition causes swelling of the lips, nose and eyelids, protrusion of the eyes, distention of the chest and abdomen and swelling of the extremities. These changes may lead to a false impression of antemortem obesity, but usually the changes pose no problems. There are, however, some subtle changes caused by decomposition that need elaboration. In decomposed bodies, the presence of bloody fluid in the mouth and nose is a frequent finding. In the presence of pulmonary edema, large quantities of such fluid may escape from the mouth and the nose. An erroneous conclusion may be drawn that the person died from massive hemorrhage. Decomposition blebs are occasionally misinterpreted as vesications from burns.

The position of a decomposing body may contribute to more disturbing artefacts as the following case illustrates:

> An autopsy on a middle-aged woman revealed bloated face with marked hemorrhages in the conjunctivae. Extensive hemorrhages were also found in the strap muscles of the neck. There was bluish discoloration resembling diffuse bruising of the vulva and vagina. Elsewhere decomposition was relatively less marked. All three forensic pathologists at the table, each with over 10 years' experience, "rushed" to the judgment that this was a case of rape and strangulation. To complicate matters, the acid phosphatase test on vaginal secretions turned out to be positive (an artefact). However, the history revealed that this woman was found dead seated on a toilet with her head hanging between the thighs. The examination of the head showed a massive intracerebral hemorrhage.

In a decomposed body a deep groove may be seen around the neck if the deceased had been wearing a buttoned shirt or blouse at the time of death. These grooves often simulate ligature marks seen in strangulation cases. Mummification can also produce a false groove around the neck in relation to the collar of the shirt or the blouse. Even in nondecomposed bodies, bands or grooves of contact flattening in the skin of the neck of obese individuals or of well-nourished infants may be seen (Fig. 17-5). Also, when the blood in the body decomposes it acquires a darker color and produces the appearance of congestion in the brain, lungs, right side of the heart, and other parts of the body, so that it becomes difficult to form a conclusion of death from asphyxia.[3] In view of these facts, the marks on the neck should be carefully interpreted.

On rare occasions one may observe rupture of the stomach or the esophagus caused by too rapid digestion of the wall of the stomach or the lower esophagus by gastric acid. In such cases, the contents of the gastrointestinal tract are found in the pleural or peritoneal cavities. One may be inclined to erroneously attribute the rupture to an antemortem injury, especially if no definite cause of death is found at the autopsy.

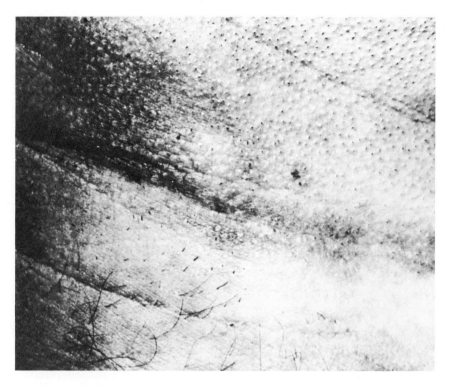

Fig. 17–5. A pseudostrangulation mark on the neck was caused by shirt collar. (See Color Plate.)

Even with minimal decomposition, in some cases marked bluish discoloration of the loops of the intestine is seen, particularly of those loops crowded together in the pelvic room (Fig. 17-6). Many pathologists too readily label this finding an infarcted bowel. Such postmortem discoloration of the bowel is one of the first decomposition changes. Awareness of this fact prevents misinterpretation of such findings.

As long ago as 1913, Chiari[4] declared that the presence of gas bubbles in the blood may be an early and even the only recognizable sign of decomposition. Correct interpretation of the finding of air in the large veins and in the right side of the heart is of great importance in medicolegal autopsies. During life, air may enter the systemic venous circulation during criminal abortions, craniotomy, urethroscopy, fallopian tube insufflation, pneumoperitoneum, aortography[20] and intravenous infusions. In cases of air embolism following abortion, air bubbles are usually found in the cavity of the uterus and its wall, the uterine and adnexal veins, the inferior vena cava and right heart, the pulmonary arteries, the left heart and the systemic arteries.[19] The presence of gas in the right side of the heart resulting from decomposition may resemble the findings in air embolism and it may be

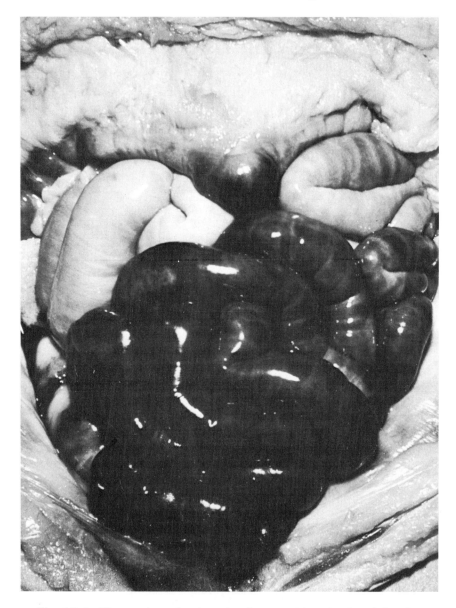

Fig. 17–6. Changes brought about by decomposition simulate infarction of the bowel.

difficult to distinguish one from the other. Zeldenhurst, *et al.*[22] suggest that the analysis of the gas may enable us to make the differentiation; the gas is collected from the heart and brought into contact with an alkaline pyrogallol solution that turns brown in the presence of free oxygen, thus giving support to the diagnosis of antemortem air embolism. Gas produced by decomposition will not produce this color change.[1] The other method that can help differentiate antemortem from postmortem air in the heart is quantitation of the air. In cases of air embolism, the volume of air is much larger than that accumulated through decomposition. Erben and Nadvornik[5] described a method for quantitative demonstration of air embolism in certain cases of fatal trauma.

Very rarely are unusual artefacts seen. Gonzales, *et al.* described postmortem separation of the sutures of a child's skull caused by the presence of putrefactive gases within the brain.[7]

The histological artefacts due to decomposition are too numerous for all to be recorded here. Passing reference is made, however, to the particularly disturbing findings observed in the pancreas. In a decomposing body the pancreas may grossly appear to be hemorrhagic; this may resemble hemorrhagic pancreatitis. Histological changes resembling pancreatic necrosis are commonly seen within a few hours after death (Fig. 17-7). In the absence of inflammatory reaction and fat necrosis these are identified as postmortem changes. Also, the sections of lungs frequently show postmortem bacterial colonies.

Miscellaneous Artefacts. *Fauna bites.* Specific changes, but confusing if unrecongnized, may be caused by animal bites, as the following case illustrates:

> A police officer investigating a death called this author one morning saying, "Doctor, we have a murder at hand." At the scene, an old man was found dead in bed in an unkempt house. Part of his scalp was missing. Examination of the injury revealed that rats in the house had eaten away part of the scalp, leaving characteristic teeth marks (Fig. 17-8).

Voight[22] described specific postmortem changes produced by larder beetles. Some cases of drowning may show evidence of the ravages of fish, crabs or shrimps. Some injuries, particularly those caused by crabs, simulate stab wounds (Fig. 17-9). In such bodies passing boats, propellers and the effects of the tides may increase the amount of damage and disintegration. The damage that ensues must be carefully differentiated from antemortem injuries or else suspicion of crime may be raised without foundation.

Postmortem hemorrhage. The finding of extravasation of blood in the tissues or even pools of blood in the body cavities does not necessarily mean that the hemorrhage was from antemortem trauma. Under normal circumstances blood in the body remains in a fluid state for a time. During this time a postmortem injury may open a blood vessel and lead to a postmortem hemorrhage. The significance of blood in the pleural cavities observed after death has been discussed by Shapiro and Robertson.[17] According to these authors, substantial bleeding may occur from wounds inflicted on the chest wall and the lung tissue postmortem. Their experiments on recently dead bodies showed that bleeding from small wounds

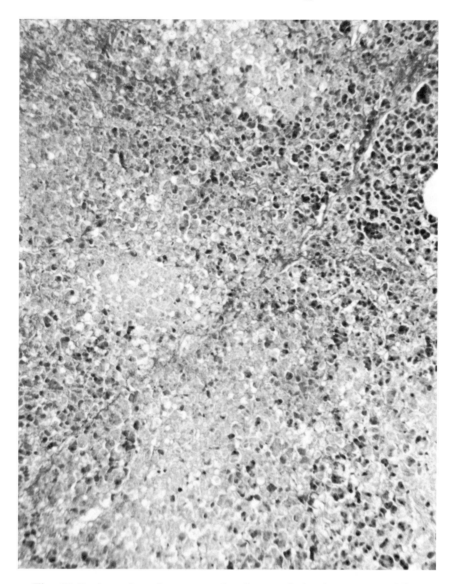

Fig. 17–7. A section of pancreas showing autolytic changes resembling pancreatic necrosis (× 125).

of the lungs may be from 50 ml. to 1 litre within 30 minutes. They suggest that in evaluating the significance of the volume of blood found in the chest cavity after death, greater attention should be paid to the injuries that may have been inflicted in the intercostal veins as opposed to the intercostal arteries, since the contribution from the latter is probably insignificant.

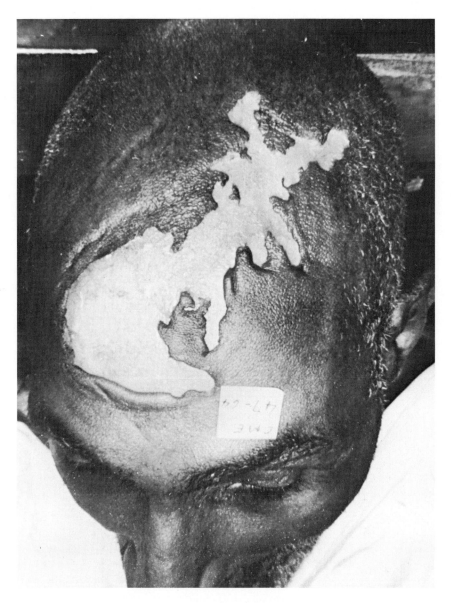

Fig. 17–8. Rat bites of the scalp with characteristic scalloping of the margins.

Flattening of the convolutions of the brain. Flattening of the cerebral hemispheres is invariably seen in cases of edema of the brain caused by pathological lesions. This flattening is generalized. However, regional flattening of the cerebral convolutions is a common postmortem artefact. The parts of the brain in contact with the cranium, particularly the dependent

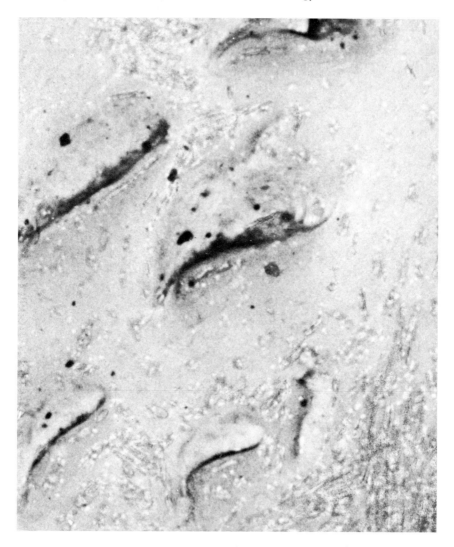

Fig. 17–9. Crab injuries simulating stab wounds.

parts, show flattening, the occipital lobes showing such flattening most frequently. A study of brains in 30 cases of sudden death from acute coronary insufficiency showed variable degrees of regional flattening in all but one case (see Fig. 17-10). The longer the body remains in one position and the longer time after death, the more marked is the flattening. To prevent additional artefactual flattening from contact with the container, the brains, in order to be fixed, should be suspended in formalin by a hook passed around the basal arteries.

Grooving of the unci. It is a widely accepted concept that the grooving

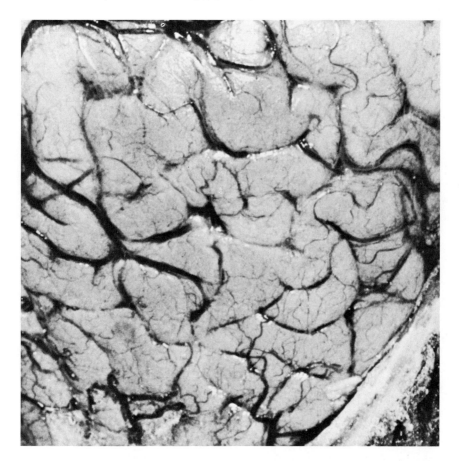

Fig. 17–10. Postmortem postural flattening of the cerebral convolutions.

of the uncus is an important accompaniment of genuine edema of the brain from cerebral lesions. The fact that this is not necessarily so needs to be stressed. Klintworth[9] reported observations on the paratentorial region of 250 brains free from cerebral diseases. He observed a well-defined sagittal uncal groove in over 95 percent of the cases. In 13 percent of his cases the furrow was unilateral. The study of 30 brains mentioned above confirmed Klintworth's findings; in 26 of these brains obvious grooving of the unci was seen (see Fig. 17-11). Thus, uncal grooving is an extremely common finding in normal brains at autopsy, and this artefact should not lead the pathologist to a misinterpretation. If the brain remains in the cranium for a long time, the uncal groove tends to be more prominent than when the brain is removed from the cranium soon after death.

Discoloration of the liver. It is fairly common to find blackish-brown discoloration of the liver at the site of contact with the large bowel. This

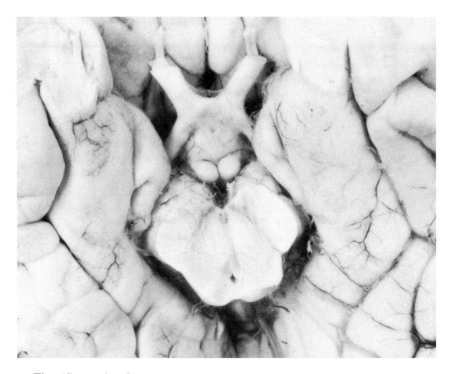

Fig. 17–11. Artefactual grooving of the unci of the brain.

is a postmortem change, the result of substances passing from the bowel to the liver and depositing sulfides in the adjacent liver tissues. Similarly, bile also causes staining of the liver surface.

Apparent growth of beard. The growth of hair stops at death but sometimes the beard appears to be more prominent than it should be. This apparent growth after death is caused by postmortem shrinkage of the skin and greater exposure of hair shafts above the epidermis.

Artefacts Introduced During Autopsy

In the head, one of the commonest artefacts is the introduction of air bubbles into the vessels at the top of the brain. In the majority of cases while the dura is being pulled in the sagittal line, air gains access to the blood vessels (Fig.17-12). Likewise, postmortem introduction of air into the veins of the neck during the reflection of the skin is also very common. In cases of suspected air embolism following attempts at criminal abortion, artefactual presence of air bubbles in the vessels of the brain and the neck may initiate confusion; the diagnosis of air embolism may be erroneously entertained.

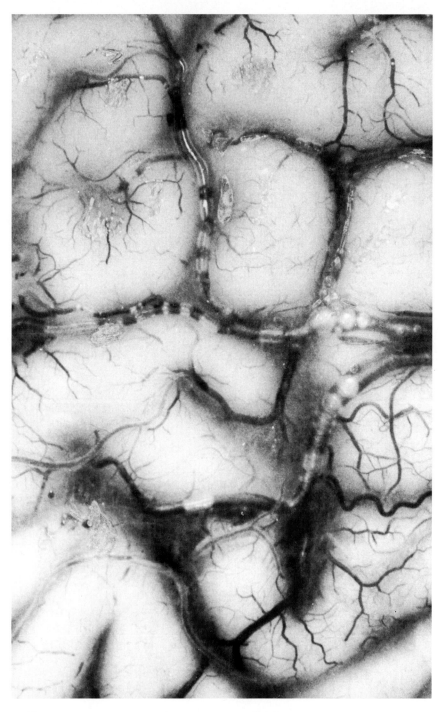

Fig. 17–12. Air bubbles in the vessels of the brain introduced during removal of the skull cap at autopsy.

While sawing off the vault of the skull during the autopsy, partial sawing and the forceful pull of the cap sometimes leads to fractures of the skull. In an already fractured skull, the antemortem fracture may be extended or additional fractures created. At times it may be impossible to differentiate a postmortem fracture from an antemortem one. Therefore, due care should be exercised if correct evaluation of the head injury is to be made. Postmortem tears of the midbrain may also be caused during the removal of the brain from the cranium.

Handling of the organs and incisions of the vessels during routine postmortem examinations often result in the extravasation of blood into the tissues, particularly in the neck. Recognition of autopsy artefacts in cervical tissues is of special importance because they simulate antemortem bruises seen in the cases of throttling and strangulation. Therefore, dissection of the neck should be meticulous, ruled by the necessity of avoiding the artefacts from seepage of blood from the neck vessels.[2] Schrader[10] first drew attention to these artefacts and suggested that the neck be drained of blood by removing the brain and the heart before reflecting the skin of the neck. Prinsloo and Gordon[13] confirmed the importance of these artefacts. They summarized their study of 51 cases by saying: "It was found that dissection artefacts of the neck were of common occurrence and could not be distinguished from antemortem bruises by a naked-eye or histological examination."

SUMMARY

An attempt is made to enumerate various artefacts observed in medicolegal autopies. The essence of the discussion is the recognition of pitfalls in the practice of forensic pathology, and separation of the significant antemortem changes from the inconsequential postmortem artefacts. In medicolegal cases misinterpretations may turn out to have disastrous effects. If a pathologist is to avoid mistakes in the performance of a medicolegal necropsy, particularly in an instance in which homicide is a possibility, he should be aware of the artefacts. If an autopsy finding is so important that it may make the difference between freedom or imprisonment, or the life or death of someone, it is the duty of the pathologist to interpret that finding correctly.

Observations and examples discussed in this chapter indicate that misinterpretations may lead to: (a) a wrong cause of death, (b) a wrong manner of death, (c) undue suspicions of criminal offense, (d) a halt in the investigation of a homicide and/or nondetection of a murder, (e) miscarriage of justice in civil suits, (f) unnecessary spending of time and effort as a result of misleading findings.

In addition, it must be stressed that a mistake made by a pathologist in the interpretation of an artefact may work to his detriment in court, for many a lawyer knows about the pitfalls and may attempt to shake the testimony of a pathologist.

REFERENCES

1. Bayer, F.: Gasanalyse. Stuttgart, Encke Verlag, 1941.
2. Camps, F. E. (ed.): Gradwohl's Legal Medicine ed. 2. Baltimore, Williams & Wilkins, 1968.
3. Casper, J. L.: Handbook of Forensic Medicine. Vol. 1. London, New Sydenham Society, 1861.
4. Chiari, H.: Handbuch der arztlichen. Sachverstandigentatigkeit. II, 1913.
5. Erben, J. and Nadvornik, F.: The quantitative demonstration of air embolism in certain cases of fatal trauma. J. Forensic Med., *10:*45, 1963.
6. Forster, B.: The plastic, elastic and contractile deformation of the heart muscle in rigor mortis. J. Forensic Med., *11:*148, 1964.
7. Gonzales, T. A., Vance, M., Helpern, M., and Umberger, C. J.: Legal Medicine Pathology and Toxicology. ed. 2. New York, Appleton-Century-Crofts, 1954.
8. Hudson, R. P.: Personal communication, 1971.
9. Klintworth, G. K.: Grooving of the uncus in the absence of overt intracranial disease. J. Forensic Med., *9:*137, 1962.
10. Maschka, cited by Forster, B.: The plastic, elastic and contractile deformation of the heart muscle in rigor mortis. J. Forensic Med., *11:*148, 1964.
11. Moritz, A. R.: Classical mistakes in forensic pathology. Am. J. Clin. Path., *26:*1383, 1956.
12. Paddock, C. E.: Antenatal rigor mortis. Am. J. Obstet., *48:*148, 1903.
13. Prinsloo, I., and Gordon, I.: Postmortem dissection artefacts of the neck: their differentiation from antemortem bruises. South Afr. Med. J., *25:*358, 1951.
14. Robertson, I., and Mansfield, R. A.: Production of postmortem bruises. J. Forensic Med., *4:*240, 1957.
15. Schauenstein, A.: Handbuch d. Gerichlichen Medicine III: 386, 1882.
16. Schrader, G.: Handworterbuch der Gerichtlichen Medizin und Naturwissenschaftlichen Kriminalistic. Berlin, Springer, 1940.
17. Shapiro, H. A., and Robertson, I.: The significance of blood in the pleural cavity observed after death. J. Forensic Med., *9:*5, 1962.
18. Simpson, K. (ed.): Taylor's Principles and Practice of Medical Jurisprudence. ed. 12. vol. I. London, J & A Churchill, Ltd., 1965.
19. Simpson, K.: Forensic Medicine. ed. 6. London, Edward Arnold Ltd., 1969.
20. Teare, R. D.: Air embolism. J. Forensic Med., *6:*15, 1959.
21. Voight, J.: Specific post-mortem changes produced by larder beetles. J. Forensic Med., *12:*76, 1965.
22. Zeldenhurst, J., Makkink, B., and Voortman, M.: Pseudo air embolism in suspected abortion. Med. Sci. Law, *3:*227, 1963.

18

Negative Autopsy

In the practice of forensic pathology it is not uncommon to come across a case of negative autopsy. One may consider that when no cause of death is found at the postmortem table the autopsy is negative. This, however, is not the true meaning of "negative autopsy." For the purpose of discussion in this chapter an autopsy is considered to be negative when all efforts, including gross and microscopic studies and toxicological analyses, fail to reveal a cause of death. Theoretically speaking, there is *always* a cause of death. However, in practice it is not possible to establish the true cause of death in every case. In the best of medicolegal centers the rate of negative autopsies ranges from 2 to 10 percent of the total cases autopsied.

A negative autopsy may result because of one of the following factors:

1. Commencement of autopsy without adequate history. There is often a situation in which the autopsy is entirely negative because the postmortem examination is begun without the knowledge of the circumstances of death. Therefore, before a necropsy is begun on any medicolegal case, a complete history of the events leading to death should be obtained. Without a history the cause of death (e.g., pneumothorax, air embolism) may be inadvertently lost or the postautopsy investigations rendered much more difficult and time-consuming. Such situations arise when a pathologist is preparing a body in the autopsy room for postmortem examination and has not received appropriate information from the investigators who worked on the case during the night and who are off duty and unavailable during the day.

In a case of drowning, for instance, if death results from laryngeal edema, no positive postmortem changes may be present. The body of a person dying from status epilepticus or vagal inhibition may not show any anatomical findings. Deaths from hypersensitivity reactions may not present enough autopsy evidence to explain the cause of death. In such cases a knowledge of the circumstances of death is important.

It is a mistake, sometimes a costly one, to perform an autopsy without prior knowledge of the full facts of the case. This fact cannot be overemphasized.

2. Lapses in external examination. Frequently the cause of death is obvious from external examination of the body. Conversely, if the external examination is not made carefully the cause of death may be missed. In the investigation of the death of a drug addict, for instance, the presence of old and fresh needle marks render a substantial lead, but these marks may not always be obvious on cursory examination. Electrocution cases demand careful external examination lest the electrical burn and the cause of death be missed. Deaths from snake bites or wasp bites cannot be explained unless the external lesions are identified.

3. Inadequate or improper internal examination. Various disease conditions that may be overlooked are described in subsequent pages. The pathologist about to commence an autopsy on a medicolegal case must be alert to the fact that the two conditions most often missed unless carefully looked for are air embolism and pneumothorax.

Air embolism. In every woman of child-bearing age dying suddenly and in individuals receiving intravenous therapy, air embolism should be suspected. The body in suspected cases of air embolism must be carefully opened. Initially, the loops of small intestine should be examined after making an abdominal incision to detect the presence of air bubbles in the mesenteric vessels. Then, the larger veins and the heart should be examined. Extreme care should be exercised to prevent cutting of larger veins; otherwise the embolized air escapes detection.

Pneumothorax. This condition should be suspected before the thoracic cavity is opened. The method to detect air in the chest cavities is described in Chapter 2. It should suffice to stress here that a negligent opening of the chest in a case of pneumothorax may result in a negative autopsy.

4. Insufficient histological examinations. Microscopic lesions which can account for death are discussed in appropriate paragraphs.

5. Lack of toxicological and other investigations. No autopsy should be declared obscure unless adequate toxicological studies have been performed. If poisoning is suspected, analyses for the agents known to be available to the decedent should first be requested. In the event that these analyses are negative, further tests for a general unknown should be carried out. Because it is impossible to identify several of the poisons in biological mterials, the findings in a case of poisoning may be negative despite exhaustive studies. Extensive research may be required to detect certain poisons as the investigation of the cases of insulin poisoning[1] and succinylcholine overdose[10] illustrate.

6. Pathologist's training. Training can be an important factor. Hospital pathologists and forensic pathologists think and work differently. There is even a great variation from pathologist to pathologist in the acceptability of certain findings as being enough to cause death. The criteria adopted by hospital pathologists in general differ from those accepted by forsensic pathologists. For instance, a hospital pathologist who has been accustomed to seeing cases of coronary thrombosis with myocardial infarction may not accept severe atherosclerosis of the coronary arteries as a cause of death. On the other hand, a forensic pathologist who deals with a great number of cases of sudden, unexpected deaths with atherosclerotic narrowing of the coronary arteries without thrombosis or infarction readily accepts sclerotic narrowing of the coronary arteries as a cause of death. Fatal arrhythmias from myocardial ischemia due to atherosclerotic narrowing (not necessarily total occlusion) of the coronary arteries are common and one should have no hesitation in labeling such a death as "acute coronary insufficiency" if other causes are meticulously excluded. In another instance, a hospital pathologist may not accept a few foci of bronchopneumonia as sufficient to cause death in an elderly person in whom there is no other anatomical cause of death, wheras a forensic pathologist may consider this an adequate and valid cause of death.

In the following paragraphs, several of the conditions that can be missed at autopsy or those that can create difficulty in interpretation are described.

Death from Fright or Shock

There is no doubt that death can result from severe emotional disturbance. When fright causes death, there may not be any anatomical findings to explain it. Such deaths are distinctly rare; this author has not seen a single genuine case of death from fright. Cases, however, have been cited in the literature. Bowden[2] reported a case in which a 16-year-old girl died from fright. When the girl came home and opened the front door of her house she saw her father standing there with his head wrapped in bandages and a policeman standing near him. As soon as she saw her father in that condition she dropped dead. The postmortem examination was entirely negative.

Concealed or Apparently Insignificant Trauma

Even trivial injuries inflicted in certain areas can cause death. Slight blows on the neck, for instance, may result in vagal inhibition and death. Similarly, a blow or blows in sensitive areas such as the precordial region, epigastrium or the area of the genital organs may precipitate death. Injuries in these regions may either be concealed and escape detection or may be so trivial as to be discarded as insignificant. Careful examination and interpretation of such injuries is essential. The cases described by Mallik[11] illustrate this point well.

A 22-year-old man was found dead in a railway compartment hanging from a bunk by the sleeves of his shirt tied around his neck. Autopsy revealed no ligature marks around the neck. Careful dissections revealed the evidence of squeezing of both testicles. This was the cause of death and the hanging was postmortem.

In another case, a 14-year-old boy who was found hanging from a branch of a tree had severe crushing injuries of the testes with no other evidence of trauma.

Obscure or concealed lesions such as concussion and atlanto-occipital joint dislocation are discussed with the lesions of the nervous system. In all such cases if the lesions are not detected or if their significance is not appreciated, the pathologist is without a cause of death.

Lesions of the Nervous System

There are certain fatal conditions in the nervous system that may be difficult, if not impossible, to detect. The conditions that can be missed are:

1. Concussion.
2. Atlanto-occipital joint dislocation with spinal cord injury.
3. Epilepsy.
4. Chronic encephalitis.
5. Fat or air embolism.
6. Delirium tremens.

Cerebral Concussion. When death results from traumatic head injury gross changes are usually obvious. Surface or deep hemorrhages and cortical contusions, if present, are readily noticeable. Sometimes, however, traumatic lesions are subtle and may not appear significant on casual evaluation. In the case of death from cerebral concussion little or no changes may be seen at autopsy.[5] If changes are present, they are usually in the form of petechial hemorrhages in the white matter of the brain. These suspected areas of damage should be examined microscopically to determine whether there is disintegration of the brain substance and changes in the nuclei of the nerve cells. Special stains may reveal increased enzyme accumulations in the disintegrated tissue.

While performing an autopsy on an automobile accident victim one should keep in mind the possibility of concussion, especially when no other significant injuries are present. Concussion is severe if the moving head is struck as is the case when a person falls from a height or is thrown around within a car during a collision. In the following case death was considered to be from cerebral concussion.

A 21-year-old man was a front seat passenger in a car which became involved in a head-on collision. After the collision the car overturned twice. The driver and the passenger were found dead in the car. The driver had sustained severe multiple injuries. The autopsy on the passenger revealed no injuries apart from a two-inch laceration on the forehead with minimum bleeding. There were many petechial hemorrhages in the white matter. There was no evidence of asphyxiation and no natural disease was found. Toxicological analysis revealed no alcohol in the blood.

Atlanto-occipital Joint Dislocation with Spinal Cord Injury. In deaths resulting from falls or automobile accidents, especially those showing no obvious injuries, the cervical spine should be carefully explored. Although fractures of the spine are easily detected the dislocation of the atlanto-occipital joint is not always clearly visible, so that sometimes it is extremely difficult to demonstrate this injury. If this type of injury is suspected, no amount of time or effort should be spared to detect it or to rule it out. The dislocation may be associated with tears of the ligaments and with the displacement of the skull from the spine. Even if ligamental tears are present their exploration is difficult, demanding considerable patience. One should not be satisfied to judge the immobility of the head over the spine merely by manual moving of the head since this can be misleading. Another misleading factor is that once displaced the skull may have returned to normal position at the time of examination.

Sudden movement of the head over the spine with displacement may be associated with injury to the spinal cord. Such an injury, if rapidly fatal, may be in the form of contusion and laceration of the cord. If death is delayed, there may be edema, softening of the spinal cord and necrosis of its tissue in the region of trauma. Microscopic examination confirms the presence of interstitial edema and foci of necrosis and may reveal changes in the myelin sheaths and axis cylinders of the nerve fibers.

With these injuries death can be rapid. If the medulla oblongata is involved, death can result in seconds. Injury to the spinal cord causes concussion similar to cerebral concussion and shock from the concussion of the spinal cord is responsible for the rapidity of death. Whiplash injuries are known to cause cerebral and upper spinal cord concussion. Therefore, while dealing with an automobile accident fatality, careful inquiry should be made concerning the possibility of whiplash phenomenon.

Epilepsy. Death can occur in status epilepticus from myocardial ischemia or asphyxia. An autopsy on a person dying from status epilepticus may be negative. If there are no signs of asphyxia and if other corroborative findings such as a bitten tongue are not present, it may be impossible to arrive at a cause of death. Occasionally, one may be able to discern on microscopic examination areas of gliosis in the Ammon's horn. Ischemic nerve cell changes may be seen in the cerebral cortex, hippocampus, basal ganglia and cerebellum, especially in children dying from status epilepticus.[12] In idiopathic epilepsy usually there are no demonstrable lesions in the brain. Therapeutic levels of long-acting barbiturates in the decedent's blood sometimes give a hint about the possibility of epilepsy. In the investigation of a death from status epilepticus the history is all-important. With an adequate history, the pathologist renders a valid opinion as to the cause of death. Without the background information, on the other hand, he finds it impossible to explain the death.

Chronic Encephalitis. In the investigation of a death in which the gross examinations are negative, violence is ruled out and poisoning is excluded, one is wise to review the histological slides again and perhaps cut more sections from various parts of the brain. These may reveal the diagnosis of chronic encephalitis. The lesions in chronic encephalitis consist of collections of chronic inflammatory cells around blood vessels with ischemic changes in the adjoining tissue (Fig. 18-1). It is thought that the etiological agent in these cases is a virus and that death is caused by cerebral anoxia.

Embolism. Fat embolism occurs after bone fractures or injury to the fatty tissues.[14] The organ most likely to cause death from fat embolism is the brain. Cerebral fat embolism leads to widespread ischemia of the brain. Grossly, the fat emboli in the brain present as dark red spots in the white matter. In a potentially negative autopsy such a finding at the autopsy table should be followed up with fat stains of the brain sections to demonstrate the emboli.

If air embolism is present and it is not identified at the autopsy table, the result may be a wrong conclusion or no conclusion about the cause of death.

Delirium Tremens. It is well-known fact that a person in delirium tremens can die suddenly and unexpectedly, although the precise mechanism of death is not known. Cerebral anoxia is probably an important factor. Other possible explantions of death are liver failure and biochemical disturbances such as hypoglycemia, hypokalemia and respiratory alkalosis. The pattern in these cases seems fairly characteristic. Victims are usually chronic alcoholics with recent history of heavy drinking. In some cases, the postmortem examination is entirely negative; in others, the only positive finding is a fatty liver. The body sometimes reveals trivial skin bruises, recent and old. Blood alcohol levels are invariably far below fatal levels. These findings when considered in conjunction with the history provide the pathologist a satisfactory explanation of death. For the purpose of certification, perhaps the most acceptable terminology to designate the cause of death is "acute and chronic alcoholism."

Lesions in the Neck

Examination of the neck organs is frequently omitted with or without reason. An autopsy on a medicolegal case cannot be considered complete if such an examination is not carried out. While dissecting the neck organs,

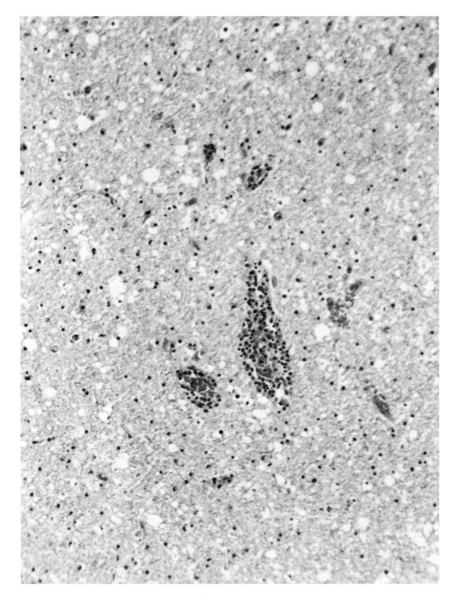

Fig. 18–1. Chronic encephalitis. Note the collections of chronic inflammatory cells around the blood vessels (× 130).

special attention should be paid to the detection of conditions causing obstruction of the air passages, traumatic lesions and disease processes.

Examination of the larynx should always be a routine part of the autopsy. An obvious cause of death such as *choking on food* is missed if the
neck organs, including the larynx, are not examined.[6] Foreign bodies such

as partial dentures, candies (sweets) and solid foods may become impacted in the larynx and cause death from asphyxia.

A 71-year-old man returned to his place of residence for lunch after he had imbibed some alcohol. He was served a steak. A few seconds after he started to eat, he turned blue and started to breathe spasmodically. His gasps weakened and he died within 15 minutes. At necropsy a large piece of unchewed meat was found completely obstructing the larynx (Fig. 9-9).

A woman, aged 48, was in a mental hospital for paranoid schizophrenia. One afternoon she was given an orange after lunch. A few minutes later a nurse saw her collapse in the hospital corridor. She died within a half hour after the collapse. Autopsy revealed a large mass of unchewed orange totally blocking the larynx.

Without careful removal and examination of the neck organs other conditions such as *inflammation and edema of the larynx* are missed. Inflammatory conditions of the larynx (e.g., diphtheria) can cause unexpected death. Inflammatory edema of the larynx in laryngotracheobronchitis may cause death from asphyxia. Similarly, swelling of the glottis and the supraglottic tissues from hypersensitivity reactions may cause rapid death.

The detection of *trauma to neck organs* is also important. Relatively minor trauma to the neck may result in fractures of the larynx leading to death. The compression or injury may cause rapid death, or the subsequent edema of the larynx may cause delayed death. It must be remembered that a person strangled to death may not show any evidence of trauma on external examination but internal examination may reveal contusions of the tissues with signs of asphyxia. The fractures of the hyoid bone with presence of antemortem hemorrhages may be present. These findings are obvious only if the neck is explored. It must be stressed, however, that there are certain traumatic lesions in the neck that may not be detected despite a careful examination. For instance, one may not be able to detect the cause of death if the fatality resulted from *laryngeal spasm*. A grip on the neck or the induction of anesthesia may be associated with laryngeal spasm with no evidence of trauma. Deaths from *reflex stoppage of the heart* or obstruction to the return of blood from the brain caused by compression of the neck may result in unconsciousness and death. In such cases no anatomical cause of death may be found. Also, asphyxial deaths such as those caused by suffocation from plastic bags covering the head and face may not show any visible postmortem changes, especially in elderly persons. In all such cases only a careful correlation of the history and investigative findings can provide correct answers to questions relating to the cause and manner of death.

In some anesthetic deaths and deaths due to therapeutic misadventures the autopsy may be entirely negative. These cases are discussed in Chapter 16.

Some of the *natural disease conditions* that are known to cause sudden death are missed if examination of the neck organs is excluded. These include thyrotoxicosis, myxedema, parathyroid tumors and carotid artery occlusions. In appropriate cases, gross and microscopic examinations should be carried out to detect these diseases.

Lesions of Cardiovascular System

The most common cause of sudden, unexpected death is cardiovascular disease. Several apparently obscure cardiovascular conditions are frequently responsible for negative autopsies. Therefore, the pathologist should pay special attention to the heart and blood vessels while dealing with a case of sudden death. Some of the conditions that are missed are:

1. Distal coronary artery occlusion.
2. Coronary spasm.
3. Pathology of the SA and AV nodes and the bundle of His.
4. Asymmetrical obstructive hypertrophy of the heart.
5. Myocarditis.
6. Periarteritis nodosa.
7. Brown atrophy of the heart.
8. Sarcoidosis.

Distal Artery Occlusion. Coronary artery disease is responsible for more sudden deaths than any other condition. In the practice of forensic pathology these cases form a large percentage. In every case of sudden death the coronary arteries should be fully explored. It is not good practice to split the coronary arteries with scissors. Serial sections at 5 mm. intervals should be made to evaluate the narrowing of the lumen and to detect the presence of hemorrhage or thrombosis. In every case the coronary arteries should be sectioned along their entire length; otherwise a thrombus or an occlusive lesion in the terminal part of the artery escapes detection. Also, the examination of the ostia of the coronary arteries should be made to detect possible ostial occlusion by atherosclerosis of the aorta.

Coronary Spasm. It is believed that coronary artery spasm can cause sudden death.[3] Spasm of the coronary arteries can occur whether the artery is diseased or healthy. Such spasm leads to cardiac arrhythmia and death. In the following case such a mechanism of death appears most likely.

> A sportsman, aged 19, was batting during a cricket match when he was struck in the precordial area by a fast ball. Immediately after this he took a deep breath, collapsed and died. Autopsy revealed no injuries. The heart weighed 275 gm. There was no valvular, myocardial, aortic or coronary artery disease. Microscopic examinations were noncontributory.

Pathology of the SA and AV nodes and the bundle of His. The lesions of the conducting system of the heart sometimes cause arrhythmias and unexpected deaths. In selected cases of sudden death with no gross or microscopic findings on routine examinations, the conducting tissues of the heart should be examined. In most cases the artery supplying the atrioventricular (AV) node arises from the right coronary artery. The sinoauricular (SA) node is sometimes supplied by the right coronary artery and other times by the left. Detection of the narrowing or occlusion of the nodal arteries, edema, hemorrhage and degeneration of the nodal tissue or inflammatory and degenerative changes in the bundle of His may explain the cause of death when none is obvious. In nine cases of sudden death in which the conducting tissue was eximined, Ferris[8] noted narrowing of the nodal artery in four cases, recanalized thrombus in the AV nodal artery with fibrosis of the nodal tissue in one, hemorrhagic destruction of the nodal tissue in one, degenerative changes in the bundle of His in two cases, and in an elderly man with a history of fainting the histological changes were consistent with heart block. The subject of the examination of the conducting tissue has been well reviewed by James.[9]

Asymmetrical Obstructive Hypertrophy of the Heart. This condition, the cause of which is unknown, is not widely recognized among hospital pathologists. However, it is more common than is generally thought. In this condition the left ventricle is usually characteristic—the anterior wall near the base is greatly hypertrophied while the thickness of the posterior wall is normal. The interventricular septum is greatly hypertrophied and actually bulges into the left ventricular cavity (Fig. 18-2). The hypertrophied areas frequently show small and large patches of fibrosis. Microscopic examination reveals hypertrophied muscle fibers in the affected areas with large hyperchromatic nuclei (Fig. 18-3). The fibrosis occasionally involves the conducting tissue in the septum.

Myocarditis. In every case in which the gross anatomical examination is inconclusive with reference to the cause of death, it is advisable to retain the whole heart. In such circumstances, a routine search for the foci of myocarditis should be made. If conventional sections fail to show any pathology, an additional 15 to 20 sections of the ventricles should be made. Occasionally, focal myocarditis may be revealed to explain the cause of death. In a series of 32 cases of isolated myocarditis described by Corby[4] the hearts were grossly normal and only histological examination revealed the cause of sudden death. The foci of infection may involve the conducting tissue. Acute or chronic lesions are the result of virus infections, principally the Coxsackie and poliomyelitis viruses. Focal myocarditis may also be caused in infants by toxoplasmosis, the Toxoplasma gondii organisms being found in the myocardium with focal areas of necrosis. With increasing incidence of drug abuse administered parenterally, such lesions in the myocardium are not as uncommon as generally believed. In young narcotic addicts with no history of the administration of a drug immediately

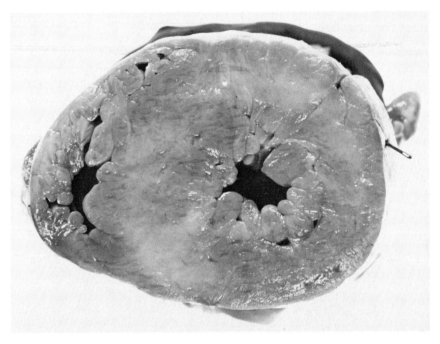

Fig. 18–2. Asymmetrical hypertrophy of the heart. (Courtesy of D. J. L. Carson, M.D.)

prior to death together with negative autopsy and toxicological studies, the finding of the foci of myocarditis, not entirely unexpected, is a valid explanation of the cause of death. The following case illustrates this.

> One afternoon, a 19-year-old drug addict was in the company of her friends. She complained of heaviness in the chest, started to sweat and within seconds she collapsed and died. One of her friends indicated that she had "injected" LSD into her arm prior to the illness. The other friends did not confirm this story. At the autopsy no fresh injection marks were visible on any part of the body. Internal examination revealed no injuries or gross pathological lesions. Comprehensive toxicological studies were negative. Histological studies revealed the evidence of chronic hepatitis and several areas of myocarditis (Fig. 18-4).

Periarteritis Nodosa. The etiology of this condition is unknown, although hypersensitivity to drugs has been indicated as one of the causes. The arteries in this condition show inflammation with hyaline degeneration and necrosis of the vessel wall. Large numbers of neutrophils and eosinophils are usually present in the wall. The involvement of the coronary arteries may lead to a rare condition of myocardial infarction and finally to death. The gross autopsy in a case of periarteritis nodosa may be negative. Hence, the value of histological studies in suspected cases is stressed.

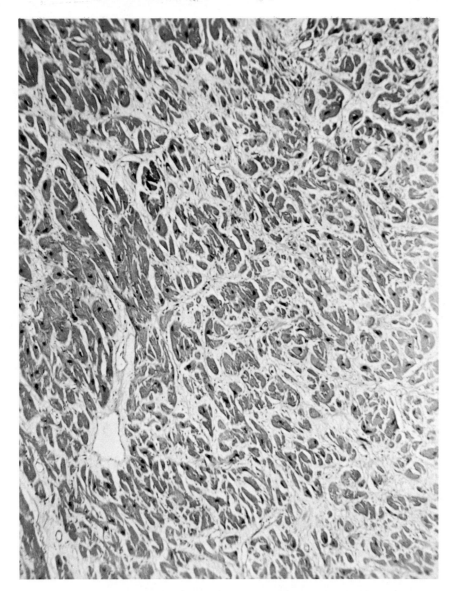

Fig. 18–3. Myocardial fibrosis with hypertrophied muscle fibers containing hyperchromatic nuclei (× 50).

Brown Atrophy of the Heart. This is an acquired condition sometimes seen in elderly people and in young adults. It may be associated with starvation and with chronic diseases such as pulmonary tuberculosis, asthma and cancer. Brown atrophy can lead to congestive heart failure and death. The pathologist looking for the cause of heart failure may over-

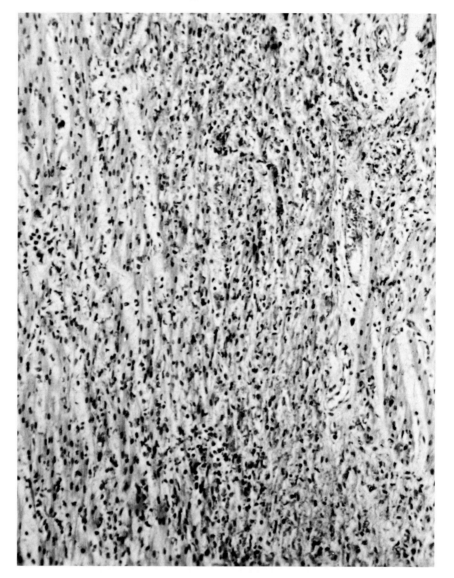

Fig. 18–4. Myocarditis in a drug addict (× 130).

look the existence of a small heart with brown muscle that can explain the cause of the heart failure. The brownish coloration of the heart is due to yellowish brown pigment, lipofuscin. On microscopic examination this pigment is found in the sarcoplasm of the muscle fibers, usually near the poles of the nuclei. Occasionally, the pigment may be found between the muscle fibers. In addition to the finding of the pigment, the myocardium may show cloudy swelling and fatty degeneration.

Sarcoidosis. The lesions of sarcoidosis in the heart can also be missed if careful histological examination of the myocardium is not made. This condition is being recognized with increasing frequency in recent years and the lesions in the heart are known to cause sudden death[13] Granulomatous inflammation resembling noncaseating tuberculosis with or without considerable myocardial fibrosis may be found (Fig. 18-5). Sarcoid lesions may also occur in the endocardium and epicardium.

Lesions of the Adrenal Glands

The cause of sudden, unexpected death may be found in the adrenal glands as a result of hemorrhage, infarction of the tissue, infection or total destruction by tumor. When the autopsy is likely to be negative, gross and microscopic examinations of the adrenal glands should not be omitted. Voight,[15] in his discussion of the adrenal lesions in medicolegal autopsies stresses, "Microscopy of the adrenals should, of course, form an integral part of the complete microscopic examination required in all obscure cases." The features that should be particularly noted are hypertrophy and atrophy of the cortex and lipid depletion, in addition to the pathological changes noted above. In the following instance the diagnosis of fatal Addison's disease was made by careful exploration of the adrenals and microscopic examination.

A 27-year-old married woman, mother of two children, was seen by several doctors over a period of months with the complaints of tiredness, weakness, loss of weight, transient aches and urinary tract infection. She even complained of her skin getting darker. The doctors considered her to be psychoneurotic and dismissed her complaints as being due to "bad nerves." During the week before she died she had an episode of hyperventilation syndrome and was treated with tranquilizers. Two days after the symptoms of hyperventilation appeared she developed new symptoms of severe headache and vomiting that lasted all night. The following morning she went to a doctor and while in the physician's office she suddenly collapsed and died. Autopsy revealed slight dehydration, marked pigmentation of skin, lymphadenopathy and slightly enlarged spleen. The adrenal glands were small. Figure 18-6 shows the adrenals from the decedent with normal adrenals for comparison. On microscopic examination the adrenal glands showed marked increase of fibrous tissue and lymphoid tissue intervening small islands of adrenal cortical cells.

The possibility of adrenal lesions as a cause of death in infants should be borne in mind. In ten cases described by Favara,[7] there were clinical signs consistent with adrenal insufficiency but clinical diagnosis of adrenal deficiency was not made in any of the cases and the gross postmortem

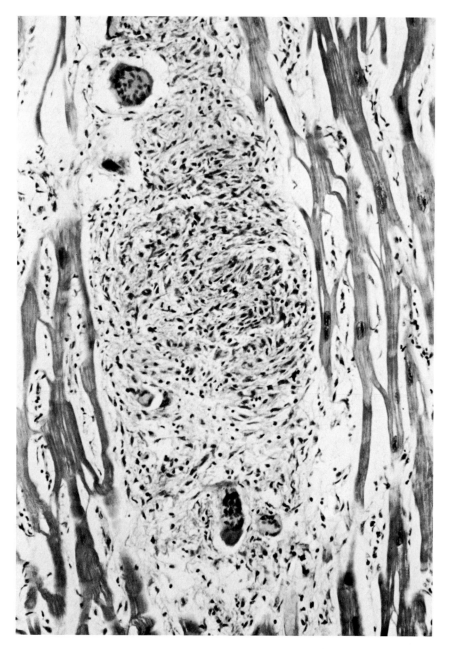

Fig. 18–5. Sarcoidosis of the heart (× 50).

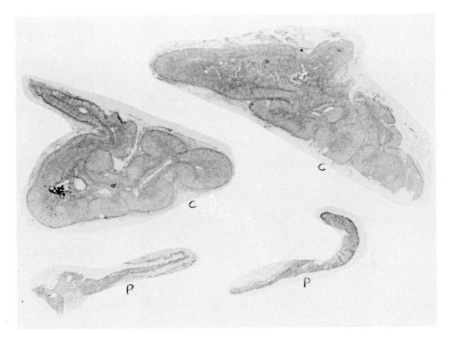

Fig. 18–6. Hypoplastic adrenal glands (P, P) in a case of Addison's disease. Normal adrenal glands (C, C) included for comparison.

examination failed to show any anatomic cause of death. However, microscopic examinations revealed miniature adrenals in nine of the ten cases and in four of these adrenal hypoplasia was considered to be the cause of sudden death.

Sickle Cell Disease

An instance of acute fatal sickling may produce a negative autopsy. The diagnosis is obvious on microscopic examination. However, until the diagnosis is made a great confusion may be created in certain circumstances. The following case, one of a type not uncommonly seen, illustrates this:

> One evening a young Negro male was arrested for being drunk and disorderly. There was some struggle between him and the arresting officers before he was put in prison. The next morning he was found dead in his bunk. The relatives charged police brutality and demanded an inquiry. At the autopsy the only findings were slight edema of the lungs and acute visceral congestion. There were no marks of violence and the blood alcohol was negative. Microscopic examination of the tissues revealed massive sickling of the red blood cells (Fig. 18-7).

In situations similar to this one determination of the cause of death readily dispels rumors and charges of negligence.

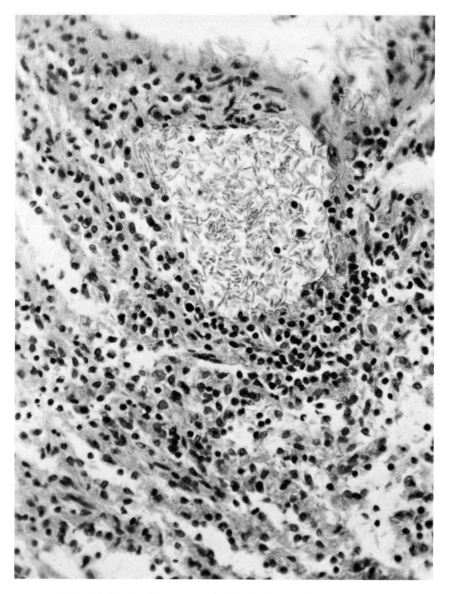

Fig. 18–7. Sickling of red blood cells in the spleen (× 340).

Decomposition

Decomposition is responsible for more negative autopsies than any other factor. With advanced putrefaction several of the natural disease conditions and even evidence of trauma are obscured. Microscopic studies and sometimes toxicological studies are rendered useless. A routine thorough investigation is all that is expected from a pathologist in such cases.

WHAT TO DO WHEN THE AUTOPSY IS NEGATIVE

One of the important purposes of an autopsy on a medicolegal case is the determination of the cause of death. In most cases, examination of the body reveals the precise cause of death. Fatal anatomic changes, disease processes and injuries are often readily discerned. In some instances only a careful histological examination reveals the cause of death. Whereas the dissection of the body and the microscopic examinations detect natural diseases and injuries, in poisoning cases thorough toxicological investigations establish the cause of death with rare exceptions. There are times when all investigations fail to reveal a cause of death and the autopsy is truly negative. In unexplained deaths no doubt certain biochemical disturbances must be operating, but the current state of the knowledge does not make it possible to identify these. In situations when the pathologist feels that everything that should be done has been done, he is completely justified in giving the cause of death as "undetermined." Medical examiners and coroners requesting the autopsy like to know the manner of death also in such cases. Although the death probably is natural, in view of the remote possibility of undetectable trauma or poison, the manner of death in cases of negative autopsies should also be listed as "unknown."

REFERENCES

1. Birkinshaw, V. J., Gurd, M. R., Randall, S. S., Curry, A. S., Price, D. E., and Wright, P.H.: Investigations in a case of murder by insulin poisoning. Brit. Med. J., 2:463, 1958.
2. Bowden, K. M.: The larynx. J. Forensic Med., 9:10, 1962.
3. Camps, F. E., and Purchase, W. B.: Practical Forensic Medicine. London, Hutchinson, 1956.
4. Corby, C.: Isolated myocarditis as a cause of sudden obscure death. Med. Sci. Law, 1:23, 1960.
5. Courville, C. B.: Commotio Cerebri Cerebral Concussion and the Postconcussion Syndrome in Their Medical and Legal Aspects. Los Angeles, San Lucas Press, 1953.
6. Fatteh, A.: Sudden death at table. Brit. Med. J., 1:120, 1964.
7. Favara, B. E., Franciosi, R. A., and Miles, V.: Idiopathic adrenal hypoplasia in children. Am. J. Clin. Path., 57:287, 1972.
8. Ferris, J. A. J.: The conduction tissue in sudden death. Abstracts, Sixth International Meeting of Forensic Sciences. Edinburgh, September, 1972.
9. James, T. N.: Anatomic relationship of a coronary occlusion to the blood supply of the sinus node and atrioventricular node in the etiology of myo-

cardial infarction. *In* James, T. N., and Keyes, J. W. (eds.): The Etiology of Myocardial Infarction. Boston, Little, Brown and Co., 1963.

10. McDonald, J. D.: No Deadly Drug. Garden City, N.Y., Doubleday & Co., 1968.
11. Mallik, C. C.: Homicide without any visible mark of injury. Abstracts. Sixth International Meeting of Forensic Sciences. Edinburgh. September, 1972.
12. Norman, R. M.: The neuropathology of status epilepticus. Med. Sci. Law, *4:*46, 1964.
13. Pascoe, H. R.: Myocardial sarcoidosis. Arch. Path., *77:*299, 1964.
14. Sevitt, S.: Fat Embolism. London, Butterworth & Co., 1956.
15. Voight, J.: Adrenal lesions in medico-legal autopsies. J. Forensic Med., *13:*3, 1966.

19

Investigation of Poisoning Deaths

Every year poisons kill thousands of people and the literature indicates that deaths from poisoning are on the rise in all parts of the world. Every death resulting from poisoning has to be investigated to establish its precise cause and to determine whether it was accidental, suicidal or homicidal. No doubt the medical examiner, coroner or the police surgeon who investigates the scene of death can contribute substantially to the determination of the questions of cause and manner of death, especially the latter. Additional help is frequently needed from the pathologist and/or the toxicologist to identify the fatal poison. Thus, a complete investigation of a poisoning fatality should consist of an adequate scene investigation, a complete autopsy and toxicological studies. There is no doubt that in some cases poisoning may not be suspected at all and the death may be certified as natural, particularly in elderly persons with some history of medical problems and no clear evidence of poisoning. In such cases, only a high index of suspicion coupled with autopsy and toxicological studies provides right answers.

EXAMINATION OF THE SCENE OF DEATH

Throughout the book the importance of the scene investigation of a death is stressed. A poisoning death also cannot be adequately investigated without the full understanding of the circumstances of death at the scene. The pathologist, therefore, should make every effort to examine the scene. Failing that he should secure full details of the facts surrounding the death from the investigator at the site of death. In some circumstances, the presence of a doctor at the scene not only helps the investigator but also prevents further tragedy.

What should the medical examiner, coroner or pathologist do at the scene of death? The general objectives of the examination of the scene have already been outlined in Chapter 1. In a suspected case of poisoning, the investigator should attempt to determine whether the death is, in fact, from poisoning or from other causes. If death appears to be from poisoning, the only way the cause can be positively established is by an autopsy and/or toxicological analysis. To aid the pathologist and the toxicologist in arriving at a rapid and accurate cause of death, the investigator at the scene should procure as much information as possible pertaining to the agent responsible and the circumstances of its administration. If the pathologist is not at the scene, the investigator should gather the following information.

1. The decedent's name, age, sex, race, past medical history; history of the use of medications and drugs, of depression and of suicide threats, and attempts; signs and symptoms prior to death (if observed).
2. Method of administration of the poison—inhalation, ingestion, injection or other
3. Agent adminstered—medicinal drug, domestic or industrial compound or gas.
4. If medicinal drug—name of the drug, estimated amount used, quantity found unused, quantity prescribed, date of prescription, date of dispensation, name of the doctor and pharmacy.
5. Presence or absence of a suicide note.
6. If accidental poisoning—name of the poison, estimated quantity used and source.
7. If suspicions of foul play—details of the circumstances of administration of poison including details about the poison and the suspect involved in the administration of poison.

In a case of poisoning in which the circumstances of death are clear and the cause of death appears obvious, it may not be necessary to perform an autopsy. However, before the body is released or embalmed, toxicological analyses should be done to establish the cause of death. The following example illustrates such a disposition of the case.

A 41-year-old man who had been depressed was found dead in his car in a closed garage at his home. One end of a rubber tube led into the car through a partially open window and the other end was connected to the exhaust pipe. The other windows of the car were closed. The car engine was not running but the ignition key was in ON position. The skin of the decedent showed pink livor. No injuries were seen on the body. The medical examiner obtained a sample of blood from the body that showed carboxyhemoglobin saturation of 70 percent. The autopsy was not necessary.

However, things are not always what they seem to be. The findings at the scene of death may mislead the investigator into drawing wrong conclusions as the following case illustrates.

One morning an elderly gentleman who had been in poor health revealed frustration to his wife and the attending nurse. He ran to the bathroom with a bottle of Seconal capsules expressing on the way that he was tired of life and was going to end it with the capsules. He locked the bathroom door on the inside. In less than five minutes the door was broken open and he was found dead lying on the bathroom floor away from the door. Several capsules were found scattered on the bathroom floor. The family members and the medical examiner accepted this as a suicide from acute barbiturate poisoning. The autopsy, nonetheless, revealed no evidence of poisoning and exhaustive toxicological studies were negative. Death was natural.

AUTOPSY ON A POISONING DEATH

The purposes of an autopsy are to determine that the death was from poisoning, to estimate the amount of poison in the body and to produce data that can help determine the manner of death.

Death from poisoning may be rapid because of a large overdose or it may be delayed from the effects of the poison in vital organs. The pathologist should bear in mind these considerations when performing an autopsy on a poisoning death.

Rapid Poisoning Death. As far as acute poisoning is concerned, cases can be broadly divided into those with positive findings and those with no gross anatomical clues. This latter variety is discussed in Chapter 18. Among cases of acute poisoning one finds negative findings more often than not. All cases of acute poisoning have one change in common—acute congestion of visceral organs. Some may show edema of the lungs, the brain and the kidneys.

Positive evidence of poisoning can be gathered by careful external and internal examination. The presence of pills, tablets or capsules in clothing, staining of lips and mouth from ingested poison, the color of livor and the presence of cyanosis should put the pathologist on guard. On internal examination, staining of the gastrointestinal tract, especially the mucosa of the esophagus, stomach or duodenum, and congestion and/or corrosion of the mucosa of the stomach may be observed, in addition to generalized congestion and edema referred to above (Fig. 19.1).

Delayed Poisoning Death. Single large doses or repeated overdoses can cause various gross anatomical and microscopic changes in the organs. Pathological changes caused by specific poisons are discussed in Chapter 20. Sometimes death occurs from complications of poisoning; at other times it is precipitated by poisoning in a person with a serious natural disease. In such circumstances, it is important to evaluate carefully the role of the poison and the natural disease in the causation of death.

Collection of Biological Specimens. An important part of an autopsy on a poisoning death is the collection of proper materials from the body. Not infrequently, pathologists retain wrong samples or insufficient quantities

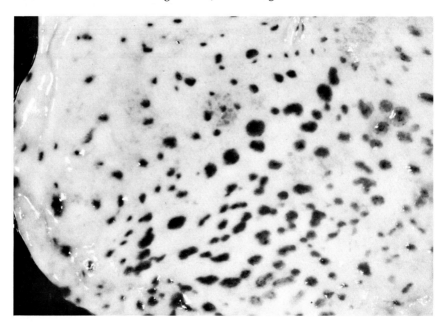

Fig. 19–1. Acute ulcers in the mucosa of the stomach. Such ulcers should arouse suspicion of poisoning by an irritant.

of samples for toxicological analyses. On one occasion a pathologist from an academic department sent one gram of liver and requested analyses for "general unknown." At times the pathologist may have clear clues as to the offending poison and may limit the collection of materials to certain items. On the other hand, if there is no inkling of the poison responsible for death, much more material may need to be retained. A brief note on what should be retained under different circumstances is added here to guide the general pathologist.

General unknown. If there is no knowledge of the type of poison and if there is likelihood that the toxicologist may have to perform multiple analyses to exclude several poisons, the following specimens should be retained. The quantities specified are the minimum required.

Blood—50 ml. (This can be drawn from the heart and great vessels with a syringe and needle to avoid contamination. If sufficient quantity is not available, more can be obtained from iliac and femoral veins by cutting the iliac veins, squeezing the thighs and letting the blood pour into a container from the cut vessels. Half of the blood should be retained in a plain tube and the other half in a container with 1 mg. of sodium fluoride per 1 ml. of blood.)
Urine—100 ml. If less, obtain all available (withdraw from the bladder with a syringe and needle).
Stomach contents—all available.
Liver—about 200Gm.
Brain—about 200Gm.

Kidney—one kidney.
Cerebrospinal fluid—50 ml. if blood is not available. (This can be easily withdrawn with a long needle inserted in the subarachnoid space through the cisterna magna.)

Specific poisons. If the pathologist has a reasonable knowledge that he is dealing with a certain kind of poison, it may not be necessary for him to collect large quantities of some of the materials listed above for the general unknown. In such circumstances it is sufficient to retain only some of the materials. Table 19-1 specifies the *minimum* quantities of various samples the pathologist should retain. In addition to the specified samples, any time a poison is suspected to be in the stomach, the stomach contents

TABLE 19-1: Amounts of Materials to be Retained for Toxicological Analyses for Various Poisons.

Poison	Amounts to be Retained in ml. (fluids), in Gm. (solids)				
	Blood	Urine	Liver	Gastric Contents	Other
Acids, organic	10		10		
Alcohol	5	5	10		
Arsenic	10	10	20	All available	Nails, hair
Barbiturates	10	10	20	All available	
Bases, organic:	10	20	20		
Amitriptyline,					
Amphetamines, Atarax,					
Darvon, Demerol,					
Librium, Methadone,					
Methapyrilene,					
Nicotine,					
Phenothiazine,					
Pyribenzamine,					
Quinine, Strychnine					
Carbon monoxide	5				
Cyanide	10			All available	
Doriden	10		20		
Fluorides	10			All available	
Halogenated					
hydrocarbons	10		20		
Heroin (Morphine)	20	20	20		Injection site
Isopropanol	5		20		
Lead	10	20	20		
Mercury		30	20		Kidney
Methanol	5				
Paraldehyde	5				
Pesticides	20		50		Lung
Phosphorus			50	All available	
Salicylates	5	5			

should be saved. Analyses can be made with amounts less than those indicated in the table but adequate material leaves room for repeat tests.

Unavailable specimens. There may be circumstances when it is not possible to get what is indicated. Advanced decomposition, for instance, may make it impossible to obtain the required sample of *blood.* Even the liver may disintegrate and disappear. In such cases the brain, even if it is liquefied, should be retained. Concentrations of poisons in the brain fairly approximate the levels in the blood. If the brain substance is also not available, *skeletal muscle* should be obtained. Fairly large portions of relatively well-preserved skeletal muscle (psoas muscle or muscles of thighs or legs) can be obtained even from bodies undergoing advanced decomposition. Occasionally, one may be able to collect some *cerebrospinal fluid* when it is not possible to obtain blood. Also, in the absence of blood, intraocular fluid can be drawn. Vitreous or aqueous humor, about 2 ml., can be conveniently obtained from each eye by inserting a small needle through the outer angle of the eye and withdrawing the fluid with the attached syringe.

Disposition of specimens. All specimens to be collected should be put in separate containers that are clean and sealable. They should be labeled immediately and initialed by the pathologist.

Once the samples are collected, they should be delivered to the toxicologist as soon as possible. If delay is foreseen, the samples should be kept refrigerated. If they are to be mailed to the toxicology laboratory, they should be sent by a carrier or by registered or certified mail with return receipt requested to maintain the chain of custody.

With the specimens identifying papers should be sent. These should include:

1. Name of the decedent, age, sex, race.
2. Date and place of death.
3. Brief summary of the circumstances of death.
4. Brief description of gross autopsy findings.
5. Identification of the material submitted.
6. Specification of analyses requested.
7. Name, address and telephone number of pathologist.

Such information will not only help the toxicologist identify the case but will also allow him to evaluate it better from the toxicological standpoint.

INTERPRETATION OF TOXICOLOGICAL RESULTS

Interpretation of the toxicological results is not a mathematical matter. Several factors are involved and each can affect the true significance of a particular concentration of the poison. The factors that deserve careful consideration in the interpretation of the results of toxicological analyses are:

1. Age and weight of the decedent.
2. Presence of a natural disease condition.
3. Presence of traumatic lesions.
4. Degree of tolerance of the individual.
5. Hypersensitivity reaction.

Individual responses to overdoses of different poisons vary enormously. Children succumb to much smaller doses than do adults. The presence of significant natural disease conditions do alter the susceptibility of a person. For instance, a man with a severe heart disease or chronic liver or lung condition dies with a lower blood alcohol concentration than does a healthy person. Likewise, a person with a significant head injury is likely to die with a smaller amount of alcohol or other poison than the amount that kills a man with no such injury. The degree of tolerance is also a very important factor. Tolerance may develop from exposure to or frequent use of a certain agent. Chronic alcoholics can consume large quantities of alcohol without being seriously affected; similar quantities if used by novice drinkers lead to disastrous effects. If a serious reaction or even death results from hypersensitivity to a particular agent, no reliance can be placed on the levels of that particular agent in the body fluids or tissues.

Despite these factors and individual variations, case studies indicate that it is possible to estimate average amounts of poisons that may prove fatal. It must be remembered, however, that it is not the amount that entered the body that is important but the actual quantity absorbed into the system. In a normal person in whom none of the above factors is operative, certain averages of fatal levels of poisons in the body fluids and tissues help the pathologist draw right conclusions. Therefore, fatal doses and fatal concentrations for several poisons are given in Table 19-2 and should be interpreted in light of the total picture of the case. (This table was compiled from various sources: Curry,[2, 3] Kaye,[4] McBay,[5] Moritz and Morris,[7] Polson,[8] and Simpson.[9])

FINAL ANALYSIS OF A POISONING CASE

By the time the scene investigation, gross and microscopic studies and toxicological analyses are completed, the cause of death is clear in most cases. However, there may be an occasional case in which it is not possible to determine whether death was from a near lethal concentration of a poison found on toxicological analysis or from a serious natural disease found at the autopsy. The subtleties of such situations will be discussed with the consideration of individual poisons in Chapter 20.

TABLE 19-2: Fatal Doses of Various Poisons and Their Minimum Fatal Concentrations in Body Fluids and Tissues.

Poison	Fatal Dose	Minimum Fatal Concentration (mg. % unless specified)		
		Blood	Urine	Liver
Acids (HCl, H$_2$SO$_4$, HNO$_3$)	5–10 ml.	30		
Alcohol (whiskey)	1–2 pts.	350	400	
Alkalies	10–20 Gm.			
Amitriptyline		1–2		5–10
Amphetamine	150 mg.	0.05	0.3	0.4
Arsenic	120–200 mg.	0.5–2	0.1–0.5	1–2
Barbiturates:				
Short-acting	15–20 g.	1–2		4–6
Intermediate-acting	20–30 g.	2–4		6–10
Long-acting	30–50 g.	6–7		15–20
Boron		4.0		
Bromides		100		
Carbon monoxide	55–60% (COHb)	55–60% (COHb)		
Chloral hydrate	7 Gm.	1–2		
Cyanide	200–300 mg.	1.0		
Demerol (meperidine)	1 Gm.	1.0		1.0
Doriden (glutethimide)	10 Gm.	2–3		30–50
Ethchlorvynol		2–3		2–10
Fluorides	3–5 Gm.	0.3		0.2
Heroin (morphine)	100–200 mg.	0.1	.5	0.1
Imipramine	600–1000 mg.	0.5	0.5–1.0	4–5
Isopropanol	200 ml.			
Lead	5–10 Gm.	0.05	0.01	0.5
Meprobamate	20.0 Gm.	3–5	15–30	10–20
Mercury	5–7 g.	20–30 μg%	10 μg%	1.0
Methadone		0.3		1.0
Methanol	75–100 ml.	80.0	100.0	
Nicotine	50–60 mg.	0.5		1.0
Paraldehyde	100 ml.	50.0		
Parathion	15–20 mg.			
Phenol	8–10 Gm.			
Phenothiazines	5 Gm.	0.5		1.0–2.0
Phosphorus	2–3 g.	traces		
Propoxyphene (Darvon)	1–2 Gm.	0.3		3.0
Salicylates	20–30 Gm.	50–100		
Strychnine	50–75 mg.	0.2		0.4

Manner of Death

One of the most important issues to be considered in the final analysis of a poisoning death is the manner of death. For obvious reasons it is vital to rule on whether the death was suicidal, accidental or homicidal.

Suicide. Most poisoning suicides are easy to interpret. The findings at the scene often make the issue clear if the scene is not disturbed. However, it must be remembered that in every part of the world suicide is a social stigma to the family. Therefore, it is not uncommon for members of the family to conceal the medications used by the decedent and to alter the scene to make the death look natural. Such an interference can easily mislead the investigator, particularly if the decedent is a middle-aged or elderly person. A high degree of suspicion, based on the behavior of the relatives and absence of a history of natural disease in the decedent, leads to the authorization of autopsy that reveals a secret suicide. At the autopsy, of course, the absence of natural disease or signs of violence and the presence of ingested poison in the stomach help the pathologist suspect poisoning in a completely unsuspected case. In every case in which the autopsy is negative as to the anatomical cause of death, careful search for evidence of poisoning should be undertaken.

Accident. The circumstances of accidental death from poisoning are usually clear, and witnesses are able to provide information about the mode of administration and the nature of the poison. Cases of industrial poisonings, domestic accidents (e.g., drinking of wrong drinks) and children swallowing medications form some of the obvious cases. If, however, a person is found dead in bed, poisoning may not be suspected. A common accident in adults is caused by the combined ingestion of alcohol and barbituates or other drugs. The danger of such a combination is not adequately recognized, and one frequently sees fatalities with moderately high but not lethal amounts of alcohol and medications. Such combinations are, in most instances, unintentional and deaths accidental. High concentrations of medications with some alcohol should, however, be carefully evaluated to rule out suicide. Deaths from narcotic drugs are invariably accidental.

Homicide. In the field of forensic medicine the investigation of a homicide by poisoning is one of the most difficult tasks. It may not be difficult to establish the cause of death, but the conclusions concerning the criminal administration of the poison can be extremely difficult. Even with the best of investigative systems, it cannot be denied that some murders by poisoning are undetected. The best a general pathologist can be expected to do is to keep in mind the possibility of homicide every time he is investigating a death from poisoning. Murder by poisoning is uncommon; experience indicates that about one percent of poisoning deaths are homicides. The most commonly used poison to commit murder is perhaps arsenic. A majority of the murder victims succumbing to arsenic poisoning have a history of illnesses indicating poisoning by arsenic on previous occasions. In Europe other agents such as phosphorus and organo-phosphates have been used. A knowledgeable person may use an unusual poison; the use of succinyl-choline by Coppolino is a good example.[6] The possibility of the administration of therapeutic agents such as barbiturates and insulin for criminal purposes should also be kept in mind.[1]

In summary, the investigation of a poisoning death can be brought to a satisfactory conclusion only if two vital elements are put to work—high index of suspicion and systematic approach.

REFERENCES

1. Birkinshaw, V. J., Gurd, M. R., Randall, S. S., Curry, A. S., Price, D. E., and Wright, P. H.: Investigations in a case of murder by insulin poisoning. Brit. Med. J., *2:*463, 1958.
2. Curry, A. S.: Advances in forensic and clinical toxicology. Cleveland, The Chemical Rubber Co., 1972.
3. Curry, A.: Poison Detection in Human Organs. ed. 2. Springfield (Ill.), Charles C Thomas, 1969.
4. Kaye, S.: Handbook of Emergency Toxicology. ed. 3. Springfield (Ill.), Charles C Thomas, 1970.
5. McBay, A. J.: Acute poisoning. New Eng. J. Med., *273:*38, 1965.
6. McDonald, J. D.: No Deadly Drug. Garden City, N.Y., Doubleday & Co., 1968.
7. Moritz, A. R., and Morris, R. C.: Handbook of Legal Medicine. ed. 3. St. Louis, C. V. Mosby Co., 1970.
8. Polson, C. J.: Clinical Toxicology. ed. 2. London, Pitman Publishing Co., 1971.
9. Simpson, K.: Forensic Medicine. ed. 6. London, Edward Arnold (Publishers) Ltd., 1972.

20

Consideration of Individual Poisons

Every pathologist is bound to encounter deaths from poisoning. In Chapter 19 general information is given on how to deal with a poisoning fatality. In this chapter individual consideration is given to those poisons that account for a large percentage of deaths from poisoning. The information on each of the poisons is intended to assist the pathologist in interpreting the findings of his investigation. The signs and symptoms of poisoning are described in brief so that the pathological and the toxicological findings can be evaluated in the right perspective. The pathological changes are, of course, discussed in greater detail. The information on poisons causing deaths on rare occasions cannot be provided in a book of this size. The reader is referred to some of the books listed on page 282 and works by Clarke,[4] Goodman, and Gilman,[17] Simpson,[42] Stewart, and Stolman,[45] and Sunshine.[48]

ALCOHOLS

Ethyl Alcohol. Alcohol is the most widely used drug in the world. In the United States as well as in many other countries, alcohol kills more people than any other poison. A study of the figures of 1970 in North Carolina showed that alcohol was responsible for 44 percent of poisoning deaths. Pertinent facts about ethyl alcohol, and information about the interpretation of findings in cases of acute and chronic poisoning from alcohol as presented below, assist the pathologist in his investigation.

Absorption. Alcohol is absorbed through all channels. Rapid absorption occurs from the gastrointestinal tract—about 20 percent from the stomach and 80 percent from the intestines. Absorption is faster if the stomach is empty and foods, especially fatty foods, slow absorption. The rate of absorption is about 90 percent of alcohol absorbed in the first hour and almost 100 percent absorbed in one and one-half hours.

Metabolism. About 95 percent of alcohol is oxidized, mainly in the liver, to carbon dioxide and water; 5 percent is eliminated by way of the kidneys and lungs. The rate of metabolism is 10 to 15 ml. of absolute alcohol metabolized every hour. The rate of the fall of alcohol concentration in the blood is about 15 to 20 mg. per 100 ml. per hour.

Acute Ethyl Alcohol Poisoning. *Symptoms.* Nausea, vomiting, vertigo, slurred speech, sweating, inability to walk, excitement with loquacity, sense of well-being, loss of emotional restraint and confusion.

Signs. Odor of alcohol in the breath, flushed skin, dilated pupils, sluggish reflexes, poor motor coordination, unsteady gait, impaired judgment, weak but fast pulse, cyanosis, acidosis, circulatory collapse, and delirium tremens during recovery.

Differential diagnosis. Conditions to be considered in the differential diagnosis of acute ethanol poisoning are head injury, hypoglycemic coma, diabetic coma, speech defects, organic tremors, epilepsy, brain tumors, parkinsonism, and poisoning from carbon monoxide, barbiturates, paraldehyde, antihistamines, morphine, atropine and hyoscine.

Autopsy findings. Common observations are dirty clothes, poor body hygiene, presence of old trivial bruises most frequently on the extremities (elbow, knees), evidence of vomiting, evidence of urination and defecation, clothing and body smelling of alcohol, generalized visceral congestion, stomach contents smelling of alcohol, edema of lungs and brain, and findings associated with chronic alcoholism (see p. 285).

Toxicological results. Results of alcohol concentrations are usually expressed in two ways: The analyses of breath from living persons are usually reported as percentages; the results of the analyses of blood and urine are reported either as percentages or milligram per 100 milliliters of the specimen analysed. A result expressed as 100 mg. per 100 ml. is the same as 0.10 percent and 50 mg. per 100 ml. is the same as 0.05 percent.

Interpretation of alcohol concentrations. In the majority of jurisdictions in the United States, a level of less than 0.05 percent or 50 mg. per 100 ml. of blood is considered to be prima facie evidence that the person is not under the influence of alcohol; a level in excess of 150 mg. per 100 ml. or 0.15 percent is considered to be prima facie evidence that the person is under the influence of alcohol for the purpose of operating a vehicle.

Fatal levels. The usual fatal alcohol concentration is above 400 mg. per 100 ml. of blood. However, there is no one level below which all persons survive and above which all persons die. Survivals with levels of 550 mg. per 100 ml. of blood are not uncommon. On the other hand, fatalities in which no other cause of death is found, blood alcohol levels of 350 to 400 mg. per 100 ml. are frequently seen. Prolonged survival in coma causes blood alcohol levels to drop because of the continuing metabolism of alcohol. With a history of drinking and a negative autopsy, blood alcohol levels of 350 mg. per 100 ml. or higher can be accepted as valid cause of death.

If only urine alcohol levels are available for interpretation, blood alcohol levels can easily be deducted. The usual urine alcohol to blood alcohol ratio is 1.3:1.0; the brain to blood alcohol ration is 0.9:1.0.

Preexisting conditions and blood alcohol levels. Certain preexisting conditions (e.g., extreme cold, fatigue, cerebrovascular arteriosclerosis) cause a person to succumb to less than the usually fatal blood alcohol concentrations. Also, in persons with serious heart conditions (e.g., coronary atherosclerosis, valvular disease or hypertension) severe pulmonary emphysema, fibrosis or bleeding peptic ulcer, alcohol levels well below 400 mg. per 100 ml. of blood may be accepted as fatal. Aspiration of the gastric contents in an intoxicated person may accelerate death and lower than fatal concentrations of blood alcohol may be found. Alcohol is frequently misused in combination with other drugs, most often with barbiturates. In such events, even with a small concentration of a drug, alcohol in moderate concentrations proves fatal. A third of the fatal dose of a barbiturate in combination with alcohol can kill, and in the same way a third of the usual fatal concentration of alcohol with sublethal concentrations of barbiturate can be lethal.

Quantitation of ingested alcohol from blood alcohol concentrations. Often a doctor is asked to relate the blood alcohol concentrations to the quantities of alcohol consumed. Under ordinary circumstances, an average-sized person attains levels falling in a certain range at certain times after drinking alcohol. Table 20-1 contains approximate blood alcohol levels

TABLE 20-1. Quantitation of Ingested Alcohol from Blood Alcohol Concentrations.

Whiskey	*Beer*	Blood Alcohol Concentration	
oz.		*mg. per 100 ml.*	*Gm. %*
1	12	20–25	0.02–0.025
2	24	50	0.05
4	48	100	0.10
6	72	150	0.15
8	96	200	0.20

corresponding to the amounts of whiskey or beer ingested.

Manner of death. With rare exceptions, a person dying from acute alcohol poisoning imbibes large quantities of alcohol with no knowledge that excessive drinking can kill. Such deaths are usually accidental. Therefore, in a case of acute alcohol poisoning, the manner of death on the death certificate should be listed as accidental, unless the circumstances clearly indicate a different manner of death.

Chronic Alcoholism. In most cases of acute alcohol poisoning some of the stigmas of chronic alcoholism are seen. Those that can prove fatal are:

1. Acute fatty liver. While dealing with deaths from chronic alcoholism, one commonly encounters a type of case in which the deceased

is found with no apparent cause of death. In such cases there is a history of heavy drinking, little or no alcohol is found in the blood, there is no evidence of violence or poisoning from other drugs and the only positive finding at the autopsy is an enlarged, severely fatty liver (Fig. 20-1). With such situations, in many centers in the

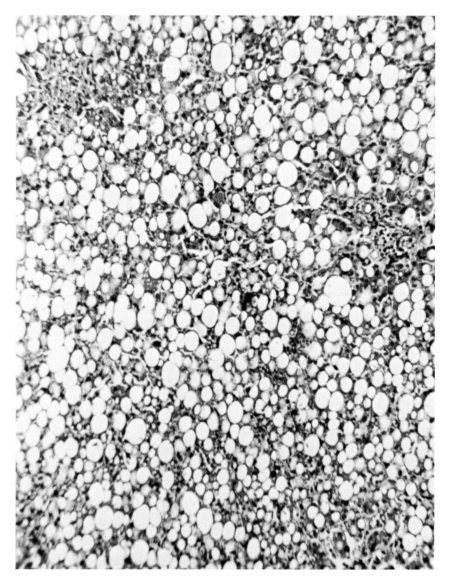

Fig. 20–1. A section showing severe fatty metamorphosis of the liver ($\times$ 50).

United States these cases are certified, for lack of better terms, as natural from "acute fatty liver." These deaths, it has been pointed out before, may be from liver failure, delirium tremens, hypoglycemia, hypokalemia or respiratory alkalosis. Research has not pointed to any one acceptable explanation of death.

2. Cirrhosis of the liver with ascites.
3. Gastrointestinal hemorrhage from bleeding esophageal varices.
4. Bleeding peptic ulcer.
5. Pulmonary tuberculosis.
6. Respiratory tract infections—bronchitis, bronchopneumonia.
7. Acute pancreatitis.
8. Aspiration of gastric contents with aspiration pneumonia.
9. Malnutrition.
10. Alcoholic cardiomyopathy, Quebec beer drinker's heart, beriberi.
11. Hypothermia.

In chronic alcoholics too, the preexisting conditions referred to in the consideration of acute alcohol poisoning accelerate death. They should be appropriately evaluated.

Chronic alcoholism and trauma. Chronic alcoholics are prone to falling. Hence, multiple bruises are frequently seen on their bodies. Occasionally, they may sustain a serious injury and may not be able to secure help because of intoxication. While investigating these deaths, in spite of blood alcohol levels within fatal limits, the possibility of internal trauma should be kept in mind. Examination of the brain should not be omitted because subdural hematoma is not an uncommon finding in such cases. With direct abdominal trauma, laceration of the spleen or rupture of an aortic aneurysm may result.

Signs of asphyxia should be looked for because suffocation from lying on the face while intoxicated, or aspiration of vomit or compression of the neck may be the cause of death.

Methyl Alcohol (Methanol, Wood Alcohol)

Methanol is cheap and easily available. It is more slowly metabolized than ethyl alcohol. It takes more than 48 hours for its total elimination. About 80 percent of methanol is excreted unchanged from the lungs and about 3 percent is excreted unchanged in the urine.

Signs and symptoms. Headache, nausea, vomiting, abdominal pain, delirium, "blind staggers," dilated pupils, depressed respirations with Kussmaul breathing, cyanosis, acidosis, optic neuritis, coma after a short latent period. Death can occur within five hours with large overdoses.

Autopsy findings. None specific. Generalized visceral congestion, sometimes marked congestion of the mucosa of the stomach. Strong smell of methanol in the stomach.

Toxicological findings. Formic acid and formaldehyde in the blood and urine. Fatal concentration in the blood: 80 mg. per 100 ml.; in the urine: 100 mg. per 100 ml.

Ethylene Glycol

Sources. Antifreeze (Prestone), paints, waxes, varnishes, lacquers, shoe polish.

Ethylene glycol is highly toxic. It is metabolized to oxalic acid in the body.

Signs and symptoms. Nausea, vomiting, diarrhea, abdominal pain, restlessness, ataxia, depression, dyspnea, sluggish or absent reflexes, oliguria, anuria, acidosis, constricted pupils, convulsions, coma.

Fatal dose. 15 to 20 ml.

Autopsy findings. Visceral congestion, edema of the lungs with or without bronchopneumonia, edema of the kidneys with nephritis, blood in the stomach, microscopic oxalate crystals in the kidneys, brain and urine (Fig. 20-2).

Toxicological findings. Elevated blood oxalate. Small amounts of formaldehyde in the urine.

Isopropyl Alcohol

Source. Rubbing alcohol.

Signs and symptoms. Nausea, vomiting, abdominal pain, excitement, confusion, poor coordination, absent or sluggish reflexes, constricted pupils, cyanosis, acidosis, circulatory collapse, coma.

Fatal dose. 200 ml.

Autopsy findings. Distinctive odor, presence of isopropanol in the stomach, congestion of the mucosa of the stomach and visceral organs, and edema of the lungs, kidneys and brain.

Toxicological findings. Isopropyl alcohol and acetone in the blood and urine.

AMPHETAMINES

With the tempo of competition getting more intense throughout the world, the amphetamines are being extensively overprescribed and widely used for central stimulation. Their use to suppress appetite and consequently to reduce weight has also been rising in recent years. Professional

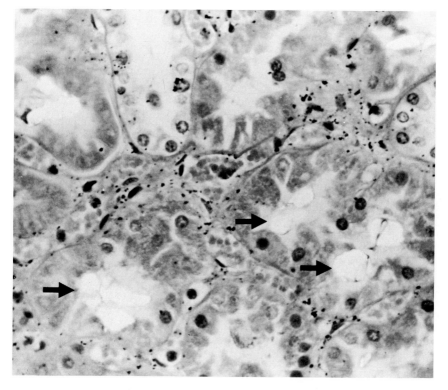

Fig. 20–2. Ethylene glycol poisoning. A section showing calcium oxalate crystals in the kidney (× 130).

truck drivers and men in competitive sports also use them. The abuse of this drug is associated with many dangers. These are well summarized by Connell.[5] The principal dangers are:

1. Overactivity leading to aggressive behavior, automobile accidents, crimes of thefts and even homicides.
2. Production of psychotic illnesses.
3. Development of addiction and habituation.
4. Shock, collapse and death due to exertion.
5. Risk of suicide.

Signs and symptoms. Alertness, mild euphoria, restlessness, agitation, inability to sleep, anorexia, nausea, vomiting, chills, sweating, diarrhea or constipation, tremors, muscle twitches, irritability, belching, tachycardia, precordial pain, irregularity of heart, palpitations, mental confusion, delirium, hallucinations, convulsions, syncope and coma can be observed with overdoses. Symptoms begin to appear within an hour after ingestion.

Pathological considerations. Deaths from amphetamine poisoning are rare but when they do occur they demand a detailed investigation. Deaths resulting from the use of weight-control pills containing amphetamines, from exhaustion and circulatory collapse following sports competition under the influence of amphetamines, and from direct or indirect involvement of amphetamines in accidents, suicides or homicides, cannot be treated lightly. Background history, clinical features and the autopsy findings should be carefully weighed with the toxicological results. The combination of other drugs, especially mono-amine oxidase inhibitors, should always be borne in mind, since such combinations are known to produce fatal results.

The autopsy may not always be rewarding. A negative autopsy should put the pathologist on the trail for the search of amphetamines and other drugs. The only gross anatomical findings one is likely to see in cases of amphetamine overdose are petechial hemorrhages in the trachea, bronchi and lungs, and gastric mucosal and subendocardial hemorrhages. Pulmonary and cerebral edema may also be present.

Amphetamines can be detected in the body fluids and tissues, and the materials that serve the best purpose for toxicological analyses are the blood, urine and brain.

ARSENIC

Fatalities from arsenic are uncommon though not rare in any part of the world. A study of the files of the Office of the Chief Medical Examiner of North Carolina on cases from half the counties of the state in the Medical Examiner System, disclosed nine deaths from arsenic poisoning in 1970 alone, three of these being homicides. Accidental and suicidal deaths may not pose a significant problem in the investigation and detection of deaths from arsenic poisoning. However, one needs to possess a high index of suspicion to detect homicides from arsenic poisoning.

Sources. Arsenic is commonly used in weed killers, food sprays, insecticides, rat poisons and fly papers. In these preparations sodium arsenite or potassium arsenite is the usual constituent. Copper arsenite is sometimes used in weed killers such as Scheele's green. Fowler's solution containing arsenic was formerly a popular remedy as a tonic but it is no longer used. Arsine gas is used only in industry. Poisoning with this gas causes severe hemolysis and leads to almost instantaneous death. Arsenic is also found in small quantities in soil, water, shellfish and tobacco.

Acute Arsenic Poisoning. The usual fatal dose of arsenic is approximately 120 mg. Massive doses can cause death within a few hours. Patients usually die of shock and peripheral vascular failure with rapid fall of blood pressure. Vomiting immediately after ingestion of the poison contributes to the degree of shock. Acute arsenic poisoning greatly resembles food poisoning. Since arsenic is a gastrointestinal tract irritant, vomiting is one of the first symptoms and with large doses retching is also observed. Vomiting may be frequently repeated and the vomit may be streaked with blood. The patient frequently complains of grittiness or roughness in the mouth and constriction in the throat. There is often difficulty in swallowing. Abdominal pain, unrelieved by vomiting, occurs. Diarrhea is another important symptom. It occurs in 5 to 24 hours and the stools have a "rice water" appearance. Thirst is a prominent symptom because of dehydration.

Chronic Arsenic Poisoning. Many of the signs and symptoms of chronic arsenic poisoning are not characteristic. Malaise, lack of appetite, loss of weight, gastrointestinal symptoms and mental irritability are observed. The patient tends to have congestion of the conjunctivae, watering of the eyes, photophobia, and chronic coryza, and complains of increased loss of hair. There is dryness of the mouth and the tongue shows a furlike white coating.

In chronic arsenic poisoning, the skin presents characteristic changes: pigmentation and hyperkeratosis. The pigmentation consists of a finely mottled brown change principally on the temples, eyelids and neck. There may be a rash that resembles a fading measles rash. The important feature of arsenical pigmentation is that it is persistent for many months. Hyperkeratosis is seen in cases with prolonged contact with arsenic. The thickening affects the skin of the palms and soles and is associated with irregular thickening of the nails.

Peripheral neuritis may also be a feature of chronic arsenic poisoning. Its onset is marked by numbness and tingling of the hands and feet that may be the presenting symptoms of subtle arsenic poisoning. There is also associated weakness and wasting of the muscles and the affected person's gait becomes unsteady. Muscle cramps occur and are usually worse at night.

Mental changes, although not always present, may be only lassitude and impaired mental energy and sometimes mental irritability. Only rarely do delusions occur. Cachexia with intercurrent infections may be observed in late stages.

Autopsy findings. In *acute* arsenic poisoning the autopsy findings may be entirely negative. In some cases the signs of irritation in the mucosa of the stomach and congestion of the organs may be the only findings. Occasionally, focal hemorrhages of the stomach or frank hemorrhagic gastritis may be seen. In cases of *chronic* arsenic poisoning, on the other hand, more reliable findings may be obtained. Externally one may observe loss of hair, with pigmentation and hyperkeratosis of the skin. There may be evidence of general malnutrition. The person may appear anemic and cachexic. Microscopic examination may show fatty degenerative changes in the liver, heart muscle and kidneys and may also disclose peripheral neural degenerative changes. In addition to these changes the gastrointestinal tract may reveal evidence of acute congestion or inflammation. Arsenic is thought to preserve the body tissues. Therefore, in bodies exhumed long after burial, one may observe unusual preservation of the tissues.

Toxicological analyses. After ingestion, arsenic is stored principally in the liver, kidneys and spleen. It takes about two weeks for the body to eliminate a single dose of arsenic from all organs except the hair and nails. Arsenic can be detected in hair within half an hour after ingestion, and with a single large dose it is detectable for a period up to three weeks. In living subjects, urine is the best specimen for detection of arsenic. In order to establish a postmortem diagnosis in acute cases, samples of the liver, kidneys, blood and urine and the gastric contents should be retained.

Prolonged administration results in the appearance of traces of arsenic, for many months after ingestion, in both the urine and feces. The storage of arsenic in the hair and nails is of particular medicolegal significance in cases of chronic arsenic poisoning. Normally, there is arsenic in the hair in amounts of less than two parts per million. If the amount exceeds three parts per million, overdose should be suspected. In cases of chronic arsenic poisoning, the analyses of liver and kidney tissues are very rewarding. However, in addition, one should also retain samples of the urine, feces, hair and nails. The estimation of arsenic in the hair and nails is done by neutron-activation analysis. The levels of arsenic in excess of 0.5 mg. percent in the liver and 0.1 mg. percent in the urine are considered to indicate serious overdose. In fatal cases, the concentration of arsenic in the liver is usually 1.0 mg. percent or over.

BARBITURATES

Barbiturates are the most popular hypnotics; some patients use them to fight insomnia and others to relieve anxieties. In the United States, it has been estimated, that over 700,000 pounds of barbiturates are prescribed each year. It is recognized that the barbiturates are at times indiscriminately overprescribed. The easy availability of these drugs explains the rising incidence of fatalities from barbiturate poisoning.

Absorption and excretion. Barbiturates are quickly absorbed from the gastrointestinal tract. Soon after absorption they are concentrated in the liver and then distributed evenly in the body tissues and fluids. Part of the barbiturates are metabolized in the liver and part excreted in the urine. Short-acting barbiturates are mainly destroyed in the liver; long-acting compounds are excreted in the urine. About 20 percent of a long-acting barbiturate is excreted in the urine in about 24 hours; and since the excretion is slow, these compounds can be found in the blood even a week after ingestion. The concentrations of short-acting barbiturates in the body fluids are usually small because they are quickly metabolized in the liver. The ultrashort-acting barbiturates are rapidly removed from the blood; hence, they may not be detectable in the blood after 12 to 24 hours.

Signs and symptoms. Short-acting compounds are used as hypnotics, long-acting for sedation and the ultrashort-acting for inducing anesthesia. In general, a minimum fatal dose is about ten times the therapeutic dose. Overdoses produce the following clinical picture:

Acute poisoning. Sleepiness, lowering of level of consciousness, depression, amnesia, Cheyne-Stokes breathing, cyanosis, ataxia, fall in blood pressure, lowering of body temperature, anoxia, urinary retention, depression of respiration, respiratory arrest, circulatory failure, dilated or contracted sluggishly reacting pupils, diminished or absent reflexes, deepening coma, pulmonary edema, pneumonia.

Chronic poisoning. Skin rash, slurred speech, cyanosis, amnesia, anorexia, ataxia, constipation, tremors, convulsions, emotional disturbances.

Postmortem appearances. The changes are usually nonspecific. In addition to generalized visceral congestion, there may be pulmonary and cerebral edema and evidence of infection. Helpful findings are the discoloration of the mucosa of the esophagus and stomach, and the presence of colored material (e.g., pink in Seconal poisoning, yellow in Nembutal overdose, bluish green in Amytal poisoning) in the stomach with remnants of capsule covers. Because the barbiturates are irritants, the stomach mucosa frequently shows corrosion with or without hemorrhages. The possibility of a combination of drugs should always be kept in mind.

In cases with prolonged survival in deep coma, there may be changes resulting from complications such as bronchopneumonia (from aspiration or immobilization), skin blisters (from anoxia of the tissue) and degenerative changes in the liver and kidneys (from toxic actions of the barbiturates).

At the autopsy specimens such as gastric contents, blood, liver and urine should be retained for toxicological analyses.

Manner of death. Consideration of the circumstances of poisoning, in most cases, helps determine the manner of death. On the one hand, suicide may leave clear evidence—a suicide note, a bottle by the bedside and findings indicating a large overdose; on the other hand there may be no clues whatsoever and the death may appear entirely natural. To determine the manner of death, the autopsy and toxicological studies that suggest ingestion of a large quantity of barbiturate should be coordinated with the detailed investigation of the background history of the decedent and the source and use of the drug. Routine screening tests for barbiturates may detect unsuspected poisonings. Accidental poisoning by barbiturates does occur. An insomniac ingesting sleeping pills after a few drinks may kill himself accidentally, not realizing the danger of the combination of alcohol and barbiturates. Another explanation of accidental death from barbiturate poisoning is the phenomenon called "barbiturate automatism." A person who has taken a few barbiturate capsules or tablets experiences amnesia and, not remembering that he has taken any drug, keeps on taking more and more, finally succumbing to an overdose.

TABLE 20-2: Common Barbiturates:
General Information.

Barbiturate	Identification	Duration of action in hours	Therapeutic Dose (mg.)	Fatal Dose (g.)	Fatal Concentration (mg. %)	
					Blood	Liver
Ultra-short acting:		< 1	100–500 (i.v. for	15–20		
Thiopentone B (Pentothal)	White powder or solution		anesthesia)			
Short-acting:		3–6		15–20	1.0–2.0	4.0–6.0
Cyclobarbitone	White tablet		200–400			
Heptabarbital			200–400			
Hexobarbitone	White tablet		300–500			
Secobarbital (Seconal)	Red capsule		75–150			
Intermediate-acting:		4–8		20–30	2.0–4.0	6.0–10.0
Allobarbitone (Dial)	White tablet		50–200			
Amylobarbitone (Amytal)	Blue capsule		100–200			
Butobarbitone (Soneryl)	Pink tablet					
Pentobarbitone (Nembutal)	Yellow capsule		100–200			
Long-acting:		8–16		30–50	6.0–7.0	15.0–20.0
Barbitone (Veronal)	White tablet		200–500			
Phenobarbitone (Luminal)	White tablet		30–120			

Cause of death. In Table 20-2 some general information is given about barbiturates and the fatal concentrations of various types. The concentrations are the minimum considered within fatal limits when no other drug is involved. If, however, the decedent's body fluids or tissues show the presence of other drugs, the significance of the concentrations changes. For instance, a person with a moderate amount of alcohol in his body dies with a third of the usual fatal concentration of barbiturate. The concentrations in different materials from the same body also vary. Liver concentrations may be much higher than blood concentrations. Curry[7] indicates that when death occurs within 3 to 4 hours after ingestion, the blood-liver ratio is up to 1:10. If death occurs at about 20 hours after ingestion, the ratio is 1:2 or 3 and after several days it is 1:2.

In barbiturate poisoning there is marked depression of the respiratory system, and paralysis of the respiratory center usually causes death. This may take a few hours. With a large overdose of a short-acting barbiturate, death may be rapid from a quick fall in cardiac output and a drop in blood pressure. Deaths within half an hour after ingestion of barbiturates have been observed.

CANNABIS (MARIHUANA)

In recent years there has been an extraordinary interest in the research on marihuana, because of its widespread use in the Western world. Thousands of references have been collected; most of these can be found in three publications (UN Commission on Narcotic Drugs; Medlar's Search; and Kwan and Rajesewaran).[27, 34, 53] Despite extensive research, little is known about cannabis. Generally acceptable methods of detection and estimation of marihuana in biological materials are not available.

Marihuana has been in use in Eastern and Far Eastern countries for centuries. It is consumed in several ways—smoked, drunk or eaten. In India the preparation that is drunk is a concoction called bhang which consists of ground cannabis leaves and fruit shoots and milk. Cakes and cookies containing marihuana are also sold in some places. Home-brewed liquors are sometimes spiked with cannabis. The most common method of use is by smoking. It is commonly smoked after the resinous matter of the cannabis plant is rolled into reefer cigarettes or a hookah is sometimes used.

Signs and symptoms. In the stage of mild to moderate intoxication the faculties are depressed, and this results in the loss of time and space orientation, exultation and euphoria, a dreamy state, lack of concentration, poor judgment, disconnected ideas, impairment of control of thought and action and in the feeling of physical and mental lifting. The user may experience vertigo and vivid dreams with the creation of unreality.

In the stage of narcosis the person feels giddy, is ataxic and experiences delirium and hallucinations. Sensations of tingling and numbness are felt and the speech is rambling. The patient feels drowsy and falls asleep. There is usually muscular weakness, and the pupils are dilated. Grand mal convulsions may occur.

Marihuana is not an addicting drug and there are no withdrawal symptoms. Recovery from intoxication occurs after a period of sleep, the patient awaking thirsty and hungry. With repeated use of marihuana there is progressive loss of appetite and weakness, tremors develop and deterioration in sexual power occurs.

Dangers of the use of marihuana. Marihuana may impair one's ability to operate a motor vehicle. An accidental death while driving under the influence of marihuana needs a careful investigation of the circumstances.

Persons using marihuana frequently use other drugs either when marihuana is not available or when they develop an urge for strong hallucinogens. The use of alcohol, barbiturates and other sedatives, stimulants and opiates as substitutes is not uncommon. Combined effects of two or more of such drugs may cause death.

Smoking of marihuana per se is not known to cause death. There is, however, a possibility that a severely intoxicated person may vomit and die by aspirating regurgitated material.

Under the influence of marihuana a person may commit criminal acts,[3] and on a rare occasion one may be called upon to investigate a homicide committed by a person under the influence of marihuana.

Toxicological problems. The only way to make positive identification of material thought to be marihuana is to search out the botanical features— plant leaves, fruits, shoots and flowering tops by gross and microscopic examination.

Identification of the material itself is possible but its identification in biological tissues and fluids is not. The cannabis plant is supposed to contain a number of compounds, the component most investigated being tetrahydrocannabinol.[51] Stone[47] has described details of experiments to recover cannabinols added to the urine and blood. Attempts to detect marihuana in the blood and urine of a person who has smoked or otherwise taken marihuana into the system are unsuccessful in most cases. The reported exception is the case described by Heyndrickx and his associates.[24] They found, in the urine of a 23-year-old man, discovered dead with large quantities of cannabis near him, a compound giving positive reactions for cannabinol. In this case there were no natural disease and no marks of violence to account for death. The authors considered this death to be from intoxication resulting from cannabis smoking.

CARBON MONOXIDE

In countries such as England using coal gas for domestic heating and cooking, carbon-monoxide poisoning causes more deaths than any other poison. In the United States, the use of harmless natural gas instead of coal gas explains far fewer fatalities.

The principal sources of carbon monoxide in industry are producer gas, Mond gas and blue gas, all used as illuminants, and in homes the sources are domestic coal gas, calor gas, fires and oil heaters burning in poorly ventilated rooms. In the United States the source of carbon monoxide responsible for a majority of the carbon-monoxide poisoning deaths is the exhaust fumes of motor vehicles.

Manner of death. Where coal gas is available for domestic use, suicides and accidents are common. A person taking his own life with coal gas frequently leaves a characteristic scene—a suicide note, if left, contains a considerate message to "Beware of gas," doors, windows and cracks are sealed to prevent the escape of gas, the suicide makes himself comfortable with pillows, clothing and cushions before turning on the gas and placing his head in the oven or near its opened door. Some suicides make more elaborate preparations.

> A young unmarried man went to a realtor pretending to want to rent a house. The realtor gave him keys to a house to let him look at it. The man went to the house, had duplicate keys made and returned the original keys to the realtor. He indicated to the realtor that he was not interested in the house. He then wrote a letter to his parents and one to a friend asking them to find him in the house he had keys for. On the front door of the house was a message "Beware of gas" and a similar message on the kitchen door. A third note on the living room door said "Play the record player." The recording explained in detail why he had decided to take his own life. He was found dead with his head in the oven in the gas-filled kitchen, the doors and windows of which were sealed with newspapers.

Accidental deaths caused by gas leaking from defective domestic appliances—cracked gas pipes, radiators and gas fires—are also common. In considering the causes of such deaths, Fiddes[13] described "the 4 D's of accidental carbon-monoxide poisoning" as "the decrepit, the diseased, the drunk and the drugged." Elderly persons with impaired sense of smell, confusion due to cerebral arteriosclerosis and poor mobility, and persons with severe coronary artery disease, chronic pulmonary disease, cerebral sclerosis and anemia are frequently victims of gas poisoning.

Automobile exhaust fumes contain carbon monoxide and defective exhaust pipes can lead to the accumulation of carbon monoxide in the car and cause poisoning. A person sleeping in the car or one drunk or drugged may succumb to such accumulations. Also, if the motor of a vehicle is running in a closed garage, the escape of exhaust fumes can cause dangerous accumulations of carbon monoxide. A common method of committing suicide with carbon monoxide is to lead the exhaust fumes into a closed car by attaching a rubber tube to the exhaust (see case history Chap. 19). The manner of death in a carbon-monoxide poisoning case should be evaluated with utmost care, since a suicide may be staged as an accidental or natural death, or a murder may be concealed by making it look like a suicide, accident or natural death. Most commonly murder by carbon-monoxide poisoning is committed by a mother who gases her children to death and then kills herself.

Signs and Symptoms. Carbon monoxide combines with hemoglobin to form carboxyhemoglobin. This combination occurs rapidly because the affinity of carbon monoxide for hemoglobin is over 200 times that of oxygen. The hemoglobin that combines with carbon monoxide is prevented from carrying oxygen. This leads to oxygen deprivation that is responsibile for the various signs and symptoms. The symptomatology for various percentage saturations of carboxyhemoglobin is:

1. 10 to 20 percent. No symptoms or mild headache. Smokers have CO levels of 2 to 5 percent. In heavy traffic one may attain a CO level of up to 20 percent.
2. 20 to 30 percent. Increased headache or throbbing in the head, malaise, dizziness, nausea, vomiting, sense of weakness, faintness, impaired reaction time, poor judgment, rapid pulse rate.
3. 30 to 40 percent. Vomiting, poor coordination, staggering, dizziness, confusion, dimness of vision, sense of faintness, severe headache, rapid pulse rate, fast respiration, fall in blood pressure.
4. 40 to 50 percent. Impaired memory, increased weakness, deterioration of coordination, mental confusion, drunken gait, slurred speech, flushing, exhaustion, dyspnea.
5. 50 to 60 percent. Fast pulse rate, syncope, intermittent convulsions, coma, incontinence.
6. Over 60 percent. Deepening coma, convulsions, respiratory arrest, death.

Autopsy findings. Carboxyhemoglobin tints the blood cherry-red and this is reflected in deaths from *acute poisoning* as pink livor of the skin. Although the pink livor is the best indicator of carbon-monoxide poisoning on external examination, it should be noted that persons dying of exposure and refrigerated bodies also show pinkish livor. Chemical tests readily detect carbon monoxide. The muscles of the body and the cut surfaces of the internal organs also show reddish pink coloration in carbon-monoxide poisoning.

The other change that is invariably seen and is common to all poisonings is generalized visceral congestion. Petechial hemorrhages may be seen on the pleural surfaces, heart and lungs. Slight edema of the brain and right ventricular dilatation may be observed.

In deaths from chronic carbon-monoxide poisoning or *delayed death* from acute poisoning, the pathological changes are better defined. Some of the lesions that can be seen are:

1. Bullous skin lesions due to anoxia.
2. Pulmonary edema and bronchopneumonia.
3. Decubitus ulcers (bed sores) from prolonged immobilization.
4. Gangrene of the legs (rare).
5. Muscle necrosis.[1]
6. Acute renal tubular necrosis.
7. Focal anoxic degeneration (heart, liver, kidneys).
8. Bilateral necrosis of the globus pallidus.
9. Petechial hemorrhages in the white matter of the brain.

Specimens for toxicological analysis. Uncontaminated blood should be obtained. In severely charred bodies it may not be possible to obtain a sample of blood. In such cases a small quantity of bone marrow is helpful.

Fatal concentration. The carboxyhemoglobin saturations of over 55 to 60 percent are usually fatal in average persons. Every person does not die at a certain level. Some attain levels of over 80 percent at death; others die with levels less than 50 percent. In persons with severe coronary artery disease, severe chronic lung disease or cerebral arteriosclerosis, carboxyhemoglobin levels as low as 20 percent may precipitate death. Individuals with moderately high blood alcohol concentrations or persons under the influence of drugs may succumb to lower than usual fatal concentrations.

CARBON TETRACHLORIDE

Carbon tetrachloride, an excellent solvent, is a highly toxic chemical. It is used in the manufacture of other chemicals, in fire extinguishers, for fumigation of grains, in the manufacture of rubber, in dry cleaning and as a degreasing agent. It is also a constituent of several cleaning agents and insecticides.

The most common mode of poisoning is by inhalation of carbon tetrachloride. The upper limit of safety is inhalation of air with 1000 ppm. of carbon tetrachloride vapors. The inhalation of about 20,000 ppm. for about an hour causes intoxication, and exposures to about 80,000 ppm. for even less than an hour are fatal. Carbon tetrachloride is absorbed through the gastrointestinal tract. A dose of 2 to 4 ml. of ingested carbon tetrachloride is within fatal limits.[29]

Signs and symptoms. Inhalation of toxic concentrations causes nausea, vomiting, headache, dizziness and irritation of eyes, nose and larynx. Prolonged exposures lead to convulsions and coma with cardiac arrhythmia, extrasystoles and ventricular fibrillation. Death usually results from toxic effects on the vital centers of the brain or from ventricular fibrillation. With survival for 2 to 3 days, evidence of liver and kidney damage appears. The delayed clinical features are abdominal pain, vomiting, diarrhea, jaundice with enlargement of the liver and hematemesis. Renal damage is accompanied by proteinuria, hematuria and cylindruria before the onset of anuria. Occasionally, optic neuritis, pancreatitis, and necrosis of the adrenal cortex may complicate the picture. The serum glutamic oxalacetic transaminase is usually markedly elevated.

With ingestion of carbon tetrachloride, almost the same clinical features result with more severe gastrointestinal symptoms and hematemesis.

Postmortem changes. Deaths from carbon tetrachloride may result from suicidal overdosage, accidental ingestion (mistaking the contents of the container for a drink, usually by children or intoxicated adults) or from industrial exposure to vapors in confined spaces. With exposures to serious concentrations or ingestion of large overdoses death is rapid. If death is rapid no gross changes may be seen apart from congestion of the visceral organs and edema of the lungs. If death results 2 to 3 days after the onset of intoxication, anatomical changes are invariably present principally in the liver and the kidneys.

On external examination jaundice with or without petechial hemorrhages in the skin may be present.

The liver is usually enlarged, sometimes up to twice its normal size. It is pale, greasy and slightly soft. It may be mottled purple if areas of necrosis are present. Subcapsular hemorrhages may be present. When sectioned fatty changes and necrotic areas, if present, are seen. Total necrosis results in acute yellow atrophy. Microscopic examination of the affected liver reveals a centrilobular type of necrosis with peripheral fatty changes (Fig. 20-3). In chronic alcoholics preexisting fatty metamorphosis and cirrhosis may be additional findings; however, it must be noted that chronic exposures to carbon tetrachloride vapors also cause cirrhosis of the liver.[19]

The kidneys are usually pale and swollen, more so the cortices. The capsules are tense and strip easily. On the surfaces petechial hemorrhages may be present. When sectioned swollen cortices bulge. Microscopic studies reveal tubular fatty degeneration; the second convoluted tubules and the ascending limb of Henle are notably affected. The picture is one of lower nephron nephrosis. Thromboses of the tubulo-venous communications may also be seen. The renal changes have been well described by Woods.[58] Rarely does chronic exposure cause nephrotic syndrome.

The lungs are edematous and may show areas of bronchopneumonic consolidations. The heart may show the presence of subendocardial hemorrhages particularly in the interventricular septum on the left side. Evidence of toxic myocarditis may be present.

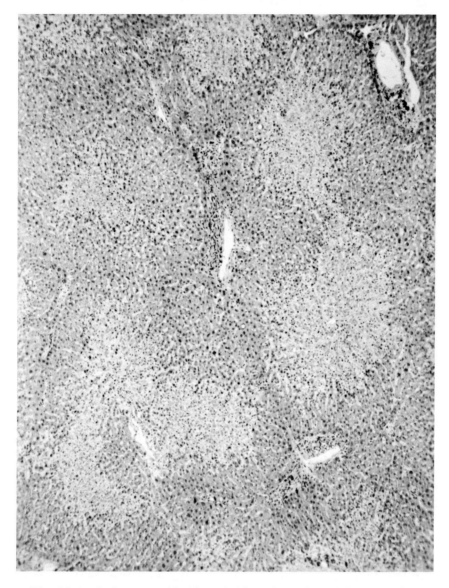

Fig. 20–3. Carbon tetrachloride poisoning. A section of liver showing centrilobular necrosis (× 130).

From a case of poisoning with carbon tetrachloride, specimens that should be retained for the toxicologist are blood, urine, brain, liver and lung. Details of the levels of various halogenated hydrocarbons have been reviewed by Curry.[8]

CYANIDES

A case of cyanide poisoning can be easily missed, not only because poisoning from cyanides is uncommon but also because there may not be any characteristic findings to rouse suspicions. A majority of the cases of cyanide poisoning are suicides with some accidental deaths. Since the autopsy findings are of limited help, a thorough exploration of the circumstances of death should be an essential part of the investigation.

Hydrogen cyanide gas is used in industry for fumigation of ships and greenhouses, and in houses to kill rats. Accidental deaths from this gas may resut if it is used in closed spaces with poor ventilation. Another cyanide compound, prussic acid (Scheele's acid), is commonly used in veterinary practice in a 2 or 4 percent solution. It is also used in electroplating and photographic processes. Because this compound is easily obtained it is sometimes chosen by suicides. The agents most commonly responsible for cyanide poisoning are the alkaline cyanides, namely, sodium cyanide, potassium cyanide, calcium cyanide and magnesium cyanide. These substances are invariably present in laboratories, widely used in industry and often by gardeners and photographers. Most of the suicides accomplished by cyanides are with alkaline cyanides, because they can be acquired most easily. Deaths from other cyanides such as sodium and potassium nitroprusside and potassium thiocyanate are extremely rare.

Absorption and action. The ingested substance is absorbed from the stomach, whereas the respiratory system is the route of absorption for inhaled gases. Cyanide can also be absorbed through the skin. Absorption from the stomach is rapid if the stomach is empty. Hydrochloric acid in the stomach combines with the ingested alkaline cyanide to liberate hydrocyanic acid. Cyanide is a cytotoxic poison. The absorbed cyanide acts by poisoning the enzyme system. There is a strong affinity between the enzyme cytochrome oxidase and the cyanides, resulting in the inhibition of oxygen metabolism. Although there is enough oxygen in the system, the tissues cannot utilize it and the person dies of anoxia.

Signs and symptoms. The ingested poison rapidly causes respiratory failure and death may occur within minutes. During the short interval between ingestion of the poison and death, one may observe dramatic signs and symptoms. The patient may complain of burning of the throat and tongue, tightness of the chest, increased salivation, nausea, vomiting, headache, vertigo, photophobia, tinnitus, dizziness and fainting. The clinician may observe cyanosis of the face, frothing at the mouth, rapid weak pulse, rapid and sometimes irregular respirations, dilated pupils and sluggish reflexes. The breath of the patient may smell of bitter almonds. Just prior to death the cyanosis becomes marked, and there are muscular twitchings and convulsions associated with incontinence of feces and urine. If the offending agent is inhaled gas, the patient experiences palpitation and difficulty in breathing in addition to nausea, vomiting, headache, salivation, watering of the eyes, irritation of the mouth and throat and giddiness. Weakness of the extremities develops rapidly and the patient collapses. Convulsions may precede coma and death.

Fatal doses. Lethal doses vary according to the mode of poisoning. There is a wide range of fatal quantities as far as ingested cyanides are concerned, because factors such as food in the stomach and the amount of gastric hydrochloric acid play important roles in the rate of absorption. The presence of hydrochloric acid in the stomach is essential for the formation of HCN; hence persons with achlorhydria can tolerate large doses of ingested cyanides. Under ordinary circumstances the following quantities prove fatal.

Hydrogen cyanide gas: 200–500 ppm. (death within ½ hour)
1500–2000 ppm. (death immediate)
Sodium cyanide: 150 mg.
Potassium cyanide: 200 mg.
Prussic acid (Scheele's acid): 1.5 to 2.5 ml. of 2 percent solution

Pathological changes. In most cases the changes are nonspecific or merely indicative of tissue anoxia. The only pathognomonic feature at autopsy, if one is able to detect it, is the distinctive odor of cyanides. This smell, not unlike that of burnt almonds, is penetrating and instantly tickles the back of the throat when the pathologist is near the body. The smell is readily dulled, and one is not able to sense it unless a few moments are spent away from the body in fresh air. The smell again hits the pathologist when he opens the victim's stomach, since the concentrations of HCN are likely to be the highest in the stomach. The other internal organs too may smell of cyanide. The pathologist should be careful in smelling the stomach contents lest he inhale an overdose. It should be noted that not all persons can smell cyanide.

Other findings to be noted on external examination are suffusion of the face with cyanosis of the lips, froth in the mouth and the bright red or brick red color of livor. This color is due to cyanmethemoglobin in the blood and in some cases it appears characteristic; in other cases of cyanide poisoning the color of livor is no different from that seen in usual cases. On internal examination of the body, a bright red color of the muscles and the cut surfaces of the organs is sometimes noted. Congestion of the mucosa of the stomach is a common finding and sometimes may be exaggerated to intense hemorrhagic gastritis. Alkaline cyanides may cause corrosion and shredding of the mucosa. Occasionally, one may find hardening of the mucosal folds.

LEAD

Lead, one of the first metals known to man, is widely used in industry. Among its various uses in industry are plumbing typesetting, smelting, shipfitting, diamond cutting, file making, painting, car welding and polishing. It is also used in the manufacture of colors and dyes, alloys, toys, insecticides and bullets. Its industrial uses have led to many cases of poisoning culminating in civil suits for personal injury to health and workmen's compensation. Poisoning can occur by ingestion of contaminated food and water, and many outbreaks from such contamination of domestic water supplies have occurred. Absorption of lead can also occur from the skin with compounds such as tetraethyl lead. The dust and vapors of lead inhaled, during the manufacture of white lead and during welding and smelting, can also cause poisoning by being absorbed from the respiratory tract.

Deaths from lead poisoning occur from time to time from overdosages or from complications of acute and chronic poisoning.

Symptoms and signs. With *acute poisoning* the patient complains of a metallic taste in the mouth, a burning feeling in the mouth and pharynx with salivation. Nausea, vomiting, gastrointestinal irritation, abdominal colic, diarrhea, malaise and anorexia develop. Occasionally, there is black lead sulphide in foul-smelling stools, with albuminuria, hematuria and oliguria. Deterioration in vision, encephalopathy, convulsions and coma are sometimes seen. Severe vomiting and diarrhea may lead to dehydration, hypothermia and circulatory collapse.

Chronic Lead Poisoning (chronic plumbism) is the commoner of the two forms of poisoning. When the absorbed lead is not excreted as fast as it is absorbed, accumulation occurs in the body over a period of time and results in chronic poisoning. The clinical features of chronic lead poisoning can be grouped as follows:

1. Alimentary system. Metallic taste in the mouth, stomatitis with foul mouth odor, blue line 1 mm. wide on gums from lead sulphide (seen in about 70 percent of the cases), constipation, rigidity and contraction of abdominal wall, intense abdominal colic (characteristically at night).
2. Hemopoietic system. Marked pallor of the skin, icteric tinge, anemia (normochronic or hypochronic), punctate basophilia, polychromasia, reticulocytosis, rarely increase in granulocytes.
3. Nervous system. Confusion, mental retardation, psychological disturbances, tremors (of eyes, tongue and fingers), incoordination,

peripheral neuritis, partial paralysis, muscular atrophy, wrist or foot drop, loss of vision, encephalitis.
4. Cardiovascular system. Vascular constriction with hypertension and arteriolar degeneration.
5. Urinary system. Polyuria, albuminuria, glycosuria, casts and red blood cells in the urine, features of renal damage.
6. General. Headache, loss of weight, malaise, weakness.

The most important of the clinical features of plumbism are: anemia, blue line on gums, colic, wrist drop and encephalopathy.

Pathological findings. A pathologist may be required to establish the cause of death in a case with a suspected overdose or to evaluate the role of chronic lead poisoning in the causation of death.

With acute overdosages, one may find ingested material in the gastrointestinal tract with evidence of irritation and foul-smelling black stools. The fatal dose of lead acetate is about 2 Gm.

In cases of chronic poisoning one may be able to confirm the clinical features. Microscopic studies may reveal renal damage in the form of swelling and dissolution of tubular epithelium with proteinaceous, and cellular components in the tubules. The sections of kidneys may show arteriolar degeneration and areas of renal sclerosis; the sections of bones showing lead lines may reveal disruption of the development of bone.

In a case of chronic lead poisoning x-rays of the bones may show lead lines.

At the autopsy samples of blood, liver, kidney, brain and bone should be retained. From clinical cases the specimens of choice are blood and urine.

Interpretation of toxicological results. Lead is normally present in the body. The average "normal" lead level in blood is 17 μg per 100 ml.; in the urine it is 35 μg per 1. The level of 60 μg per 100 ml. of blood is considered the upper limit of normal (American Public Health Association, 1964). Eighty to 90 percent of the lead is in the erythrocytes. In chronic accumulations lead is mainly concentrated in the bones. Normal and abnormal concentrations of lead in various biological materials are given in Table 20-3.

LSD (D-LYCERGIC ACID DIETHYLAMIDE)

A brief discussion of this drug is included here not only because a death from LSD poisoning, although rare, may be encountered but also because this drug is likely to lead to deaths indirectly. The pathologist may be required to answer questions pertaining to its role in a particular death. In

TABLE 20-3. Comparison of Average Lead Concentrations in "Normal" and Poisoning Cases.

Fluid or Tissue	"Normal" Lead Level	Levels of Lead in Plumbism
Blood	15–40 μg per 100 ml.	1050 μg per 100 ml.
Urine	80 μg per l.	0.2 mg. per l.
Bone	4 to 12.5 μg per Gm. of ash	200 μg per Gm. of ash
Hair	5 mg. per 100 Gm.	28.2 mg. per 100 Gm.
Feces	Up to 0.3 mg. per day	> 0.3 mg. per day

Compiled from Curry,[6] Goldwater and Hoover,[16] Gossmann and Heilenz,[18] Kopito, et al.,[26] Simpson,[43] and Varley.[54]

the past the use of LSD was restricted to research and to religious practices. Now its use by the young generation for hallucinogenic effects is not only creating social chaos but also confronting the men of law and medicine with difficult problems. Despite legal restrictions in the United States and the British Isles, its use has been increasing uncontrollably.

Actions of LSD. The drug is mainly used for self-exploration, to experience varied hallucinations and to get out of day-to-day boredom. Unfortunately, it does more than that—it leads to fatal accidents and serious crime. The hallucinating person has no control over his actions. The feeling of being able to fly under the influence of LSD can lead users to jump out of windows, and fatalities from such actions have been reported. The hallucinations may result in murders. In a case described by Ungerleider and Fisher,[52] a young man who ingested LSD for the first time in his life was convinced that he had to offer a human sacrifice. He was to throw his girlfriend off the roof of a Hollywood hotel and had to be prevented from doing so.

The most harassing aspect of the effects of LSD is the reappearance of hallucinations days, weeks or even months after the ingestion of a dose. No biochemical or physiological explanation is available for this phenomenon. It must be noted that these delayed recurring symptoms may lead to bizarre behavior, suicide or even homicide.

Materson and Barrett-Connor[33] have described the occurrence of hepatitis after intravenous use of LSD. The reader is referred to excellent reviews of the unfavorable reactions to LSD.[39, 44] LSD is also known to cause genetic abnormalities such as teratogenic effects and chromosomal aberrations.

Investigation of a death. Proven deaths from overdose of LSD are rare. The psychotic reactions are more frequently responsible for accidental deaths than simple overdoses. Also, frequently seen are complications such as bronchopneumonia and hepatitis.

The usual dose of LSD for hallucinogenic purpose is about 100 μg. and the LD_{50} for humans is about 14 mg.[39] Biological half-life of LSD in man is 3 hours.

In the investigation of a case involving LSD, the task of the forensic toxicologist is a difficult one. No methods are available to detect and identify LSD in biological materials. However, the bulletin of the International Association of Forensic Toxicologists reports that after acute poisoning from LSD, blood levels are about 1 ng. per ml. and a time lapse of 4 hours after ingestion makes the detection of LSD in blood impossible.[23, 57]

MORPHINE (HEROIN)

Although the true incidence of deaths from intravenous narcotism cannot be determined, there is little doubt that in recent years it has increased throughout the world, especially in urban areas. In New York City alone there were 2500 deaths in a 15-year period between 1950 and 1964.[22]

Most deaths from intravenous narcotism are sudden, unexpected fatalities in young persons with little or no medical history. While in some instances the explanation of the cause and manner of death is obvious, in others a careful detailed investigation may be necessary to establish these facts. A brief procedural review of the various aspects of deaths from intravenous narcotism is presented here.

Scene investigation. At the scene of death, some features are characteristic and can help the pathologist draw conclusions from the preliminary examination of the scene and the body. Some of the commonly observed characteristics are:

1. *Decedent.* Usually a young adult (most often less than 30 years of age), male (more often a Negro male in the United States), laborer or unskilled worker.
2. *Site of death.* Usually a concealed spot with maximum privacy, a closed room, lavatory or bathroom, hallway; the decedent is usually on a bed, floor, sofa or chair.
3. *Addict's paraphernalia.* Commonly found at the scene of death are disposable plastic syringe previously used and disposed of, medicine dropper with tip fitted to hypodermic needle, tourniquet, matches, spoon, bottle cap, cotton, water. (Addicts put the powdered drug in a spoon with water, warm it by lighting the match and suck the drug into the syringe through cotton which serves as a filter.)
4. *Drug.* The powdered drug is frequently mixed with lactose, mannitol or quinine before use.

External examination of the body at the scene of death. The investigator will encounter some of the following features on the body.

1. Fresh needle punctures on antecubital fossa (most common); on arm, forearm, hands, femoral area, buttocks, jugular area (occasionally); on feet (rarely).
2. Contusions around recent needle punctures.
3. Dark brown pigmented scars and keloids due to needle punctures in the past (sometimes in a row) on antecubital fossa, arm, forearm, hand, femoral vein area, buttocks or on jugular area (paregoric addict).
4. Tattoos at the sites of needle punctures or scars (imprinted to conceal injection sites).
5. Ropelike thickened veins with or without knots caused by thrombi at the injection sites.
6. Subcutaneous abscesses at the injection sites.
7. Palpable enlarged lymph nodes—axillary, cervical or inguinal.
8. Froth (occasionally blood-tinged) in the nostrils and mouth.
9. Cigarette burns or scars on upper chest.
10. Jaundice.
11. Evidence of malnutrition.

Internal examination of the body. It must be stressed that the internal examination of a narcotic victim may be entirely negative, with the exception of generalized visceral congestion. However, a careful examination may reveal one or more of the following findings.

1. *Injection sites.* Fresh needle punctures concealed under blood spots or tattoos, with subcutaneous hemorrhages and needle tracts (skin should be incised to explore these features and to see needle punctures in veins); subcutaneous fibrosis and abscess; thickening and thrombosis of veins previously used for injecting (portions of these should be excised for microscopic examination).
2. *Generalized findings.* Generalized visceral congestion, dark red blood, signs of septicemia and systemic necrotizing angiitis.[56]
3. *Lungs.* In rapid deaths enlarged and heavy with intense congestion and marked edema, focal hemorrhages and areas of atelectasis; slight acute emphysema; froth in the trachea and bronchi; aspirated material (especially milk which some addicts use as "antidote") in the mouth, stomach, trachea and main bronchi and variegated acute changes in the lungs—"narcotic lungs."[40]
4. *Heart.* Marked dilatation of right ventricle; bacterial endocarditis commonly from Staphylococcus aureus; septic embolism; abscesses and infarction.

5. *Liver.* Congestion; hepatomegaly; acute hepatitis; postnecrotic cirrhosis; portal fibrosis.
6. *Lymph nodes.* Enlargement of axillary, hepatic and subpyloric (around the head of pancreas) lymph nodes.[41]
7. *Brain.* Cerebral edema; congestion; softening due to septicemia.
8. *Kidneys.* Congestion; softening and swelling due to septicemia.
9. *Spleen.* Enlargement; congestion; softening.
10. *Complications.* If death does not occur from overdose of the drug or from hypersensitivity reaction, it may occur from one of the following complications: septic endocarditis, viral hepatitis, postnecrotic cirrhosis, tetanus (organisms in subcutaneous tissues), miliary tuberculosis, bronchopneumonia, lung abscess, pulmonary fibrosis, malnutrition.

Microscopic examination. Histological studies will confirm the gross anatomical findings and may reveal the following additional changes.

1. Microabscesses in various organs such as the brain, heart, spleen, liver, kidneys, lymph nodes secondary to septicemia; systemic necrotizing angiitis.
2. Chronic hepatitis (a constant finding)—lymphocytic infiltrate of portal and periportal areas with occasional neutrophils; acute hepatitis with necroses and acute inflammatory cell infiltration.
3. Edema and lymphocytic hyperplasia of lymph nodes.
4. Interstitial pulmonary fibrosis; pulmonary tuberculosis; scattered granulomas of foreign-body type. (Polarized light useful to see foreign material—usually talc or starch. X-ray diffraction can be used to identify the foreign material.)[2]
5. Foreign body granulomas in skin around blood vessels; thrombophlebitis; organizing thromboses of veins.

Specimens to collect and analyses to request. The following specimens should be collected from a suspected case of intravenous narcotism.

1. Tissues from injection site—excise skin with injection marks, subcutaneous tissues and portions of underlying muscle.
2. Blood
3. Urine
4. Liver

In a suspected case of narcotism the analyses for morphine should, no doubt, be done. However, tests for mannitol, quinine, cyanide and nicotine may give positive results because the addicts tend to mix some of these substances for various reasons. The analysis for alcohol should, of course, be done as a routine.

Interpretation of the findings. The scene of death frequently presents convincing evidence of death from intravenous narcotism. The autopsy and toxicological studies not only help establish the cause of death, but they may also indicate the mechanism of death and throw light on previous usage of the drug. Death may be sudden from hypersensitivity reaction or overdose of the drug, or delayed from complications of drug abuse. The analyses of the tissues from the site of injection and of the body fluids and tissues may not show the presence of the narcotic drug. Victims who are found with a needle still in a vein sometimes die from hypersensitivity reaction. In these persons the toxicological studies may be negative. Therefore, even if the toxicological results are negative, one is justified in certifying death from intravenous narcotism, provided there is evidence of recent and past drug abuse and no other anatomical cause of death is found. In deaths from overdose the usual concentrations of morphine are 0.1 mg. per 100 ml. of blood, 0.5 mg. per 100 ml. of urine and 0.1 mg. per 100 Gm. of liver.

ORGANOPHOSPHATES (PARATHION)

Compounds commonly producing organophosphate poisoning are Parathion (diethyl-para-nitrophenyl monothiophosphate) and Malathion. Occasionally, DFP (diisopropyl fluorophosphate), HETP (hexaethyltetraphosphate), TEPP (tetraethylpyrophosphate), OMPA (octamethylpyrophosphoramide), Disyston, Diazinon, methyl parathion, Guthion, Thimet, Azodrin, Phosdrin may cause poisoning. These substances are widely used by farmers for crop dusting, hence, they and other agricultural workers are particularly liable to exposure to these poisonous agents. These pesticides are also used to kill insects in yards and gardens. Therefore, the presence of organophosphate insecticides in homes and in agricultural districts is not uncommon.

In every nation of the world where these pesticides are used poisonings and deaths occur. Accidental poisoning is common among agricultural workers involved in spraying crops, at times with fatal outcome. In Europe organophosphates, especially parathion, are not only used to commit suicide but also to accomplish murder. In the 40 fatal cases of acute parathion poisoning studied by Vercruysse and Deslypere,[55] 19 were suicides, 13 accidents and 8 homicides. Whether it is a suicide, an accident or a murder by parathion the investigation must be thorough. Vercruysse and Deslypere warn that the "pathologist must bear in mind that parathion is detected only when, its use being suspected, it is specifically looked for by the chemist."

Action. Organophosphates can be absorbed through the skin, from the lungs and also from the stomach. Organophosphates are powerful inhibitors of cholinesterase. They act by stopping the enzyme acetylcholine esterase from performing its function of destroying acetylcholine at the neuromuscular junction. Acetylcholine is not hydrolyzed at its site of activity and this results in the nicotine and muscarine effect. Symptoms of parathion poisoning, thus, are similar to those from overdosages of physostigmine, pilocarpine and muscarine.

Signs and Symptoms. Symptoms of poisoning become evident with alarming rapidity, usually within 30 minutes after the ingestion of even a few drops of the poison or after a brief exposure to a cloud of insecticide spray. With large overdoses death is rapid. Symptoms usually appear if the cholinesterase level falls to 25 to 30 percent of the normal. With smaller overdoses the symptoms experienced are nausea, vomiting, headache, diarrhea, profuse perspiration, salivation, lacrimation, visual disturbances, weakness, abdominal cramps and tightness of the chest. The signs usually detectable are vasodilatation with flushing and sweating, increase in the temperature of the skin, miosis, muscular fasciculations, increased secretions, areflexia, twitchings, tonic and clonic convulsions, urination and defecation and, in terminal stages, shock and coma. Poisoning in children may not be associated with some of these dramatic signs and symptoms and one may observe only convulsions that are followed by deepening coma. However absence of the signs and symptoms does not rule out the possibility of organophosphate poisoning. Various diagnostic problems have been well discussed by Davis and his colleagues.[10]

Autopsy findings. Neither the gross changes nor the microscopic appearances in cases of parathion poisoning are in any way pathognomonic. One may be able to detect an odor similar to that of gasoline, turpentine, xylol or rancid butter. Occasionally, softening of the brain is detected. When the poison is inhaled, there is invariably edema of the lungs. There may also be evidence of aspiration of regurgitated material.

A histological staining method can be used to diagnose organophosphate poisoning. Petty and Moore[37] have demonstrated with the help of a histochemical method that in cases of poisoning with organic phosphate compounds, the activity of cholinesterase is markedly less at the motor end-plates than at similar sites in normal individuals. The advantages of this method are that the procedure is simple, practical and foolproof, and cholinesterase activity at the myoneural junctions can be detected in spite of decomposition or embalming of the body.

For chemical analyses the specimens of choice are gastrointestinal contents, the blood, liver, kidney and urine. Tests for identifying organic phosphate insecticides in gastric lavage fluid, dermal residues, tissues and urine have been described.[14, 30]

Interpretation of toxicological results. Every case of parathion poisoning must be confirmed by chemical tests. The use of a rapid screening test to determine cholinesterase levels in blood indicates the need for further work. A simple screening procedure is described later.

Normal cholinesterase levels in red blood cells (RBC) and whole blood as measured in micromoles of acetylcholine hydrolyzed (Data from Camp)[3] are

Males
RBC   0.74 to 2.38
Whole blood   0.78 to 3.88
Females
RBC   0.90 to 2.33
Whole blood   1.33 to 3.32
Children
RBC   0.72 to 2.25
Whole blood   1.52 to 2.88

With exposure to parathion, plasma cholinesterase falls more rapidly than RBC cholinesterase. Therefore, if exposure is not serious there may be a fall in the plasma cholinesterase level and not in the RBC cholinesterase. In the recovery stage the reverse is true. In the stage of acute serious poisoning, the cholinesterase levels in both plasma and RBC are low, having fallen to more than 25 percent of the normal. With the onset of recovery from poisoning, the cholinesterase levels begin to rise and reach normal levels in one to two weeks.

Fortunately, the cholinesterase levels are not affected in postmortem material even after decomposition sets in. Therefore, it is never too late to perform histological studies of the myoneural junctions or determine cholinesterase levels in the blood. Even in bodies exhumed after a prolonged burial, these tests may turn out to be rewarding.

In parathion poisoning p-nitrophenol is excreted in the urine; therefore, urine should be tested for this additional information. All one needs to do is steam distillate urine and add sodium hydroxide. This gives a strong yellow color indicating the presence of p-nitrophenol. A rapid visual method for the estimation of cholinesterase activity in the blood using acetylcholine as substrate and based upon the color change of bromothymol, has been described by Fleisher and his associates.[15]

PROPOXYPHENE HYDROCHLORIDE (DARVON)

Propoxyphene hydrochloride was made available in the United States in 1957. It soon became a widely prescribed drug. The drug is now one of the most popular analgesics and is used principally for symptomatic relief of mild to moderate pain. It has also been extensively misused; in combination with alcohol it has had fatal results. Propoxyphene hydrochloride is also used occasionally by suicides.[59]

Signs, symptoms and pathological features. Adverse reactions of propoxyphene hydrochloride consist of nausea, vomiting, abdominal pain, dizziness, headache, euphoria, somnolence, paradoxical excitement, insomnia, skin rashes and in some, constipation. Manifestations of overdosage resemble those of narcotic overdosage and include circulatory collapse, respiratory depression, convulsions and coma. The combination products containing salicylates may give the clinical picture of salicylism or may induce hypersensitivity reaction.

Pathological changes are nonspecific. Skin rashes and hemorrhages in the gastrointestinal tract may be seen.

Interpretation of toxicological results. McBay[31] believes that the lethal dose of propoxyphene hydrochloride for adults is between 1 and 2 Gm. Such doses produce concentrations of 0.3 mg. per 100 ml. of blood and 3.0 mg. per 100 Gm. of liver. In McBay's 12 cases in which death was attributed to propoxyphene hydrochloride, concentrations in the blood ranged from 0.3 to 1.5 mg. per 100 ml., and in the liver they were 5.5 to 30 mg. per 100 Gm. In the 17 cases described by Thompson and his associates,[49] the concentrations of propoxyphene hydrochloride in the liver ranged from 3.1 to 12.6 mg. per 100 Gm. with a median of 6.7 mg. per 100 Gm. One issue of *Toxicology and Applied Pharmacology* was devoted entirely to the discussion of propoxyphene hydrochloride; for additional information the reader is referred to it.[11]

PSYCHOSEDATIVE DRUGS

Phenothiazines

Phenothiazines are used commonly as tranquilizers in the treatment of psychoses and parkinsonism, and as antiemetics and antihistamines. These varied uses have led to widespread distribution of the drugs in the general population, so that accidental ingestion by children is not uncommon. Commonly used preparations are Thorazine* (chlorpromazine), Stelazine* (trifluoperazine), Phenergan† (promethazine), Sparine† (promazine), Compazine* (prochlorperazine), and Mellaril‡ (thioridazine). Occasionally, suicides are committed using these drugs.[12] Accidental deaths in adults

---

* Trademark, Smith Kline & French.
† Trademark, Wyeth.
‡ Trademark, Sandoz.

may occur because of peculiar ability of these drugs to cause sudden, unexpected death.[28]

Signs and symptoms. Even the normal therapeutic doses of chlorpromazine of 100 to 800 mg. per day are sometimes associated with symptoms. Patients complain of weakness and drowsiness and frequently experience palpitations and faintness. The complaint of feeling cold is not uncommon. These drugs also cause mild depression, tremors, convulsions and coma. Some of the important toxic effects of chlorpromazine include postural hypotension, cardiac arrhythmia, obstructive jaundice, aggranulocytosis and urticarial rash. It is well known that the routine administration of phenothiazines is associated with hypotension,[38] and increased therapeutic doses may result in a serious drop in blood pressure causing death. Virtually all phenothiazines, it has been shown, cause alteration in the electrocardiogram of a patient under treatment; and it is believed that in some instances death may result from serious arrhythmias caused by phenothiazines.[25] Hepatic damage appears to be the commonest and most serious of the complications, it occurs in 2 to 4 percent of the patients receiving phenothiazines and becomes evident in 2 to 6 weeks after the start of the treatment. Phenothiazines cause swelling of the parenchymatous liver cells and sometimes severe centrilobular necrosis of the hepatic cells. Intrahepatic biliary obstruction may also occur. Blood dyscrasia, especially aggranulocytosis, may result from a hypersensitivity reaction that may prove fatal.

Autopsy findings. Deaths resulting from large overdoses rarely show any characteristic autopsy findings. All one may be able to see is congestion of organs and edema of the lungs and brain. If death results from prolonged treatment or if the person dies as a result of hypersensitivity reaction, several pathological changes may be observed. Skin rash and jaundice may be present. The liver shows swelling and necrosis of cells in the centrilobular zones, and intrahepatic biliary obstruction.

For toxicological analyses the specimens of choice are the blood, urine, liver, bile and lung.

Interpretation of toxicological results. Curry[7] believes that if the levels are in excess of 0.1 mg. per 100 ml. of blood they indicate a large overdose. He indicates that a dose of 1 Gm. of chlorpromazine (Thorazine) can give a blood level of about 0.1 to 0.2 mg. per 100 ml. Concentrations in the liver are usually much higher than in the blood.

Meprobamate (Miltown, Equanil)

A popular tranquilizer for anxiety states, meprobanate has properties similar to those of barbiturates. It relaxes the muscles in spasm. Because of its popularity as a tranquilizer it is occasionally responsible for an accidental or suicidal death. Meprobamate is excreted slowly, about 10 percent being excreted unmetabolized in the urine. Toxic effects include sleepiness, poor motor coordination, impaired reaction time, collapse of cardiovascular and respiratory systems, fall in blood pressure, pinpoint pupils and coma. Meprobamate is also known to cause allergic and hematological manifestations. The therapeutic doses are in the region of 400 mg. per day. Such doses give blood levels of about 0.5 mg. per 100 ml. of blood. Fatal concentrations vary a great deal but are usually above 3 mg. per 100 ml. of blood and 10 mg. per 100 Gm. of the liver.[32]

Imipramine (Tofranil), Amitriptyline (Elavil), Desipramine (Pertofrane)

Imipramine is used exclusively for the treatment of depression. Although in normal persons it causes weakness, in affected persons it leads to excitement and euphoria. Occasionally, patients experience hallucinations. The toxic effects of a therapeutic administration of imipramine include dryness of the mouth, palpitations, constipation, blurred vision, tachycardia, urinary retention, sweating, dizziness, nausea, vomiting, insomnia and tremors. More serious side effects such as aggranulocytosis, bone marrow depression and eosinophilia have been reported. Severe, sometimes fatal, hypotension, apnea, severe oliguria, hyperpyrexia, convulsions and cardiac arrest are known to occur with overdoses. In rare instances obstructive jaundice results from the use of imipramine.

The *therapeutic doses* of imipramine and amitriptyline range from 100 to 300 mg. per day and of desipramine from 50 to 200 mg. per day. Since the absorption of these drugs is rapid, concentrations in the blood following therapeutic doses are low, usually less than 0.1 mg. per 100 ml. of blood. Adults may succumb to doses as small as 625 mg., although recovery following ingestion of 5375 mg. of imipramine has been reported.[20]

Autopsy findings. Usually no specific changes are seen. In delayed deaths cerebral edema with degenerative changes in the cortex may be seen. Jaundice, obstructive type, with gross and microscopic liver damage may be present. A diagnosis of poisoning by any of these anti-depression drugs must be made by toxicological analyses.

Toxicological findings. These vary a great deal in fatal cases. Values of 0.2 to 3 mg. per 100 ml. of blood have been observed.[124] Liver concentrations are several times greater than the blood levels.[9] In the absence of any significant disease conditions, imipramine concentrations in excess of 0.5 mg. per 100 ml. of blood should be considered fatal.

SALICYLATES

Aspirin is one of the most commonly used drugs in the world. It is sold everywhere without any restrictions because it is a "safe" drug. Since every household is likely to have it, poisoning due to therapeutic or accidental overdose is extremely common.

Salicylates are absorbed from the stomach and intestine and excreted in the urine. The absorption of aspirin begins within half an hour. Most cases of poisoning receive combative treatment before serious damage is done. For this reason the number of deaths compared with the number of poisonings is very small. Nevertheless, deaths from salicylate poisoning are not uncommon. In fact in world incidence salicylates can be listed with the ten leading poisons responsible for a high incidence of fatalities. The majority of serious poisonings and deaths occur in children who take overdoses accidentally, either mistaking salicylates for candies or simply because they like the taste of the salicylate preparations. Occasionally, suicides use salicylates. A therapeutic accident may occur if the person is hypersensitive to aspirin.

Signs and symptoms. The prominent feature of salicylate poisoning in the earlier stages is dyspnea due to stimulation of the respiratory center. Later, depression of the respiratory center occurs and death results from respiratory arrest. Patients with moderate overdoses perspire heavily, complain of dimness of vision and tinnitus and are cyanotic. Vomiting is common, leading to dehydration, and is frequently blood stained. Cerebral stimulation causes delirium, disorientation, muscular twitchings and convulsions. There is usually cutaneous vasodilation (flushing) and hyperpyrexia. Melena may be present. Convulsions are followed by gradually deepening coma and death. The combination of the symptoms and signs of sweating, cyanosis, vomiting, delirium, tinnitus, hyperpyrexia and hyperventilation is characteristic of salicylate poisoning.

If a person is sensitive to salicylates, even small doses may cause dramatic symptoms. Soon after ingestion the patient becomes dizzy and faints. There is massive sweating and the skin becomes pale. Nausea, vomiting and tinnitus are common. The patient breathes with air hunger and slumps down.

Fatal dose. The lethal dose of sodium salicylate in infants is 2 to 5 Gm., in older children 5 to 10 Gm. and in adults 20 to 30 Gm. The fatal dose of methyl salicylate is smaller—5 to 10 ml. in children and 15 to 30 ml. in adults.

Autopsy findings. No gross changes may be seen in some cases. Salicylic acid causes irritation of the mucosa of the stomach and the upper intestinal tract. This irritation may be reflected as acute congestion of mucosa, hemorrhagic gastritis or as necrosis of the mucosa. There may be altered blood in the rest of the gastrointestinal tract. If large doses are ingested, masses of white unabsorbed material may be still present in the stomach. Petechial or confluent hemorrhages may be present in the pleural and pericardial surfaces as well as in the surface of the heart. The kidneys are edematous and they also sometimes show petechial hemorrhages in the surface. The brain may show some degree of edema. In delayed deaths bronchopneumonia and renal damage may be seen.

From a case of suspected salicylate poisoning the doctor should retain blood, urine, stomach contents, and the liver and kidneys for toxicological analyses.

Fatal concentrations of salicylates in the blood are usually in the range of 50 to 100 mg. per 100 ml. If death is delayed the levels are lower.

REFERENCES

1. Bowen, D. A. L.: Acute renal failure in carbon monoxide poisoning. J. For. Med., 7:78, 1960.
2. Burton, J. F., Zawadzki, E. S., Wetherell, H. R., and Moy, T. W.: Mainliners and blue velvet. J. Forensic Sci., 10:466, 1965.
3. Camps, F. E. (ed.): Gradwohl's Legal Medicine. ed. 2. Baltimore, Williams & Wilkins, 1968.
4. Clarke, E. G. C. (ed.): Isolation and Identification of Drugs. London, The Pharmaceutical Press, 1969.
5. Connell, P. H.: The amphetamines. I and II. Med. World (Lond.), 96:18, 1962.
6. Curry, A. S.: Advances in Forensic and Clinical Toxicology. Cleveland, Chemical Rubber Company, 1972.
7. Curry, A. S.: Poison Detection in Human Organs. Springfield (Ill.), Charles C Thomas, 1963.
8. Curry, A. S.: Poison Detection in Human Organs. ed. 2. Springfield (Ill.), Charles C Thomas, 1969.
9. Curry, A. S.: Seven fatal cases involving Imipramine in man. J. Pharm. Pharmacol, 16:265, 1964.
10. Davis, J., Davies, J. E., and Fisk, A. J.: Occurrence, diagnosis and treatment of organophosphate pesticide poisoning in man. Ann. N.Y. Acad. Sci., 160:383, 1969.
11. Dearborn, E. H. (ed.): Toxicology and Applied Pharmacology, vol. 19, no. 3. New York, Academic Press, 1971.
12. Fatteh, A.: Death from chlorpromazine poisoning. J. Forensic Med., 11:120, 1964.
12A. Fatteh, A.: Death from imipramine poisoning. J. Forensic Sci., 13:124, 1968.
13. Fiddes, F. S.: Accidental carbon monoxide poisoning; dangers of inadequate ventilation. Br. Med. J., 2:697, 1956.
14. Fisk, A. J.: Czercoinski, G. R., and Kenhart, J. H.: A rapid screening technique for the identification of organic phosphate insecticides in gastric lavage fluid or dermal residues. J. Forensic Sci., 10:473, 1965.
15. Fleisher, J. H., Woodson, G. S., and Simet, L.: A visual method for estimating blood cholinesterase activity. A.M.A. Arch. Ind. Health, 14:510, 1956.
16. Goldwater, L. J., and Hoover, A. W.: An international study of "normal" levels of lead in blood and urine. Arch. Environ. Health, 15:60, 1967.

17. Goodman, L. S., and Gilman, A.: The Pharmacological Basis of Therapeutics. New York, McMillan, 1970.
18. Gossmann, H. H., and Heilenz, S.: Lead content of human bone tissue. Dtsch. Med. Wochenschr., *92:*2267, 1967.
19. Harden, B. L.: Carbon tetrachloride poisoning—a review. Indust. Med. Surg., *23:*93, 1954.
20. Harthorne, J. W., Marcus, A. M., and Kaye, M.: Management of massive imipramine overdosage with mannitol and artificial dialysis. New Eng. J. Med., *268:*33, 1963.
21. Hecke, V., Derveaux, W., and Hans-Berteau, M. J.: A case of criminal poisoning by Parathion. J. Forensic Med., *5:*68, 1958.
22. Helpern, M., and Rho, Y.: Deaths from narcotism in New York City; incidence, circumstances and postmortem findings. N.Y. State J. Med., *66:*2391, 1966.
23. Hessel, D. W., and Modglin, F. R.: The detection of LSD in human blood and bile. Bull. Int. Ass. Forensic Toxic., *7*(3) : 2, 1970.
24. Heyndrickx, A., Scheiris, C., and Schepens, P.: Toxicological study of a fatal intoxication by man due to cannabis smoking. J. Pharm. Belg., *7:*371, 1969.
25. Hollister, L. E., and Kosek, J. C.: Sudden death during treatment with phenothiazine derivatives. JAMA, *192:*1035, 1965.
26. Kopito, L., Byers, R. K., and Shwachman, H.: Lead in hair of children with chronic lead poisoning. New Eng. J. Med., *276:*949, 1967.
27. Kwan, V. H. Y., and Rajeswaran, P.: Recent additions to a bibliography on cannabis. J. Forensic Sci., *13:*279, 1968.
28. Leestma, J. E., and Koenig, K. L.: Sudden death and phenothiazines, a current controversy. Arch. Gen. Psychiatry, *18:*137, 1968.
29. Lewis, C. E.: The toxicology of carbon tetrachloride. J. Occup. Med., *3:*82, 1961.
30. Luckens, M. M.: Screening tissues and urine for pesticides. J. Forensic Sci., *11:*64, 1966.
31. McBay, A. J.: Personal communication, 1973.
32. Maes, R., Hodnett, N., Landesman, H., Kananen, G., Finkle, B., and Sunshine, I.: The gas chromatographic determination of selected sedatives (ethchlorvynol, paraldehyde, meprobamate and carisoprodol) in biological material. J. Forensic Sci., *14:*235, 1969.
33. Materson, B. J., and Barrett-Connor, E.: LSD mainlining a new hazard to health. JAMA, *200:*202, 1967.
34. Medlars Search. Brit. Med. J., *3:*430, 1967.
35. Merkus, F. W. H. M.: Thin layer chromatography of cannabis constituents. Pharm. Weekbl., *106:*49, 1971.
36. Occupational Lead Exposure and Lead Poisoning. American Public Health Association, New York, 1964.
37. Petty, C. S., and Moore, E. J.: Histochemical demonstration of cholinesterase—application to forensic pathology. J. Forensic Sci., *3:*510, 1958.
38. Rosati, D.: Hypotensive side effects of phenothiazine and their management. Dis. Nerv. Syst., *25:*366, 1964.
39. Schwartz, M.: D-lysergic acid diethylamide (LSD-25)—a survey of the literature. Milit. Med., *132:*667, 1967.
40. Siegel, H., and Bloustein, P.: Continuing studies in the diagnosis and pa-

thology of death from intravenous narcotism. J. Forensic Sci., *15:*179, 1970.

41. Siegel, H., Helpern, M., and Ehrenreich, T.: The diagnosis of death from intravenous narcotism, J. Forensic Sci., *11:*1, 1966.

42. Simpson, C. K. (ed.): Taylor's Principles and Practice of Medical Jurisprudence. London, J. & A. Churchill, 1965.

43. Simpson, K.: Forensic Medicine. ed. 6. London, Edward Arnold (Publishers) Ltd., 1972.

44. Smart, R. G., and Bateman, K.: Unfavorable reactions to LSD. A review and analysis of the available case reports. Can. Med. Assoc. J., *97:*1214, 1967.

45. Stewart, C. P., and Stolman, A. (eds.): Toxicology, Mechanisms and Analytical Methods, vol. 1, 1960, vol. 2. New York, Academic Press, 1961.

46. Stone, H. M.: An investigation into forensic chemical problems associated with cannabis. UN Secretariat ST/SOA/SER5/18, August, 1969.

47. Stone, H. M., and Stevens, H. M.: The detection of cannabis constituents in the mouth and on the fingers of smokers. J. Forensic Sci. Soc., *9:*31, 1969.

48. Sunshine, I. (ed.): Handbook of Analytical Toxicology. Cleveland, The Chemical Rubber Company, 1969.

49. Thompson, E., Villaudy, J., Plutchak, L. B., and Gupta, R. C.: Spectrophotometric determination of d-propoxyphene in liver tissue. J. Forensic Sci., *15:*605, 1970.

50. Tompsett, S. L.: Lead poisoning. *In* Curry, A. S. (ed.): Methods of Forensic Science vol. 3. New York, Interscience Publishers, John Wiley & Sons, 1964

51. Turk, R. F., Forney, R. B., King, L. J., and Ramachandran, S.: A method for extraction and chromatographic isolation, purification and identification of tetrahydrocannabinol and other compounds from marihuana. J. Forensic Sci., *14:*385, 1969.

52. Ungerleider, J. T., and Fisher, D. D.: The problems of LSD-25 and emotional disorder. Calif. Med., *106:*49, 1967.

53. United Nations Commission on Narcotic Drugs Document E/CN7/479. The question of cannabis. Cannabis Bibliography. September, 1965.

54. Varley, H.: Practical Clinical Biochemistry. ed. 4. London, Hienemann, 1967.

55. Vercruysse, A., and Deslypere, P.: Acute parathion poisoning. J. Forensic Med., *11:*107, 1964.

56. Wetli, C. V., Davis, J. H., and Blackbourne, B. D.: Narcotic addiction in Dade County, Florida. An analysis of 100 consecutive autopsies. Arch. Path., *93:*330, 1972.

57. Widdop, B.: The detection of LSD in biological fluids. Bull. Int. Ass. Forensic Toxic., *7:*(4):6, 1970.

58. Woods, W. W.: The changes in the kidneys in carbon tetrachloride poisoning, and their resemblance in the "crush syndrome." J. Path. Bact., *58:*767, 1946.

59. Young, D. J.: Propoxyphene suicides: report of nine cases. Arch. Intern. Med., *129:*62, 1972.

21

Artefacts in Forensic Toxicology

INTRODUCTION

When the forensic pathologist or toxicologist goes to a court of law to testify concerning the analyses and findings, he may be "grilled" in the witness box. The attorneys will try to shake his testimony by detecting errors in obtaining or interpreting the final results. The usual attack routes are related to the handling of the material to be analyzed, particularly its chain of custody and the details of analytical procedures. Occasionally, the central issue revolves around the introduction of an artefact that materially alters the end result. Since the results of the analyses in medicolegal cases are frequently required to be presented in courts, forensic pathologists and toxicologists must be aware of various artefacts that are likely to be encountered in their practice.

The definition of "artefact" has been stated in Chapter 17.

The subject of artefacts in forensic toxicology has been only scantily discussed in the medicolegal literature. A clear appreciation of what constitutes an artefact in medicolegal cases perhaps will help the toxicologist, the pathologist and the lawyer in drawing correct conclusions. Therefore, a review of various artefacts that a pathologist or a toxicologist is likely to come across is presented. This review is limited to the discussion of artefacts in the materials removed from dead bodies.

TWO GROUPS OF TOXICOLOGICAL ARTEFACTS

Toxicological artefacts can be broadly divided into two groups: those introduced between death and the postmortem examination; and those introduced during the autopsy.

Artefacts Introduced Between Death and the Postmortem Examination

The factors that can cause artefacts prior to the performance of the postmortem examination are:

1. Decomposition of the body.

2. Burning of the body.

3. Contamination that occurs in embalming the body and/or during interment and exhumation of the body.

Decomposition of the Body. In the practice of forensic pathology and toxicology, decomposition is responsible for the most common and perhaps the most significant of artefacts.

Decomposition of the biological materials often causes apparent alteration in the constituents of the tissue. This is the reason why a considerable amount of effort has been expended to study the usual constituents of decomposed tissue.[1] Such knowledge has been helpful in identifying artefacts. For instance, it is generally known that alcohol is produced postmortem because of the putrefaction (enzymatic decomposition, especially of proteins, with the production of foul-smelling compounds) of the tissues and the fact that many of the bacteria can produce alcohol. However, it must be emphasized that the levels of alcohol generated by putrefaction are usually less than 100 mg. percent. If the levels are above 100 mg. percent, this should arouse suspicion of alcohol ingestion prior to the death of the individual. Decomposition is also known to cause other higher alcohols. According to Curry, gas chromatographic examinations of ether extracts of the distillates of putrefying tissues always yield several volatile compounds.

Decomposition is also known to cause an increase in the concentration of carboxyhemoglobin in the blood; Markiewicz[4] reported an increase up to 19 percent. According to Markiewicz, Porttheine found that a "24 hour period of delay in carrying out the determination of COHb (carboxyhemoglobin) content of blood can increase the results by as much as 25 percent, especially in summer." Other workers seem to concur with this possibility.[2]

Cyanide is produced by decomposition in toxicologically significant amounts; levels up to 10 mg. percent have been found in three-month-old blood.[1]

Many substituted phenols (extremely poisonous compounds generally derived from coal tar) have been found in decomposing tissues. The ones that cause disturbing interference in the analysis of weak acid fractions are related to p-hydroxyphenyl derivatives. In "normal" tissues, substances such as isopentylamine (an aminohydrocarbon), piperidon phenylethylamine (ethylated aniline), thymine, and others have been described as "artefacts."[1]

Burning of the Body Tissues. Combustion of body tissues and other materials associated with the burned body produces several gases. Olsen and his colleagues[6, 7] investigated gases generated in experimental fires. They demonstrated the presence of ammonia, carbon monoxide, hydrogen cyanide, hydrogen sulphide, nitrogen, oxides of nitrogen, and sulphur dioxide. Combustible materials, like silk and wool, produce high concentrations of several of these gases because their nitrogen content is high. Some of the gases may be detected in the body tissues. In such cases, the results of toxicological analyses may raise false alarms.

The occurrence of cyanide in the blood of fire victims has been reported by Wetherell.[9] He made a study of 53 fire victims and observed small but significant amounts of cyanide in the blood of the majority of the burned bodies. The levels observed were between 17 mg. and 220 mg. per 100 ml. Such a finding may lead to the suspicion of an overdose of cyanide. Therefore, it is important to make accurate determinations of the blood levels and to exclude the presence of cyanide in the stomach in such circumstances.

Contamination. Contact with contaminants may occur prior to the autopsy on the body. One of the first interferences can be the embalming of the body. Embalming fluids generally contain formaldehyde, methyl alcohol, and sometimes other interfering compounds. In cases of suspected methyl alcohol poisoning, embalming of the body adds to the difficulties of interpretation. Interment leads to exposure of the body to the contaminants of the soil and draining water. Contamination by arsenic in the soil has been known to be of significance.[8] The following case illustrates this:

> In a body exhumed from a grave in Cornwall, England in 1930, the analyses of the tissues showed arsenic in amounts far more than necessary to cause death. The clinical history also indicated the possibility of arsenic poisoning. One of the suspects was charged with murder. During the trial, evidence was introduced establishing the fact that the soil around the coffin had contained arsenic in significant amounts. The defense contended that the arsenic in the soil could have reached the body by seepage. The weight of this contention was largely responsible for the acquittal of the defendant.

Artefacts Introduced During Autopsy

The artefacts that may be added during the performance of the autopsy may be caused by:

1. Faulty technique in collecting samples.
2. Faulty technique in storage.
3. Use of preservatives.

Faulty Technique in Collecting the Samples. Many times, particularly in cases where an autopsy is not to be done, blood samples are drawn from the heart with a long needle. In the process, the sample contaminated with gastric contents may be obtained. Tests, particularly for alcohol, in such instances may be misleading. In traumatic deaths such as those due to automobile accidents, the stomach may rupture and lead to the added likelihood of contamination. Also, alcohol is known to diffuse in significant amounts from the stomach to the pleural and pericardial cavities. During an attempt to draw blood from the heart, pericardial and pleural fluid may be withdrawn, giving unreliable results.

Faulty Technique in Storage. Artefacts may also be introduced by cutting the organs with instruments contaminated by stomach contents or by putting the samples of tissue in contaminated containers. It is common practice to store portions of several organs in one container. Such a practice is apt to cause alterations in the true levels of poison, because the diffusion or drainage of blood or fluid from one organ to another may lead to an altered concentration of the poison.

Use of Preservatives. The use of preservatives can add artefacts. It should be emphasized that preservatives such as EDTA (ethylendiamine tetraacetic acid) formalin, heparin, and methenamine give a positive test for methanol and that these should not be used as anticoagulants for blood if an analysis for methanol is required. The following case illustrates this point:

> A 30-year old drug addict, found comatose at home, was admitted to the hospital. Blood was drawn soon after admission for toxicological studies. A tube containing EDTA powder was used. The analyses by a hospital toxicologist showed the presence of 170 mg. percent of methanol in addition to barbiturates and salicylates. The woman died shortly after the blood was drawn. Repeat tests on her blood excluded the presence of methanol. The false-positive methanol result caused by EDTA might have resulted in instituting wrong treatment for the patient if she had survived for a time.

The contamination with Zenker's fluid (a fixative solution containing corrosive mercuric chloride, potassium bichromate, and glacial acetic acid or formalin) in the autopsy room may alter the significance of the determination of mercury in postmortem material. The following case is an excellent example of the significance of artefacts caused by the contamination, in the autopsy room, of samples for toxicologic studies.[5]

> A woman was thought to have died of poisoning because cyanide was thrown in her face. At the trial of the accused, the pathologist admitted that he had used the same knife to obtain samples of tissue for toxicological analyses that had been used to cut the presumably contaminated skin of the upper chest. Since the test for cyanide in the blood was equivocal, the presence or absence of cyanide in the lungs became vital. The defense contended that the finding of cyanide in the lung was due to contamination. This was one of the principal arguments that led to the acquittal of the accused.

DISCUSSION AND SUMMARY

The essence of the recognition of various artefacts in forensic toxicology is the separation of genuine evidence of poisoning from inconsequential findings. Lack of knowledge of the artefacts may lead to misinterpretations that may result in identifying a wrong cause of death and/or a wrong manner of death. False-positive or false-negative results may arouse undue suspicions of criminal offense or may indicate a halt in the investigation of a homicide ending in nondetection of murder. Misleading findings may culminate in unnecessary spending of time and effort, and may cause miscarriage of justice in civil suits.

If the pitfalls are not recognized, a pathologist or a toxicologist may make a mistake that can haunt him in court and he may suffer gnawing embarrassment at the hands of a cross-examining lawyer. For these reasons, various factors that can cause artefacts are discussed. Kaempe[3] has presented a review of interfering compounds and artefacts in the identification of drugs in autopsy material. He has discussed methods for separating the interfering substances that are coextracted during analyses.

REFERENCES

1. Curry, A.: Poison Detection in Human Organs. ed. 2. Springfield (Ill.), Charles C Thomas, 1969.
2. Dominguez, A. M., Halstead, J. R., and Domanski, T. J.: The effect of postmortem changes on carboxyhemoglobin results. J. Forensic Sci., 9:330, 1964.
3. Kaempe, B.: Interfering compounds and artifacts in the identification of drugs in autopsy material. *In* Stolman, A. (ed.): Progress in Chemical Toxicology. vol. 4. New York, Academic Press, 1969.
4. Markiewicz, J.: Investigations on endogenous carboxyhemoglobin. J. Forensic Med., 14:16, 1967.
5. Moritz, A. R.: Classical mistakes in forensic pathology. Amer. J. Clin. Path., 26:1383, 1956.
6. Olsen, J. C., Brunjes, A. S., and Sabetta, V. J.: Gases produced by the decomposition of nitrocellulose and cellulose acetate. Photographic Films. Ind. Engin. Chem., 22:860, 1930.
7. Olsen, J. C., Fergusson, G. E., and Scheflan, L.: Gases from the thermal decomposition of common combustible materials. Ind. Engin. Chem., 25:599, 1933.
8. Stewart, C. P., and Stolman, A.: Toxicology: Mechanisms and Analytical Methods. vol. 1. New York, Academic Press, 1960.
9. Wetherell, H. R.: The occurrence of cyanide in the blood of fire victims. J. Forensic Sci., 11:167, 1966.

22

Analytical Procedures: Simple Tests for Pathologists

In this chapter some of the analytical procedures that a pathologist can perform in a hospital laboratory or in an autopsy room are described. These tests can be performed with minimum experience and without elaborate equipment. Pathologists who have no ready access to forensic science laboratories can use these analytical procedures with great advantage. There are times when rapid tests are necessary as aids to a medicolegal investigation. These tests may be required to establish the cause of death, or to confirm or negate certain suspicions. For such situations the procedures outlined in this chapter are useful. Technical procedures for the following tests are described: Alcohol, heavy metals (arsenic, bismuth, antimony, mercury), barbiturates, carbon monoxide, cyanide, diatoms, ferrous sulfate, gunpowder, isopropyl alcohol, lead, methyl alcohol, parathion, phenothiazines, salicylates, spermatozoa, strychinine.

Alcohol

Potassium dichromate method

1. Mix 1 ml. of blood or urine with 1 ml. of saturated aqueous potassium carbonate solution in the base of a Cavett flask.
2. In the hanging cup put 0.5 ml. of 0.1N potassium dichromate in 60 percent v/v sulfuric acid solution.
3. Seal the flask and put it in an oven at about 50°C.

A change of color from orange to green indicates ethanol levels of 50 mg. percent or over.

Modification of the microdiffusion technique[6]

1. Put 1 to 2 ml. of saturated potassium carbonate in the outer upper groove of the rim of microdiffusion cell.
2. Add 2 ml. of Anstie's reagent to the center chamber. (To prepare Anstie's reagent, dissolve 3.70 gm. of potassium dichromate in 150

ml. of water. Then add 280 ml. of sulfuric acid with constant stirring. Dilute to 500 ml. with distilled water.)

3. Spread 1 ml. of blood or urine to be tested in the outer chamber.
4. Spread 1 ml. of saturated potassium carbonate in the outer chamber on the opposite side.
5. Put the lid in place, gently twist to obtain liquid seal and swirl the unit to mix the blood and potassium carbonate.
6. Allow diffusion for one hour at room temperature.
7. Remove the lid and observe the color of the Anstie's reagent.

A canary yellow color indicates a negative result. A color change of yellow yellow-green indicates ethanol level of about 80 mg. percent, yellow-green about 150 mg. percent, green yellow-green about 230 mg. percent and blue-green about 300 mg. percent.

Heavy Metals (Arsenic, Bismuth, Antimony, Mercury)

Reinsch test

1. Place 10 ml. of urine, gastric contents, macerated kidney or liver in a flask.
2. Place a copper foil or wire, rubbed clean, in the flask with 2 ml. of concentrated hydrochloric acid.
3. Cover the flask and heat gently for one hour.

If the test is positive deposits will form on the copper foil or wire. Details of the results are summarized in Table 22-1.

TABLE 22-1. Summary of the Results of Reinsch Test.

Heavy metal	Appearance of Copper	Nature of Deposits	Sensitivity of the test in mg./ 10 ml.
Arsenic	Grayish black	Octahedral crystalline sublimate	0.010
Antimony	Dark purple	Amorphous powder sublimate	0.020
Bismuth	Shiny gray	Amorphous powder	0.020
Mercury	Shiny silver	Metallic globules of mercury sublimate	0.050

Further differentiation of the deposits can be made as follows:[7]
Arsenic. Place the grayish black copper in a test tube and add 15 drops

of 10 percent potassium cyanide. The deposit caused by arsenic will dissolve but that from antimony or bismuth will not.

Bismuth. Place the shiny gray copper in a test tube and add 15 drops of 5 percent sodium sulfite and 1 ml. of 15 percent nitric acid. The deposit from bismuth dissolves but those from arsenic and antimony do not. Add 1 ml. of water and 1 ml. of bismuth test reagent (prepared by dissolving 1 Gm. of quinine sulfate in 100 ml. of 0.5 percent nitric acid and then dissolving 2 Gm. of potassium iodide into the solution) to the dissolved bismuth solution. Orange turbidity will develop. This test is specific for bismuth.

Antimony. Deposits remain unchanged by both the tests for arsenic and bismuth.

Barbiturates

Modification of the Koppanyi method[6]

1. Obtain 50 ml. of urine or gastric contents in a funnel. Test with litmus paper. If alkaline, barely acidify with sulfuric acid.
2. Add 100 ml. of ether and shake for several minutes.
3. Let the layers separate. Discard the aqueous layer; barbiturate is in the ether layer.
4. Filter the ether into a beaker and evaporate it to dryness on a steam bath.
5. Add 10 drops of chloroform to redissolve the barbiturate residue that must be dry.
6. Take a few drops on a white porcelain spot plate and add 1 drop of cobalt acetate (1 percent in absolute methyl alcohol) and 2 drops of isopropyl amine (5 percent in absolute methyl alcohol).

Barbiturates give a purple-lilac color.

Carbon Monoxide

Simple autopsy room screening tests

1. Dilute 2 drops of blood in 20 ml. of water in a test tube. In another test tube dilute 2 drops of normal control blood (without carboxyhemoglobin). Hold both tubes against the light. The tube with carboxyhemoglobin will reveal a distinct pink tinge, whereas the control blood will be reddish brown.
2. Dilute two drops of blood with 10 ml. of water in a test tube. Also dilute control normal blood similarly. To each tube add 5 drops of 10 to 20 percent sodium hydroxide. Quickly shake the tubes. The control tube will show a brownish yellow color immediately after

shaking. If the blood to be tested contains more than 20 percent carboxyhemoglobin, the pink color seen after dilution will persist for several seconds. After about a minute the pink color will change to brownish yellow.

Conway-Feldstein-Klendshoj microdiffusion technique[6]

Place 2 ml. of 10 percent sulfuric acid in the small groove of the rim of the microdiffusion cell. Place 2 ml. of palladium chloride in the center chamber. Spread 1 ml. of blood in the outer chamber. Then spread 1 ml. of 10 percent sulfuric acid on top of the blood and rapidly seal with the lid. After the lid is placed in position gently twist to get liquid seal. Gently rotate the whole unit to mix the specimen and the liberating agent. This starts diffusion. Allow diffusion for one hour at room temperature. If carbon monoxide is present, a positive reaction of a grayish black shiny film of palladium will be seen.

Cyanide

Autopsy room screening test[1]

1. Immerse squares of filter paper in saturated picric acid and let them dry.
2. Place a drop of material (blood, gastric contents) on a piece of paper and let the material dry.
3. Then put one drop of 10 percent sodium carbonate in the center of the material to be tested.

If cyanide is present, a reddish purple color will chromatograph out from the material. The higher the concentration of cyanide, the more intense will be the blue color.

Modification of microdiffusion technique[7]

1. Place 2 ml. of 10 percent sodium hydroxide in the center chamber.
2. Use 2 ml. of 10 percent sulfuric acid as a sealer by placing it in the small groove of the rim.
3. Spread 1 ml. of material (blood, gastric contents) in the outer chamber. Overlay immediately with 1 ml. of sulfuric acid and put the lid in place. Obtain a liquid seal by gently twisting the lid. Swirl the entire unit to mix the specimen and the liberating agent.
4. Let it diffuse for one hour at room temperature.
5. Remove the lid and add 20 percent ferrous sulfate.
6. Remove the brown precipitate by adding 1 to 2 ml. of concentrated hydrochloric acid.

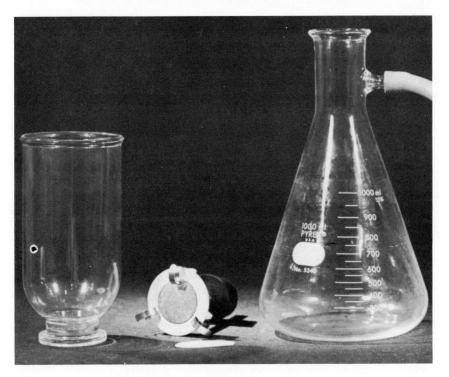

Fig. 22–1. Millipore filtering apparatus.

Cyanide will give an intense blue color.

Diatoms

Technique for diatom detection[5]

The following technical steps are for detection of diatoms in the blood.
1. Centrifuge 5 or more ml. of blood with distilled water at 3000 to 5000 rpm. Discard the supernatant fluid. Repeat this 4 or 5 times, each time removing the supernatant fluid. At the end a "button" of dark red material will be left at the bottom of the centrifuge tube.
2. Add 10 ml. of concentrated nitric acid to the "button" and heat the tube *gently*. A light yellow colored fluid will be obtained.
3. Use Filter Funnel* or similar apparatus (Fig. 22-1). Dilute the light yellow fluid in the centrifuge tube with about 1000 ml. of distilled water and pour into the funnel that forms the upper part of the

* Filter Funnel (No. F3021) Scientific Products, 1430 Waukegan Road, McGaw Park, Illinois 60085.

funnel. Place a filter membrane,† or similar millipore filter with 8 micron pores, between the funnel and the flask. (Almost all of the diatoms are 10 microns or more in size.)

4. Let the fluid in the funnel filter through the filter membrane. All the diatoms will settle on the filter.

5. Remove the filter membrane and allow it to dry under a protective cover.

6. After the membrane is dried, place it on a glass slide with 4 or 5 drops of immersion oil between the slide and the membrane. Place a coverslip on it. The preparation is ready for microscopic examination.

If solid tissues (e.g., liver, lungs, bone marrow) are to be examined, first digest the material in nitric acid (25 ml. of nitric acid to 1 Gm. of tissue) by heating. Centrifuge the digested material and remove the fat collected at the top with a clean spatula. Then follow the same steps as for detection of blood with the material at the bottom of the centrifuge tube.

This method has distinct advantages. Repeated centrifugations of blood remove most of the fat without the loss of the diatoms. The remaining dark red "button" digested by nitric acid results in a more or less clear fluid with diatoms. With this method the examination of the blood or the tissues does not entail the use of sulfuric acid. This eliminates most of the artefact of crystalline precipitate. The procedure of the transfer to the funnel of the centrifuged fluid, with sediment diluted with a large quantity of distilled water, ensures the transfer of all the diatoms from the centrifuge tube to the funnel. Further, the distilled water passing through the filter membrane leaves all the particulate matter caught up in the filter membrane. This guarantees the recovery of all the diatoms. The transfer of the filter membrane with the "catch" of all the diatoms directly on the slide further reduces handling of the material and consequently minimizes contamination. This method allows the use of relatively large amounts of material, and yet all the diatoms in the material are obtained on just one or two slides. The final preparation is always clear with no dark brown coloration as seen with other methods. There are practically no fat particles or crystals. The diatoms with such a preparation stand out distinctly.

Ferrous Sulfate

1. Dilute the stomach contents with water and filter to obtain 5 ml. of fluid.

2. Add two drops of hydrochloric acid to 5 ml. of filtered fluid in a test tube.

† Millipore Corporation, Bedford, Mass.

3. To this mixture add 1 ml. of potassium ferricyanide.
   Even traces of ferrous sulfate give a Prussian blue color.

Isopropyl Alcohol

Test for isopropanol in the blood[6]

1. Mix 5 ml. of blood with 5 ml. of 10 percent zinc sulphate.
2. Add 5 ml. of 0.5N sodium hydroxide and mix again.
3. Filter through filter paper after complete coagulation of proteins.
4. Put 5 ml. of clear filtrate in a centrifuge tube and add 5 ml. of Deniges' reagent. (Deniges' reagent can be prepared by adding 2 Gm. of yellow mercuric oxide in 16 ml. of water and mixing with 8 ml. of sulfuric acid, and then stirring to dissolve with extra 16 ml. of water.)
5. Cork and gently heat on a steam bath.

Isopropanol, acetone and tertiary butyl alcohol give a yellowish white fine precipitate. A negative test excludes the presence of isopropanol.

Lead

Tests for lead can be done using blood or urine.

Simple laboratory tests for lead[10]

1. Add dilute sulfuric acid to the specimens. A white precipitate will develop. This precipitate is insoluble in nitric acid and soluble in hydrochloric acid or ammonium acetate.
2. Add sulfuretted hydrogen to the specimen. A black precipitate will develop. This precipitate is insoluble in ammonium sulfide and soluble in hot nitric acid.
3. Add potassium iodide to the specimen. A bright yellow precipitate will develop. This precipitate is soluble in hot water. On cooling the mixture brilliant yellow crystals will develop.

Coproporphyrin test for lead in urine[7]

1. Mix 5 ml. of fresh urine with 10 drops of acetic acid and 5 drops of 3 percent hydrogen peroxide in a test tube and shake gently with 5 ml. of ether.
2. Let the layers separate and then discard the urine layer.
3. Add 1 ml. of 1N hydrochloric acid to the ether and observe under ultraviolet light (Wood's filter).

A pinkish red fluorescence indicates a positive test and a bluish green fluorescence is negative.

Methyl Alcohol

Test for methyl alcohol in blood[6]

1. Add 4 ml. of 20 percent trichloracetic acid to 2 ml. of blood and shake.
2. Filter to collect a clear filtrate.
3. Add 4 drops of potassium permanganate reagent (3 Gm. of potassium permanganate + 15 ml. of orthophosphoric acid + water to make 100 ml.) to 1 ml. of filtrate in a test tube and wait for 2 minutes.
4. Decolorize the excess potassium permanganate with some crystals of sodium bisulfite.
5. Add a pinch of chromotropic acid (EK # p-230) and shake.
6. Run down the side of the test tube 2 ml. of concentrated sulfuric acid.

The presence of methyl alcohol gives a dark purple ring at the interface.

Parathion

þ-nitrophenol test[6]

1. Steam distill 10 to 15 ml. of vomitus, gastric contents or urine and collect 10 ml. of distillate.
2. Add 2 pellets of sodium hydroxide and gently heat on a water bath.

þ-nitrophenol, a metabolite of parathion, gives a yellow color.

Phenothiazines

Forrest and Forrest[3] tests for phenothiazines in the urine

1. Add 6 drops of concentrated sulfuric acid and 2 drops of 10 percent ferric chloride to 2 ml. of urine. A light pink to purple color indicates positive reaction for a phenothiazine compound.
2. Prepare FPN reagent by mixing 5 ml. of 5 percent ferric chloride, 45 ml. of 20 percent nitric acid, and 50 ml. of 50 percent nitric acid, all w/v.

Add 1 ml. of FPN reagent to 1 ml. of urine. Chlorinated derivatives give a lilac color, fluorinated derivatives a flesh color, sulfurated derivatives a blue color and sparine an orange color. Color develops immediately and fades rapidly.

Salicylates

Phenistix test

Ferric chloride test. Add 1 ml. of 10 percent ferric chloride to 2 to 3 ml. of urine. A deep purple color develops if salicylic acid is present in the urine. If the test is positive, boil the sample of urine and repeat the test. A purple color indicates the presence of salicylic acid. This test can be positive with the ingestion of only 5 g. of aspirin. It is positive for salicylates as well as phenol derivatives. A negative test excludes the presence of salicylates.

Test for serum salicylates[7, 8]

Qualitative. Place 0.01 ml. of serum in a small evaporating dish and add one drop of 1 percent ferric nitrate in 0.07N nitric acid. Salicylates give a purple color.

Quantitative. In each of two test tubes place 0.2 ml. of serum and 0.8 ml. of water. To one tube (blank) add 1 ml. of 0.07N nitric acid. To the second tube (unknown) add 1 ml. of 1 percent ferric nitrate in 0.07N nitric acid. Mix by shaking and let the tubes stand for 5 minutes. Then read in a spectrophotometer at 540 mμ.

For preparing standard, add in one test tube (blank) 1 ml. of water and then 1 ml. of 0.07N nitric acid. To the other test tube add 0.8 ml. of water and 0.2 ml. of standard and then 1 ml. of 1 percent ferric nitrate. Salicylate standard: 25 mg. percent.

$$\frac{\text{Absorbance unknown}}{\text{Absorbance standard}} \times 25 = \text{mg. of salicylate per 100 ml.}$$

Spermatozoa: Acid Phosphatase Test

Whenever a sexual attack is suspected, the body should be examined for evidence of injuries to the genital organs. Foreign materials such as hair, fabric, dirt and vegetation in the areas of the buttocks, back, genital organs and extremities should be collected. As soon as the body is found, materials should be collected to detect the presence of prostatic fluid and spermatozoa.

Collection of specimens and examination

Obtain samples of vaginal contents as follows. If anal or oral intercourse is suspected obtain specimens from the anus and the mouth.

1. Obtain a drop of vaginal fluid with a pipet and place it on a slide. Put on a coverslip and examine microscopically. As an alternative the specimen may be obtained by means of a dry cotton swab. If a swab is used, make smears on slides just as for routine cytological examinations and examine. The material may be fixed by any of the commercial sprays for permanent record. (In the first 1 to 2 hours after intercourse, motile sperms can be seen. If the material is to be examined for motility of sperms, the swab or the aspirate should be placed in a small quantity of normal saline.)

2. Make another smear from the vaginal aspirate or from the cotton swab. Allow the smear to dry. Then stain it with methylene blue and examine microscopically.
3. Use some of the vaginal aspirate for the acid phosphatase test. If the quantity of the aspirate is small, dilute it with about 4 to 6 ml. of normal saline. Follow the method described by Shinowara, *et al.*[9] to perform the acid phosphatase test. A positive result is significant. Negative results are obtained if the victim is examined more than 12 hours after the alleged sexual attack.[2] The enzyme creatine phosphokinase, in high concentrations in seminal fluid, can be easily detected for at least 6 months even in azoospermic human ejaculate. The estimation of creatine phosphokinase can be used as an additional method for identification of seminal stains.[4]

Strychnine

Fading purple test for strychnine[6]

1. Dilute a small quantity of gastric contents with 10 ml. of water. Alkalinize this with ammonium hydroxide.
2. Shake the mixture and extract with 25 ml. of chloroform. Allow the chloroform layer to settle and then separate it.
3. Dissolve the residue in several drops of concentrated sulfuric acid and transfer it to a glass slide.
4. Place a single small crystal of potassium dichromate into the acid solution and streak the crystal with a glass rod.

If strychnine is present even in traces, the track of the crystal will be purple, changing to red orange and finally to yellow.

REFERENCES

1. Camps, F. E. (ed.): Gradwohl's Legal Medicine. ed. 2. Baltimore, Williams & Wilkins, 1968.
2. Enos, W. F., Beyer, J. C., and Mann, G. T.: The medical examination of cases of rape. J. Forensic Sci., *17*:50, 1972.
3. Forrest, I. S., and Forrest, F. M.: A rapid urine color test for imipramine. Am. J. Psycho., *116*:840, 1960.
4. Griffiths, P. D., and Lehmann, H: Estimation of creatine phosphokinase as an additional method for identification of seminal stains. Med. Sci. Law, *4*:32, 1964.
5. Hudson, R. P., Fatteh, A., and Whitehurst, L.: An Improved Technique for Diatom Detection. Unpublished Observations, 1971.
6. Kaye, S.: Handbook of Emergency Toxicology. Springfield (Ill.), Charles C Thomas, 1970.

7. Kaye, S.: Rapid, simple, reliable tests for poisons. Lab. Med., *3:*28, 1972.
8. Natelson S.: Microtechniques of Clinical Chemistry. ed. 2. Springfield (Ill.), Charles C Thomas, 1961.
9. Shinowara, G. J., Jones, L. M., and Reinhart, H. L.: The estimation of serum inorganic phosphatase and "acid" and "alkaline" phosphatase activity. J. of Biol. Chem., *142:*921, 1942.
10. Simpson, K.: Forensic Medicine. ed. 6. London, Edward Arnold (Publishers) Ltd., 1972.

23

The Pathologist As a Witness

The pathologist or medical examiner involved in the investigation of medicolegal cases can expect to be summoned to court to testify in some instances. The types of cases that may require the medicolegist's attendance in court are either criminal with indictment for homicide, or civil with action for wrongful death or damages. In some jurisdictions the pathologist is routinely called to present his findings and opinions in the coroner's courts in all cases he investigates. Many higher courts, on the other hand, accept written reports of the pathologist or the medical examiner, and they do not summon the doctor unless it is thought that questions may be raised about his reports, or that his presence would assist in the just disposition of the case. In some instances the doctor may be asked to give a deposition in order to eliminate the necessity for his personal attendance.

The physician may be called as a lay witness, witness of fact or as an expert witness. He may be required to testify at a preliminary investigation by magistrate, grand jury investigation, coroner's inquest, workman's compensation board or at trials in civil and criminal courts.

Subpoena

The medical examiner or pathologist usually receives his first notice to appear in court when he is contacted by a police officer, a court official or a lawyer who is in the process of working up the case for trial or settlement. The notice may be in the form of a legal subpoena or a telephone call followed later by a subpoena. In some instances the subpoena may arrive just a few hours prior to the trial. But in most instances the lawyer for the party who desires the physician's attendance notifies him well in advance of the trial that his presence may be required.

Subpoenas are usually made out for all witnesses to appear in court at the time the trial begins. Frequently, much time is consumed in procedural matters such as picking a jury and settlement of dockets after the court convenes. Therefore, *it is not always necessary to appear in court at the specified time on the subpoena.* It is advisable for the physician to contact the summoning party to determine the exact time for *his* appearance in court. Most attorneys alert the physician some time before his attendance is needed on the day of trial and try to put him on the witness stand promptly when he gets to court.

Preliminaries

Initial questions. The doctor who receives a subpoena should gather essential information related to the case. He must make sure whether the summoning party is a lawyer for the prosecution or for the defense and whether the case is civil or criminal. He should find out whether he can give a deposition to eliminate the need for his personal appearance. If it is necessary to go to court the doctor must locate the court and ascertain when his presence is required.

Pretrial conference. A pretrial conference is an ethical procedure. Both the lawyer and the physician witness should seek to make arrangements for the discussion of the doctor's testimony before he comes to court. Through such pretrial discussions, the physician gets a clear idea what he will be asked by the attorney calling him. The attorney also is able to advise the doctor about the anticipated content of cross-examination. Such discussions give the doctor an opportunity to find out what records will be required of him. He can point out to the lawyer salient features of the case and advise him about any visual aids such as photographs and x-rays that may be helpful for his testimony.

Fees. In some jurisdictions statutory fees and allowances are laid down for attendance in court. If set fees are nonexistent, it is perfectly in order for the physician to discuss the question of his fees with the attorney calling or consulting him. The physician can expect to be reimbursed for his professional time spent in the preparation of the case, consultations with the attorney and appearance in the court. He should, therefore, keep records of the time that he spends on the case, including travel time.

Preparation of the case. The medical witness must study the details of the case records, photographs and x-rays a few days before he goes to court. It is advisable to review the records again immediately before going to court. He should make certain that he is conversant with all the information relevant to the case. In some cases it may be necessary to study the literature on the subject about which he is likely to be cross-examined. This is particularly important if the doctor is going to testify as an expert. He should not attempt to testify as an expert witness unless he is satisfied that he is qualified in the subject that is likely to be the focus of questioning.

Materials to be carried to court. The attorney calling the witness will have received copies of the doctor's records and other materials before the trial. The doctor must carry with him copies of the records, photographs and so on so that he can refresh his memory while he is on the witness stand. The records should include the report of the investigation; autopsy report; copy of the death certificate; x-rays; drawings or diagrams; toxicology reports; special reports on swabs or smears, culture studies, serology and blood type studies; and various receipts to prove the chain of custody of the items of evidence. An identification photograph of the decedent's face should also be carried. If the doctor has any other items of physical evidence (e.g., decedent's clothes, bullets) that he is likely to be questioned about, he should carry them with him.

It is prudent to carry to court the original set of reports and photographs as well as copies of them. Frequently the records and other items of evidence are received in evidence as exhibits. Once they are so received, they become the property of the court and the witness may not get them back. A great many cases, particularly criminal cases, are appealed and there is always a possibility that a new trial may be ordered. One set of records retained by the witness will be invaluable in such circumstances.

Court Attendance

On arrival at the court. Once the time of appearance in court is arranged, the physician should arrive on time with all the necessary records. He should signify to the party who summoned him that he is ready to testify. Whenever it is possible the attorneys arrange to put the physician on the witness stand promptly, and many times even alter the sequence of appearance of other witnesses. If undue delay is caused inadvertently, the physician should courteously make a reference of it to the attorney.

There may be situations when all the witnesses except the one on the stand are "excluded from the courtroom" prior to their testimony. This is done by the judge upon motion of one of the parties in order that the various witnesses may not hear one another's testimony. The witnesses are also cautioned not to discuss the case with one another while they are waiting to testify. On arrival at the court the physician should find out whether the witnesses have been excluded. If they have been excluded, he should signify his arrival to the attorney who called him and then join the other witnesses.

On the witness stand. What makes a good medical witness? According to Tracy the "attributes of a good medical witness are that he be frank, honest, modest but not timid, have a thorough knowledge of his field of practice, talk to make himself heard, and be able to explain abstruse subjects in language that can be understood by a layman."[3]

Following are some simple basic rules that a medical witness must remember if he is to make a good impression as a witness. These will enhance the effectiveness of his testimony and make his courtroom experience pleasant.

1. Wear neat, conservative clothes.
2. Be relaxed and calm and not frightened or nervous.
3. Do not begin answering until the question is completed.
4. Answer only the question asked and confine yourself to the case on trial.
5. Do not volunteer information uncalled for from the witness stand.
6. Do not answer a question to which an objection has been raised until the judge announces his ruling. If it is overruled, proceed with the answer, but if it is sustained await another question from the attorney who may rephrase the question or abandon it.
7. Address the answers to the jury.
8. Speak clearly and loud enough for the jurors to hear.
9. As far as possible use layman's language to explain your testimony.
10. Speak with assurance. Be confident but not overconfident or arrogant. Maintain your composure. Do not lose your temper. Do not argue.
11. Be interested in what is being said. Do not appear bored. "Testifying is similar to a performance on the stage."[2]
12. Do not answer if the question is not understood. Request the attorney to repeat the question or explain it.
13. Be frank, modest and honest. Tell the truth. If you do not know the answer to a question, do not hesitate to say "I do not know." Do not evade a question.
14. Keep the opinions within the realm of reasonable medical certainty. Make reasonable deductions. Be fair.
15. If an error has been made in the testimony do not hesitate to correct it.
16. Be pleasant, polite and courteous to the lawyer.
17. Do not underestimate the medical knowledge of the attorneys.

After the witness' name is called, he proceeds toward the witness stand. Before he sits in the witness chair he is sworn in by the clerk of the court. Immediately after this, direct examination commences.

Direct examination. This consists of questions put by the attorney who summoned the doctor as a witness. Initial questions are designed to obtain the witness' name, place of residence and occupation. Thereafter, the witness is asked questions bearing upon his qualifications. The medical witness should be prepared to give information about the medical school from which he graduated, his internship and residency training, specialty board certifications, hospital affiliations, research, publications and membership of medical societies. After establishing the qualifications of the witness, the attorney will ask questions to determine the witness' relation to the case. Once these routine preliminary questions are completed, the attorney will then launch into a more specific line of questioning to bring out the facts and opinions which he considers to be important to his case. This examination will be made without the use of leading questions, that is, questions that suggest their own answers. While answering these questions the witness may consult his records but should refrain from reading from them verbatim. As far as the pathologist is concerned the questions usually relate to identification of the decedent, salient autopsy findings and cause of death. The attorney may ask the witness to identify and describe various items of evidence such as reports, photographs, bullets and clothes. If a multipage report is presented for identification, every page of it should be examined before a comment about identification is made.

If a pretrial conference was held the questions and answers of the direct examination will have been rehearsed, and the pathologist will have no difficulty on the witness stand. Therefore, at least a telephone conference between the attorney and the witness should be arranged prior to the trial.

Cross-examination. After the direct examination is completed the opposing attorney will begin questioning the witness. The purpose of this cross-examination is to get the witness to amplify his statements so that the cross-examining attorney can test his memory, and probe the reliability and credibility of his testimony. Many medical witnesses dread cross-examination, often without justification because usually no subject may be discussed on cross-examination which has not been opened during the preceding direct examination. Therefore, it is unusual for a physician-witness in a routine medicolegal case to have any problems during cross-examination. The cross-examining attorney may try to impeach the witness in order to diminish the weight of his testimony, by exposing lapses in the investigation or by detecting discrepencies in the statements made during the direct and the cross-examination. So, if the investigation of the case has been proper and the witness has presented forthright factual testimony on direct examination, he need not fear a vigorous cross-examination.

After the cross-examination is completed, there may be *redirect examination.* On redirect examination the lawyer who calls the witness usually tries to give him opportunity to explain his answers given during cross-examination. If any new issues are introduced during redirect examination, the opposing attorney may pursue a *recross-examination.* Details of these examinations are well discussed by Beeman.[1]

After both parties have completed their direct and cross-examinations and all the evidence which may be desired from the witness has been introduced, he will be excused from the witness stand. At this stage the witness should ask the judge to be excused from the case totally. Such a request is usually granted and the physician is then free to leave the court.

In summary, it must be reemphasized that if the pathologist makes prior arrangements with the attorney about the precise time of appearance in the court, he is not likely to spend unnecessary time there. Further, if the pathologist prepares the case properly and confers with the calling attorney before testifying, his task in the court will be rendered easy. Finally, most trial lawyers conduct themselves as gentlemen; hence a truthful, prepared witness should have nothing to fear in the court.

REFERENCES

1. Beeman, J.: The Pathologist As a Witness. Mundelein, (Ill.), Callaghan & Co., 1964.
2. Liebenson, H.: You, the Medical Witness. Mundelein, (Ill.), Callaghan & Co., 1961.
3. Tracy, J. E.: The Doctor As a Witness. Philadelphia, W. B. Saunders, 1957.

Index

Abdomen, examination of, 16
  injuries of, 77
Abortion, 255
Abrasions, 66
Accidents, auto-erotic sexual activity,
  6
  automobile, 208
  drowning, 155
  firearms, 117
  hanging, 146
  strangulation, 143
Acid phosphatase test, 333
Acids, 280
Adipocere, 25
Adrenal glands, lesions of, 267
Age, determination of, 39
Aircraft accidents, 219
  follow-up investigations, 221
  medico-legal investigation, 220
  organization of investigation, 220
Air embolism, 16, 160, 255
Alcohol, 283
  ethyl alcohol, 283
  ethylene glycol, 288
  isopropyl alcohol, 288
  methyl alcohol, 287
  test for, 325
Alcoholism, chronic, 285
Alimentary system and sudden death,
  191
Alkalies, 280
Allergy, 230
Allobarbitone, 294
Amitriptyline, 315
Amperage, 177
Amphetamines, 288
Amylobarbitone, 294
Amytal, 294
Anaphylaxis, 230
Anemia, in lead poisoning, 304

Anesthetic, agents, 226
  deaths, 224
  local anesthetics, 228
    autopsy findings, 227
    toxicological analyses, 228
Aneurysm, berry, 191
  traumatic, 213
Anoxia, 131
Antimony, test for, 326
Arborescent markings, 181
Arsenic, 290
  acute poisoning, 290
  chronic poisoning, 291
  test for, 326
Artefacts, 235
  agonal, 236
  burned bodies, 175
  classification, 235
  decomposition, 240
  definition, 235
  embalming, 238
  exhumation, 239
  gunshot wounds, 123
  interment, 239
  misinterpretation of, 252
  resuscitation, 236
  toxicological, 320
Asphyxia, traumatic, 150
Asphyxial deaths, 131
  autopsy findings in, 133
Auto-erotic sexual activity, 6, 143
Automobile accidents, 209
  objectives of autopsy, 210
  reconstruction of events, 211
  role of alcohol, 218
Autopsy, authorization for, 11, 17
  exhumed body, 17
  medico-legal, 11
  negative, 254
  poisoning death, 275

Autopsy (*continued*)
  preliminary procedures, 11
  protocol, 18
  special procedures, 11

Barbitone, 294
Barbiturates, 292
  fatal concentrations, 294
  fatal doses, 294
  test for, 327
  types, 294
Barr bodies, 37
Battered child syndrome, 199
Bismuth, test for, 326
Bite marks, identification by, 43
Blood, identification by, 46
  method of collection, 9
  transfusion, complications, 230
    incompatibilities, 227
  types (groups), 46
Blue line, in lead poisoning, 304
Blunt force injuries, 66
  regional, 73
Body, description of, 4
  diagrams, 13
Boron, 280
Bromides, 280
Bruises, 67
  medico-legal significance of, 68
Burns, 166
  autopsy findings, 167
  medico-legal investigation, 166
Butobarbitone, 294

Cadaveric spasm, 23
Caliber, 101
Cannabis, 295
Carbon monoxide, 296
  tests for, 327
Carbon tetrachloride, 299
Carboxyhemoglobin, 170
Cardiovascular system, 190
  lesions of, 262
Cartridges, 100
Cell-sex, 46
Centers of ossification, 32
Cerebral concussion, 74, 257
  contusion, 74
  laceration, 75
Chemical changes, in aqueous fluid, 28

  in blood, 27
  in cerebrospinal fluid, 27
  in drowning, 161
  in vitreous fluid, 28
Chest injuries, 76
Chloral hydrate, 280
Chlorides, 161
Choking, 150, 260
Chronic alcoholism, 285
Clock, postmortem, 28
Clothes, identification from, 33
Concealed trauma, 256
Concealment of crime, 215
Concussion, cerebral, 74, 257
  spinal, 258
Congestion, 137
Contrecoup bruises, 74
Contusion, cerebral, 74
Cooling of body, 20
Coronary, occlusion, 262
  spasm, 262
Coroner system, 2
Cot death, 196
Court attendance, 338
Craniofacial traits, 61
Crib death syndrome, 196
Crossexamination, 340
Cutthroat, homicidal, 89
  suicidal, 87
Cutting and stabbing wounds, 82
  autopsy, 84
  scene investigation, 82
  types, 86
Cyanides, 302
  tests for, 328
Cyanosis, 137
Cyclobarbitone, 294

Darvon, 312
Dead, identification of, 5
Death, cause(s) of, 5, 190
  circumstances of, 4 11
  manner of, 5
  pronouncement of, 3
  signs of, 3
  sudden and unexpected, 189
  time of, 7
  types of, 1
  at wheel, 211
Decomposition, 24

Decompression sickness, 160
Defense wounds, 89
Delirium tremens, 259
Demerol, 280
Dental chart, 39
Dental identification, 37
Dental plates, identification by, 42
Dentures, 40
Desipramine, 315
Dial, 294
Diagnostic procedures, complications of, 231
Diatoms, 161
    technique for detection, 329
Direct examination, 339
Disease, iatrogenic, 229
Disease and trauma, 193
D-lycergic acid diethylamide, 305
Documentation of facts, 2
Doriden, 280
Drowning 154, 207
    appearances of lungs, 158
    electron microscopy, 163
    external appearances, 156
    fresh water, 158
    internal examination, 158
    salt water, 158
    scene investigation, 154
    special investigations, 161

Elavil, 315
Electric mark, 179
Electrocution, 177
Embolism, air, 16, 160, 259
    fat, 259
Encephalitis, chronic, 259
Epilepsy, 258
Epiphyses, appearance and fusion of, 49
Equanil, 314
Ethyl alcohol, 283
    acute poisoning from, 284
Ethylene glycol, 288
Evidence, chain of custody of, 7
    collection of, 7
Examination, external, 12
    internal, 14
    regional, 15
Exhumation, 17
Exit wounds, 107, 113

Explosion, anesthetic, 227
Extremities, injuries of, 80

Facts, documentation of, 2
    record of, 4
Fauna bites, 245
Fees, for court testimony, 337
Ferrous sulphate, test for, 330
Findings, record of, 4
Fingerprints, identification by, 33
Fluorides, 280
Footprints, 34
Formulae, determination of stature from, 62
Fright, death from, 256

Genital tract, examination of, 16
Gunpowder, examination for, 127
Guns, pistols and rifles, 101
    shotguns, 100
Gunshot wounds, 97
    accidental, 117
    concealed, 117
    entrance, 104, 107
    exit, 107, 113
    homicidal, 117
    histological examination of, 127
    method of investigation, 97
    suicidal, 113
    unusual, 117
    x-ray examination, 123

Hair, apparent growth of, 250
    identification by, 35
Hanging, 144
    accidental, 146
    homicidal, 148
    suicidal, 144
Head, examination of, 15
    injuries, 73
Heatstroke, 184
    autopsy findings, 185
    clinical features, 184
Heavy metals, test for, 326
Hemorrhage, extradural, 75
    in middle ears, 159
    petechial, 134
    postmortem, 245

Hemorrhage (*continued*)
  subarachnoid, 75
  subdural, 75
Heptabarbital, 294
Heroin, 307
Hesitation wounds, 86
Hexobarbitone, 294
His, bundle of, 262
Hit and run, 214
Homicide, using automobile, 214
Hypostasis, 22
Hypothermia, 186

Iatrogenic disease, 229
Identification, of body, 5, 31
  by external stigmata, 34
  by fingerprints, 33
  by hair, 35
  by internal examination, 45
  by personal effects, 33
  by teeth, 37
  of automobile driver, 217
Imipramine, 315
Incised wounds, accidental, 91
  homicidal, 89
  suicidal, 86
Incision, primary, 14
Index, sciatic notch, 51
Infant deaths, 195
Injuries, abdominal, 77
  blunt force, 66
  chest, 76
  delayed complications of, 78
  external, 13
  head, 73
  involving extremities, 80
  regional, 73
  spinal, 78
Insecticides, 310
Investigation, kit, 2
  scene, 1
Investigator, medical, 1
Isopropyl alcohol, 288
  tet for, 331

Kit, investigation, 2

Laceration, 70
Laryngeal spasm, 159

Larynx, edema of, 261
  inflammation of, 261
  spasm of, 261
Lead, 304
  tests for, 331
Length of fetus, 32
Ligature strangulation, 138
Lightning, 181
Liver, discoloration of, 249
Lividity, 22
Livor mortis, 22
Local anesthetics, 228
Long bones, examination of, 54
  relative lengths of, 61
LSD, 305
Luminal, 294

Manual strangulation, 140
Marihuana, 295
Medical investigator, 1
  role of, 2
Meperidine, 280
Meprobamate, 314
Mercury, test for, 326
Methadone, 280
Methyl alcohol (methanol), 287
  test for, 332
Miltown, 314
Misadventure, therapeutic, 229
Mishaps, therapeutic, 224
Morphine, 307
Mummification, 25
Myocarditis, 263

Natural death, 189
  causes of, 190
  of infant, 196
Neck, examination of, 15
Negative autopsy, 254
  reasons for, 254
Nembutal, 294
Nervous system and sudden death,
  191
  lesions of, 257
Neutron activation analysis, 37
Nicotine, 280

Obscure cases, drowning, 159
Operative deaths, 224

Organophosphates, 310
Ossification centers, 32
Overdoses, 230
Overlying 150

Palm prints, 34
Paraldehyde, 280
Parathion, 310
    test for, 332
Pathologist, as witness, 336
    training of, 255
Pelvis, sexing of, 53
Pentobarbitone, 294
Pentothal, 294
Periarteritis nodosa, 264
Personal effects, identification from, 33
Pertofran, 315
Pesticides, 310
Phenobarbitone, 294
Phenistix, test, 332
Phenol, 280
Phenothiazines, 313
    test for, 332
Phosphorus, 280
Physical evidence, collection of, 7
Pistols, 101
Plumbism, chronic, 304
Pneumothorax, 16, 255
Poisoning death, 207, 273
    autopsy, 275
    collection of biological specimens, 275, 277
    final analysis of a case, 279
    fatal concentrations, 280
    fatal doses, 280
    general unknown, 276
    interpretation of toxicological results, 278
    result of, acids, 280
        alkalies, 280
        amitriptyline, 315
        amphetamines, 288
        arsenic, 290
        barbiturates, 292
        boron, 280
        bromides, 280
        cannabis, 295
        carbon monoxide, 296
        carbon tetrachloride, 299
        chloral hydrate, 280
        cyanides, 302
        Darvon, 280
        Demerol, 280
        desipramine, 315
        d-lycergic acid diethylamide, 305
        Doriden, 280
        ethyl alcohol, 283
        ethylene glycol, 288
        fluorides, 280
        heroin, 307
        imipramine, 315
        isopropyl alcohol, 288
        lead, 304
        LSD, 304
        marihuana, 295
        meprobamate, 314
        Methadone, 280
        methanol, 287
        methyl alcohol, 287
        morphine, 307
        nicotine, 280
        organophosphates, 310
        paraldehyde, 280
        parathion, 310
        phenol, 280
        phenothiazines, 313
        phosphorus, 280
        propoxyphene hydrochloride, 312
        psychosedative drugs, 313
        salicylates, 315
        wood alcohol, 287
    scene investigation, 273
Postmortem, changes, 20
    chemical, 25
    physical, 20
    clock, 28
Preanesthetic medications, 226
Precipitin test, 46
Pretrial conference, 337
Procedure in autopsy room, 12
Propoxyphene hydrochloride, 312
Psychosedative drugs, 313
Public symphysis, changes in, 52

Race, determination of, 60
Racial traits, craniofacial, 61
Record of facts and findings, 4
Rectal temperature, 21
Reinsch test, 326
Resistance, electrical, 178

Respiratory system and sudden death, 190
Revolver, 102
Rifled guns, 101
Rifles, 104
Rigor mortis, 23

Salicylates, 315
tests for, 332
Saponification, 25
Sarcoidosis, 267
Scars, 34
Scene, alteration of, 7
investigation, 1
air craft accidents, 220
asphyxial deaths, 131
automobile accidents, 209
battered child syndrome, 201
cutting and stabbing wounds, 82
drowning, 154
poisoning deaths, 273
statements at, 10
Sciatic notch index, 51
Scuba diving, 160
Secobarbital (seconal), 294
Shock, deat from, 256
Shotgun(s), 100
wounds, close-range, 105
contact, 104
long-range, 105
Sickle cell disease, 269
Skeletal remains, 48
aging of, 49
key questions, 48
sexing of, 51
Skin diving, 160
Skull, sexing of, 60
Smothering, 149
Soneryl, 294
Soot, in air passages, 170
Spermatozoa, 333
Spinal injuries, 78
Stab wounds, homicidal, 93
suicidal, 93
Stature, determination of, 63
Stigmata, external, 34
Still birth, 195
Still birth vs. live birth, 195
Strangulation, 137, 206
accidental, 143

by ligature, 138
manual, 140
suicidal, 143
Strychnine, test for, 334
Subpoena, 336
Sudden death, 189
causes of, 190
Suffocation, 149, 205
Suicidal wounds, elbows, groin, wrists, 86
neck, 87
Suicide, 7
automobile, 216
cutthroat, 87
gunshot wounds, 113
hanging, 144
poisoning, 281
strangulation, 143
Surgical procedures, complications of, 232
Suture closures, 51

Tattoos, 34
Teeth, eruption of, 32, 38
identification by, 40
Temperature, rectal, 21
Tentative wounds, 86
Test firing, 127
Tests for, alcohol, 325
antimony, 326
arsenic, 326
barbiturates, 327
bismuth, 326
carbon monoxide, 327
cyanide, 328
diatoms, 329
ferrous sulphate, 330
isopropyl alcohol, 331
lead, 331
mercury, 326
methyl alcohol, 332
parathion, 332
phenothiazines, 332
salicylates, 332
spermatozoa, 333
strychnine, 334
Therapeutic, misadventure, 229
mishaps, 224
Thiopentone B, 294
Thorax, examination of, 16

Time of death, 7
  estimation of, 20
  formulae for, 21
Tofranil, 315
Toxicological artefacts, 320
Transfusion, complications of, 230
  incompatibility of blood, 227
Transportation fatalities, 209
Trauma and disease, 193
  concealed, 256
Traumatic asphyxia, 150
Trotter and Gleser formulae, 62
Trunk, examination of, 16

Uncal grooving, 248
Unexpected death, 189
Unnatural deaths of infants, 199
Urine, method collection, 9
Urogenital system, 191

Vagal inhibition, in drowning, 159
  in strangulation, 144

Veronal, 294
Vital reaction, in burns, 169
  in wounds, 85
Voltage, 177

Witness, 336
  pathologist, 336
  preliminaries for, 337
  rules for, 339
Wood alcohol, 287
Wounds, accidental, 91
  cutting and stabbing, 82
  defense, 89
  gunshot, 97
  incised, 86
  procedure of investigation, 82
  suicidal, 86

X-rays,
  in cases of batterd child syndrome,
    202
  in cases of burns, 173
  in cases of gunshot wounds, 123
  identification by, 45